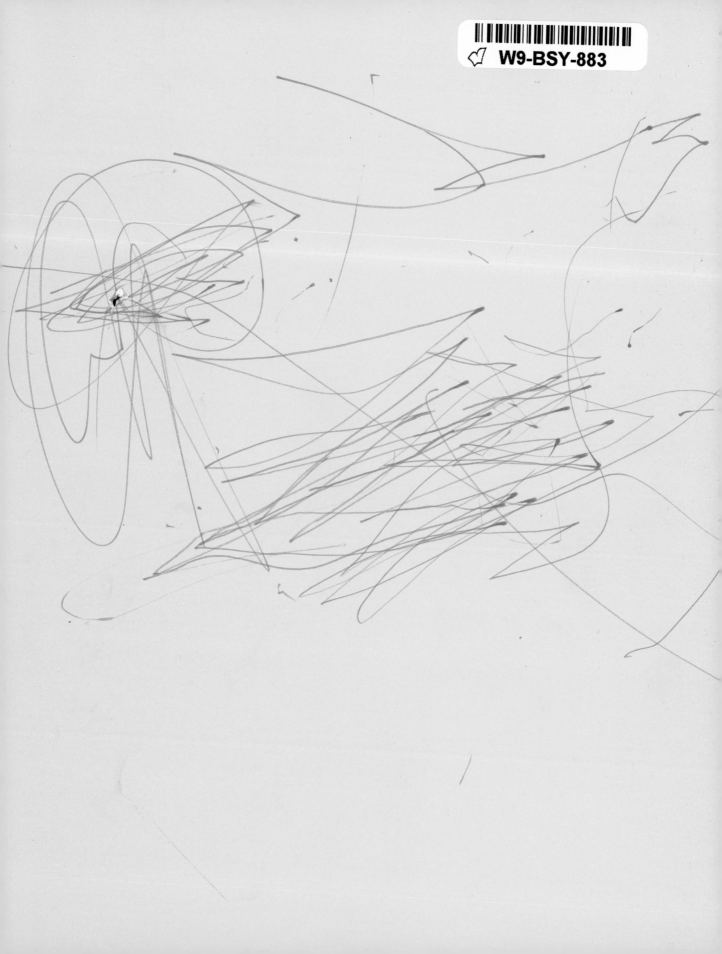

"*The Most Effective Natural Cures on Earth* is packed with useful information. Jonny Bowden has fresh insights into the healing process make a valuable contribution to the field."

—Leo Galland, M.D.,
Director of the Foundation for Integrated Medicine and
author of *The Fat Resistance Diet*

"A must-read for everyone wishing to take control of their health!"

—Larry McCleary, M.D.,
pediatric neurosurgeon and author of *The Brain Trust Program*

"Dr. Jonny Bowden, one of the nation's top experts on nutrition and natural medicine, has done it again. A must-have guide for anyone considering natural treatments."

—Cathy Wong, N.D., C.N.S.,
author of *The Inside-Out Diet* and about.com's Alternative Medicine Guide

"*The Most Effective Natural Cures on Earth* is another great contribution to the field of natural healing and I believe it will be quite helpful to all the people looking for simple guidance for improved health."

—Elson M. Haas, M.D.,
author of *Staying Healthy with Nutrition* and *The New Detox Diet*

". . . a well-researched, informative, and practical guide to natural medicine. . . "

—Alan R. Gaby, M.D.,
author of *Natural Medicine, Optimal Wellness* and past-president
of the American Holistic Medical Association

"A must-read for anyone interested in natural approaches to health. I strongly recommend you read this book!"

—Richard N. Firshein, D.O.,
author of *Your Asthma-Free Child* and Medical Director of
the Firshein Center for Comprehensive Medicine

"Not only is Jonny edgy and current, his information is impeccable, especially when it comes to the most effective natural cures on earth. I love his humor and his writing. What a gift—both he and this book."

—Ann Louise Gittleman, Ph.D., C.N.S.,
author of the *New York Times* Best Seller, *The Fat Flush Plan*

"Jonny Bowden has distilled for all of us the science behind natural cures for many diseases in a comprehensive review that is readable and understandable. This should be required reading for anyone interested in their health."

—Mark Houston, M.D., M.S., S.C.H., A.B.A.A.M., F.A.C.P., F.A.H.A.,
author of *What Your Doctor May Not Tell You About Hypertension:
The Revolutionary Nutrition and Lifestyle Program to Help Fight High Blood Pressure*
and Director of the Hypertension Institute in Nashville

THE MOST EFFECTIVE

NATURAL CURES on EARTH

The Surprising, Unbiased Truth About What Treatments Work and Why

JONNY BOWDEN, PH.D., C.N.S.

Best-selling author of *The Most Effective Ways to Boost Your Energy*

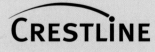

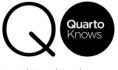

Brimming with creative inspiration, how-to projects, and useful information to enrich your everyday life, Quarto Knows is a favorite destination for those pursuing their interests and passions. Visit our site and dig deeper with our books into your area of interest: Quarto Creates, Quarto Cooks, Quarto Homes, Quarto Lives, Quarto Drives, Quarto Explores, Quarto Gifts, or Quarto Kids.

Text © 2008 Jonny Bowden

This edition published in 2018 by Crestline,
an imprint of The Quarto Group
142 West 36th Street, 4th Floor
New York, NY 10018 USA
T (212) 779-4972 F (212) 779-6058
www.QuartoKnows.com

First published in the USA in 2008 by Fair Winds Press,
an imprint of The Quarto Group, 100 Cummings Center,
Suite 265D, Beverly, MA 01915-6101

10 9 8 7 6 5 4 3 2 1

Crestline titles are also available at discount for retail, wholesale, promotional, and bulk purchase. For details, contact the Special Sales Manager by email at specialsales@quarto.com or by mail at The Quarto Group, Attn: Special Sales Manager, 401 Second Avenue North, Suite 310, Minneapolis, MN 55401, USA.

ISBN-13: 978-0-7858-3589-9

Printed and bound in China

Book production: Megan Cooney
Photography: Glenn Scott Photography

The information in this book is for educational purposes only. It is not intended to replace the advice of a physician or medical practitioner. Please see your health-care provider before beginning any new health program.

Fair Winds Press would like to thank Conley's pharmacy of Ipswich, Massachusetts, for its generosity and assistance in helping with the photos for this book.

Pill sizes, shapes, and colors may vary among manufacturers.

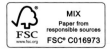

To Anja

Who, for me, makes almost anything possible

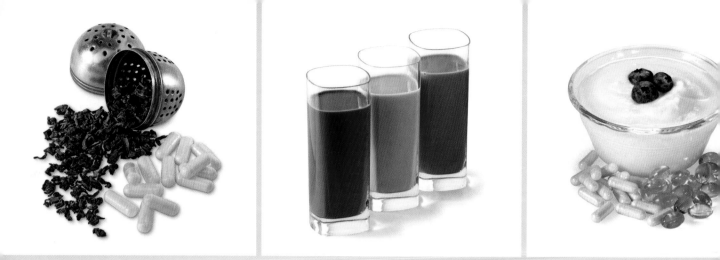

"The natural healing force within each of us is the greatest force in getting well."

—Hippocrates

"Western medicine doesn't hold all the answers. Healing cannot always be described in numbers."

—Mehmet C. Oz, M.D.

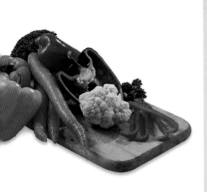
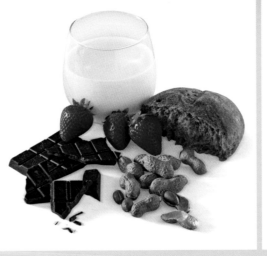
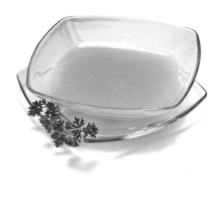

CONTENTS

INTRODUCTION

Let me be perfectly honest with you—*Natural Cures* was not, at first, my favorite title for this book.

"Cure" is a word I don't like to use when talking about natural treatments. Natural medicine—or nutritional medicine—works by treating the whole body as a system. It's not a philosophy based on taking a pill to suppress a symptom; it's about healing the condition that caused the symptom in the first place. And this generally involves an entire prescription for healing that can be as simple as a taking a few vitamins, but more typically, combines lifestyle, nutritional, physical, psychological, and even spiritual components, not your conventional "cure."

I also don't want to denigrate the power and usefulness of nutritional medicine by opening myself up to charges of hucksterism, so let me be perfectly clear from the outset: A vitamin doesn't "cure" cancer. A mineral doesn't "cure" diabetes, and there's no "natural cure" for Alzheimer's. These are serious conditions with many overlapping facets and problems, and they can't be "cured" by a pill.

However, a big "but" goes with that disclaimer.

The natural treatments in this book—vitamins, herbs, minerals, foods, plants, "designer" nutrients, acupuncture, stress reduction, image therapy, reflexology, or any of the many specific treatments or combinations of compounds—*can* make a huge difference in your health. No kidding. They can address certain metabolic conditions and blocked pathways that can contribute to your illness. They can clear up some of the obstacles that stand in the way of your healing. They can jump-start the body's amazing, natural curative powers. In some cases, following these prescriptions can actually "cure" a condition, or at least make it so minor that it doesn't bother you anymore. In some cases, they may not completely *eliminate* the condition, but you may find that you're able to significantly reduce your dependence on medication. In still other cases, they may give you a partial improvement and relieve a good portion of your suffering.

BODY, HEAL THYSELF

Natural medicine—in fact, all traditional systems of healing from traditional Chinese medicine to shamanism to herbalism—subscribe to a basic philosophy that seems to be curiously absent in conventional Western medicine, and it's this: *The body has an almost wondrous ability to heal itself.* My friend, naturopathic physician Sonja Petterson, N.M.D., points out that in sanatoriums they used to put people on fasts, hose them down, and make them walk around in the cold clean air. It sounds barbaric, and it probably was, but the philosophy behind it—now long lost in high-tech medicine—was to get patients to rally their bodies' own amazing resources and capacity for healing.

"My best friend in med school was a vet," Petterson says, "and that's what they always do when an animal is sick. They withdraw food and let them sleep. That's what an animal does in the wild, and that's what your dog does if he's sick. He stops eating and sleeps a lot. He instinctively knows that's what it takes to heal."

As in many areas of life, we can learn a lot from our dogs.

The lesson here is that your body has a *natural tendency* to heal itself, a fact that many of us seem to have forgotten. Natural medicine simply helps that process along. Nourish your body with the nutrients it needs to perform the metabolic processes involved in getting rid of viruses, bacteria, and other toxins. Support its immune responses. Stop overwhelming it with poisons, bad food, stress, polluted air, and toxic relationships. Allow it plenty of time to sleep and repair. Give it some sunshine and, yup, some tender loving.

Sound granola-ish? Maybe. But if that's one extreme approach to healing and the other end of the spectrum is heavy medication for symptoms, maybe we could look for something that's a little more of a compromise. Maybe we could begin to take advantage of the body's own miraculous ability to repair and heal by giving it natural substances that support it in that journey.

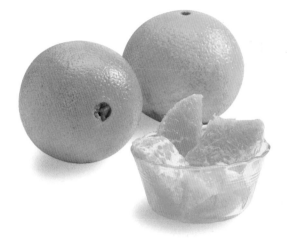

And that, in a nutshell, is the purpose of this book.

How Natural Cures Help You

One of my friends, Joseph Brasco, M.D.—interviewed for this book for his expertise in all things gastrointestinal—told me about his "rule of thirds," something that applies to the majority of the natural treatments and "cures" I write about in this book.

"One-third of the people I treat with natural medicine [like diet and supplements] will get 100 percent better—effectively cured," he told me. "One-third will improve considerably—they may be able to go off meds, or reduce meds substantially, or their symptoms will lessen, or they'll have measurably less pain and suffering. And one-third, unfortunately, won't be helped very much at all."

I agree with this, but I'd go one step further. Even for the one-third of the population whose condition might not be terribly responsive to a given treatment or "cure," chances are that *some* area of their health will be or could be improved by following the natural prescription for their

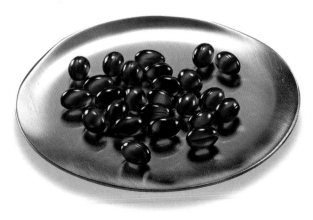

condition outlined in this book. And that could make a big difference in their overall well-being.

For example, the Paleo Diet might not entirely clear up acne in every single person who has acne, but it will almost always have an important positive effect on blood sugar and weight. And while the "kidney stone cure" of magnesium and vitamin B6 might not relieve every single case of kidney stones, the ingredients in it work together in dozens of ways in the body to improve mood and well-being. (In fact, they're two of the three key ingredients in my PMS cocktail on page 164). And omega-3 fatty acids, which are a part of a number of "combo cures," have a positive effect on so many areas of health and well-being that it's hard to imagine how anyone on the planet wouldn't benefit from them.

So the "cures" in this book will never hurt anyone, and I like to think they will help most people—at least a little, if not substantially. Best of all, not one ingredient in any of the "cures" is addictive, and not one of them has the remotest potential for abuse or for death by overdose. Though it's certainly possible to take a "toxic"

dose of a vitamin or herb (just as it's theoretically possible to have a "toxic" overdose of water) in real life, it's just not very likely. The "cures" in this book present substantially less risk to your health than prescription medications do, and the likelihood of any negative side effects from any of the natural prescriptions listed in this book— taken as directed—are incredibly small.

Remember, though, this is not "faith healing." You're not going to throw away your crutches in a single moment and proclaim, "I'm healed, I can walk again!" and go skipping out of the revival tent. No, in that narrow sense, the treatments and prescriptions in this book are not technically "cures." But they sure are powerful helpmates on your road to health. And they may *feel* like lifesavers to a lot of people. For everyone else, they *will* get you healthier, and they *will* make a difference.

And I'm pretty sure that, for some folks, they will make *all* the difference in the world.

WHY THIS BOOK IS DIFFERENT

If there's one thing that sets *The Most Effective Natural Cures on Earth* apart from the spate of other "natural cure" books it's this: research.

Let me explain.

The major objection the average person is likely to hear from establishment doctors about "natural medicine" is that there's "no good research showing it works." We hear this constantly about vitamins, antioxidants, herbs, and all sorts of non-medical healing traditions (from acupuncture to shamanism). (Later I'll go into *why* we hear this refrain constantly and the reason the media tends to report on vitamin studies so negatively.)

The point is that it's not true.

There's a *ton* of research on vitamins, minerals, phytochemicals, amino acids, fatty acids, and other nutritive substances. (Want proof? Go to the National Library of Medicine/National Institutes of Health online library, www.pubmed.gov, and put any vitamin you can think of in the search engine.) The problem isn't that there's an absence of research—it's that a great deal of this research flies under the radar screen of those whom we turn to for health advice (more on this later).

But the research exists. I've found it, *you* can find it, and your *doctor* can find it. You just have to be open to looking at it. You'll find dozens and dozens of references to published studies throughout the text of this book.

Now let me be fully frank—I wish the research were more definitive. But research in vitamins and minerals and other "natural" substances doesn't lend itself to the same kind of design as research on drugs, and therein may be one of the many problems with getting this information out there. We're used to having a symptom, taking a drug, and seeing the symptom disappear. Nutrients work differently. For one thing, they generally work in combination, much like the way they're found in nature. For another, they work more slowly and more subtly, repairing the mechanisms that caused the symptom in the first place. But that said, the substantial research on the vast majority of ingredients in *The Most Effective Natural Cures on Earth* should cause even the greatest skeptic to consider the possibilities that these noninvasive, gentle treatments could help heal a vast array of conditions and bring health to a vast number of people.

So why, you might ask, doesn't my doctor know about these treatments?

Ah, grasshopper, that is an excellent question.

To understand why this information is buried or discounted or simply ignored, you have to understand just a bit about the nature of medicine in the United States today, a subject I'm all too happy to discuss with you. Of course, if you could care less and would prefer to move on to the "good" parts, that's fine, too. But if you're interested in why so much of this information doesn't reach your doctor or—if it does—why he tends not to pay much attention, then read on.

Medicine in the U.S. Today

From the time medical students enter med school to the time they retire, their lives (and continuing education) are influenced by pharmaceutical companies. The companies buy them lunch when they're starving residents putting in ninety-hour weeks and can barely afford cafeteria fare. They give them gifts. (Take a look at the prescription pad your doctor uses or the paperweight on his desk. That's just the tip of the iceberg.) They sponsor and fund the research they read *and* the journals that publish it. They send perky and attractive pharmaceutical "reps" to the office, bringing samples, gifts, and sales pitches (carefully selected research) showing why their product is the best there is. (And if you think your local car salesman is good, you ain't seen nothin' 'till you've seen a professional pharmaceutical rep in action!)

"Pharmaceutical companies spend more than $15 billion each year promoting prescription drugs in the United States. One-third of that amount is spent on 'detailing'—an industry term for drug company representatives' one-on-one promotion to doctors," writes investigative reporter Mike Adams on NewsTarget.com.

At least eight studies in peer-reviewed journals have documented that the marketing of drugs to physicians via drug reps, honorariums, enticements, seminars, and samples has a profound influence on both their prescribing behavior and their tendency to buy "hook, line, and sinker" what the drug companies tell them about their products. One study—published January 19, 2000, in no less than the ultra-conservative *Journal of the American Medical Association*— concluded that "the present extent of physician-industry interactions appears to affect prescribing and professional behavior." Ya think? Let's file that conclusion under "duh!"

A 1992 study in the medical journal *Chest* examined all-expense-paid trips for physicians to popular Sunbelt vacation sites where pharmaceutical firms hawked their wares and spun their science to their hearts' content. The article dryly observed significant alterations in prescribing patterns by doctors after they attended these events "even though the majority of physicians … believed that such entitlements would not alter their prescribing patterns." (You can find a full list of the studies investigating the phenomenon of pharmaceutical industry influence on doctors' attitudes and behavior at www.nofreelunch.org.)

The Public Library of Science journal *Medicine* in 2007 published a damning paper called "Following the Script: How Drug Reps Make Friends and Influence Doctors." In it, coauthor Shahram Ahari—a former pharmaceutical sales rep for Eli Lilly—wrote: "It's my job to

The average doctor has a limited tool kit, and that tool kit consists exclusively of drugs. Asking the average doctor to recommend a natural treatment or supplement is like asking your piano teacher to recommend a tennis racket.

figure out what a physician's price is. For some it's dinner at the finest restaurants, for others it's enough convincing data to let them prescribe confidently, and for others it's my attention and friendship … but at the most basic level, everything is for sale and everything is an exchange."

High prescribers are identified from the Physician Masterfile database maintained by the American Medical Association, which pharmaceutical companies license for their own use. Reps work hard to maintain relationships with the highest prescribers. "The highest prescribers are every rep's sugar mommies and daddies," writes Ahari.

The article further detailed how a sales force of 100,000 drug reps (one drug rep per 2.5 targeted physicians) provides "rationed doses of samples, gifts, services, and flattery" to those physicians who are likely to prescribe the rep's drug.

"Every word, every courtesy, every gift, every piece of information provided is carefully crafted," say the authors, "not to assist doctors or patients, but to increase market share for targeted drugs." Should physicians refuse to meet with a rep, "their staff is dined and flattered in hopes that they will act as emissaries for a rep's message."

The Drug Company Solution

Doctors are taught that the solution to every illness or condition is a drug, and the competition over which drug to use is fierce. Little if any curriculum is devoted to nutrition or to any complementary medical practices in most medical schools. Medicine, at least in this country, is a business—and if you're in the business of selling lawn mowers, you don't talk much about golf carts.

The result of all of this is that the average doctor has a limited tool kit, and that tool kit consists exclusively of drugs. Asking the average doctor to recommend a natural treatment or supplement is like asking your piano teacher to recommend a tennis racket.

It gets worse. Unless your doctor has made a point of getting his own nutritional education, either academically or in continuing education seminars and workshops throughout the country, you can pretty much assume he knows next to nothing about nutrition. In fact, he gets his information from the same place you do: the

"Any secretary who's been on a diet knows as much about nutrition as the average doctor in this country."

—Jean Mayer, Ph.D.,
nutritionist and former president of Tufts University

media. He learns about supplements and vitamins from watching Sanja Gupta on CNN or reading *New York Times* nutrition columnist Jane Brody, an establishment apologist who seems to have never encountered an "official position" she didn't like.

The world-renowned nutritionist and former president of Tufts University Jean Mayer, Ph.D., was famously quoted as saying, "Any secretary who's been on a diet knows as much about nutrition as the average doctor in this country."

In other words, it's a good bet that your doctor—upon whom you rely for health information—knows no more about natural treatments or nutritional medicine than you do.

But that's not the problem.

The problem is that he *thinks* he does. Friends of mine have gone to their doctors to ask about supplements I've recommended, and the answers they frequently come back with are almost mind-numbing in their combination of wrong-headedness and arrogance.

Doctors are not nutritionists any more than plumbers are carpenters. Many are absolutely great at what they do—but they are *not* great at what they *don't* do. And unfortunately, either by temperament or training, they are not humble about what they don't know, and are frequently willing to dispense advice and information about nutrition with absolute authority even when they have absolutely no idea what they're talking about.

Which, unfortunately, is more often than you might imagine.

Is it changing? You bet it is. More young doctors are exploring holistic and integrative therapies, and more know about nutrition than ever before. And if you think I'm anti-doctor, let me immediately correct that impression: I'm anti-*uninformed* doctor. Look at the acknowledgment section of this book and you'll see enough M.D.'s and N.D.'s and Ph.D.'s to make a respectable-size "friends" list on a MySpace page. I know some of the smartest, best- informed, most open and knowledgeable doctors in America. But unfortunately, they're in a minority, and they're swimming upstream— because the medical model of health and disease in this country is stacked against a holistic view.

It's important to understand this climate so that you can fully appreciate what we're up against when trying to inform the public about treatments and interventions that don't have the "official" medical profession seal of approval. It's an uphill battle, but not an unfamiliar one.

Those of us who argued against the U.S. Department of Agriculture's (USDA) food pyramid and against the officially sanctioned high-carbohydrate, high-sugar diet have experienced this kind of resistance before. It's pretty hard to get a fair hearing for a low-carbohydrate diet when a good portion of the U.S. economy is based upon the very foods we were telling people to eat less of—corn, wheat, soy, and sugar, for example.

But I digress.

WANTED: A NEW MODEL FOR HEALING

The conventional medical model of disease is what scientists call a paradigm— a way of looking at illness. And that way of looking at illness and of healing is short-sighted. It's not wrong, it's just incomplete. And the result of this incomplete model is that many valuable healing modalities—including the ones in this book— get the short end of the stick when it comes to getting a fair hearing in the marketplace of ideas and options.

The main casualty of the current orthodox medical model of disease is the concept of the person as a *system*. We need a paradigm shift that conceptualizes illness not as a collection of dysfunctional molecules that happen to reside in a body, but as a condition of the "whole person." And this means an entirely different kind of treatment, one that *may* include drugs, but is not *limited* to them, and may in some cases not include them at all. When I discuss "natural cures" or "natural prescriptions" in this book, what I'm talking about is basically this: Things you can do that don't involve drugs.

It's that simple.

Some of the "natural prescriptions" in this book don't even use supplements (let alone drugs). The Relaxation Response for stress, for example. Or reflexology for PMS. Or the phenomenally effective EMDR (eye movement desensitization and reprocessing) technique for post-traumatic stress disorder. And some cures (like the Health Recovery Center program for alcoholism) combine an array of supplements with spiritual and psychological techniques. Though there are a dozen or so listings of single supplements or herbs under the chapter heading "pure cures," truth be told those "pure" cures are even more effective when combined with lifestyle interventions. Krill oil, for example—a "pure cure" for PMS—works even *better* if you reduce stress, caffeine, sugar, and junk food at the same time.

These are treatments that address the *whole person*, not just the disease.

See the difference?

Natural Healing: A Hard Sell That's Worth It

For most of my career, I've been advising people—first in private practice, then in books, lectures, CDs, workshops, and the like—on weight loss. And, as you may know from your own personal experience, weight loss is an uphill battle for most people. It involves making long-term, often difficult, lifelong changes that often

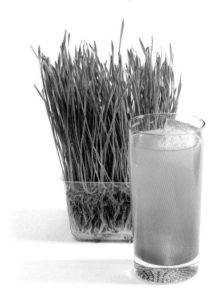

include a wholesale overhaul of the way you eat, the way you think and feel about food, the way you think and feel about exercise, your priorities, your future, and your belief in yourself. It's made even more difficult by the fact that the results are almost never immediate. This goes against everything we've come to expect from our fast-track lives, which are built around immediacy—instant gratification and instant results.

This sensibility is nowhere more apparent than in the way we take care of ourselves. It's way easier to pop an antacid when you have heartburn than it is to repair, improve, and support your body's ability to digest food. (For a "natural cure" approach to heartburn, see page 134.) But while an antacid may bring instant relief, it only masks the deeper issue, which will continue to get worse. We are like athletes who take a cortisol injection so they can ignore the pain of a torn ligament in the knee. That athlete may indeed be able to get through the game, but the damage to his knee will only get worse as he continues to pound away on it. Later, the payment will come due, and it won't be fun. Collectively, when it comes to our health care, we are like the guy whose smoke alarm makes too much noise, so he disconnects the battery.

Natural medicine is rarely quick and easy and doesn't always bring instantaneous relief. To use a money analogy, natural care is much more like a long-term 401k than it is like an "impulse purchase" on your maxed-out credit card. But like all long-term investments, it pays off in dividends much greater than the temporary "high" of dealing only with the immediate.

Is it harder and slower? Sure.

Is it worth it? You be the judge.

Super-Specialize Me

Natural medicine is also a "hard sell" because, as you'll see in this book, it addresses the whole person as a system. (Not for nothing is it called *holistic* medicine.) That "whole person" sensibility is conspicuously absent in conventional high-tech medicine, where extreme hyper-specialization is now the norm.

For example: Liver specialists rarely talk to skin specialists. Gastroenterologists know little about endocrinology. Orthopedic surgeons are clueless about psychiatry. Add to that the fact that most of today's doctors spend more of their time filling out paperwork and arguing with insurance companies than they do treating patients and you have a perfect storm for information overload. In today's medical marketplace,

it's unrealistic to expect your plastic surgeon to know much about bone diseases, or your ear, nose, and throat specialist to know much about OB-GYN.

So how could we expect *any* of them to know about naturopathy, acupuncture, or vitamins?

> *Collectively, when it comes to our health care, we are like the guy whose smoke alarm makes too much noise, so he disconnects the battery.*

In an age in which more than 17,200,000 published studies are available in the online database of the National Library of Medicine, and literally thousands more published every year, it's brutally difficult to stay up to date in your own specialized field, let alone someone else's.

This super-specialization leads to a very partisan approach to healing illness, the very opposite of the holistic, "bipartisan" approach of integrative medicine and of "natural" treatments in general. When all you've got is a hammer, every problem looks like a nail.

Add to this the politics of medicine, and the picture becomes even murkier.

Don't Take Me To an Herbalist

Now do not—please—get me wrong. I believe Western medicine is absolutely without parallel when it comes to emergency medicine. I have said many times—and will continue to say—that if, God forbid, I am in a car accident, do not take me to an herbalist. There is nothing like Western medicine, especially as practiced in the

A Sordid History

The American Medical Association (AMA) has an especially shameful history when it comes to accepting or embracing anything or anyone that is not in the "union." In the early part of the century it lobbied brutally against homeopaths. Its sister organization, the American Psychiatric Association, fought tirelessly against psychologists (we're talking Ph.D.'s here), arguing that they were not equipped to perform psychoanalysis because they were not M.D.'s. (It took Freud himself, the founder of psychoanalysis, to argue, in an essay called On The Question of Lay Analysis, that the medical doctors were full of it.)

The AMA's fight to make chiropractic disrespectable and brand it "quackery" was similarly reprehensible. "For over 12 years and with the full knowledge and support of their executive officers, the AMA paid the salaries and expenses for a team of more than a dozen medical doctors, lawyers, and support staff for the expressed purpose of conspiring [overtly and covertly] with others in medicine to first contain, and eventually, destroy the profession of chiropractic in the United States and elsewhere," writes journalist Kenny Ausubel in *When Healing Becomes A Crime*.

As an organization, the AMA is just not very nice. As investigative reporter Mike Adams writes on the excellent website NewsTarget, " ... history shows that the AMA has worked diligently to block much in the way of real progress in order to control medicine and shut out competition." Over the years, as an organization, its actions seem far more motivated by the desire to protect its members than to protect the health of America. (Doubt this? Check out its position on universal health care.)

The result is that our current medical/pharmaceutical model has created a default position on how to approach disease, and regrettably, most of us have bought into it. It goes like this: You have a symptom, you go to the doctor, she gives you a pill, the symptom is gone. Got asthma? Suck on an inhaler. Got allergies? Get a shot. Got cancer? Get chemo. Got a headache? Take an aspirin. Depressed? Have I got an SSRI for you.

Given this commonly accepted meaning of cure, I didn't want to use the word without explaining what I meant by it. And what I mean by "cure" is this: shorthand for a natural prescription that can help you heal the underlying problem, not a synonym or a substitute for a pharmaceutical intervention that only addresses the symptom.

best hospitals in America, for taking care of what is called an *acute* condition—something that is happening *right now*, is severe or extreme, and needs immediate attention. Western medicine is the absolute champion of triage. It knows how to keep your heart beating and your lungs breathing—without which, not much else matters. If I have a condition that needs that kind of attention, I'm going straight to Cedars-Sinai, thank you very much, and that's that.

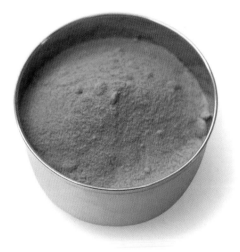

But good as it is with acute conditions, Western medicine is very bad at what are called *chronic* conditions. And it is woefully, pathetically *incompetent* when it comes to prevention. Chronic conditions are what might be called ongoing states of unwellness that are not emergencies, but last for months, years, or lifetimes. They can progress into acute emergencies, but are, for the most part, the sicknesses and conditions we live with, in varying degrees of severity. Asthma, fibromyalgia, diabetes, hypertension, fatigue, allergies, depression, low libido, heartburn, gastroesophageal reflux disease, indigestion, constipation, and muscle pain, among others, all fall into the category of stuff we need to "manage" or live with.

And it is here that natural medicine really shines.

If you're willing to rebuild your health from the ground up, so to speak, natural and nutritional medicine can help you do it. If you're simply looking for a Band-Aid to put over an annoying symptom so that you can continue about your business and allow your health to deteriorate without your really noticing, then this book is not for you. But then, if that *were*

you, you wouldn't have read this far anyway.

You're reading this far for one reason only—because the standard model of "fixing" disease by taking a drug and calling it a day isn't working for you. You want more out of your health and you want more out of your life.

GUIDING PRINCIPLES OF NATURAL MEDICINE AND NUTRITION

There really isn't an equivalent of the Hippocratic Oath for natural or nutritional medicine, but if there were it might go like this: *Treat the whole person, not just the disease.*

Whether you label them *holistic* practitioners, practitioners of *functional medicine*, *nutritional medicine*, or *integrative medicine*, what all healers who come from these traditions have in common is that they recognize the profound importance of *synergy* in treatment. You've heard that the attitude of a patient can make a huge difference in his health outcome, and it's true. But it's not the *only* thing that matters. But by the same token, neither are the drugs he's given. Nor the nutrients, especially if they're given one at a time. What *does* matter is how everything works together. The best practitioners not only recognize this, they make full use of synergy in designing treatment plans. Mind and body form a giant feedback loop in which ultimately the effects of one are indistinguishable from the effects of the other. Holistic practitioners—including those with M.D.'s—tend to recognize this. Others—not so much.

I had a personal experience of this mind-body feedback loop—and the cumulative effect of different "interventions"—the other day in the dentist's chair, of all places. Allow me to share it with you.

First thing you should know about me is that I'm a wuss when it comes to dental pain. For the procedure I was about to undergo, I decided to get nitrous oxide, a gentle and mild analgesic (painkiller) known to have a relaxing effect. So here's what happened:

First the dentist put the mask over my face and I inhaled the nitrous. Since no one is completely sure how nitrous works in the brain, I can only tell you that however it works, it felt great. Within minutes, a feeling of general relaxation came over me. But while it felt good, my anxiety was far from gone. And although I felt relaxed, had a gunman at that moment burst into the office and told everyone to put their hands up and empty their wallets, the feeling would have left me instantly, even if I remained "wired up" to the gas mask. Anxiety would have broken through the effect of the drug. The drug by itself was not enough to make me relaxed about root canal. I mention this because of what happened next.

The nurse pushed the button on the chair that gently tilts it backward so that I was almost prone. I immediately felt my body relax even further.

Then, the nurse put on some Mozart. As the classical music began playing through the speakers, I felt even *more* relaxed, my breathing deep and measured and my pulse slowing.

Finally, the dentist came into the room and started talking in his deep, comforting voice, telling me to relax, that nothing was going to hurt, and that everything was going to be fine. He happens to have a particularly reassuring bedside manner and a very sonorous, trustworthy voice. I felt myself relax even further.

He also gently put his hand on my arm while speaking. Touch. Ten more degrees of relaxation.

Now I was ready for my procedure, and, largely because of my physical and mental state, it went easily and without a hitch.

So now here's the question: Was I relaxed and calm and feeling good because of the nitrous? Because of the music? Because my body was in a restful, prone position not associated with fight or flight? Because of the reassurances of my dentist and the confidence I felt in him? Because of the reassuring physical touch? Because of the "placebo" effect?

I maintain the following argument: *It is impossible to know.*

All elements contributed mightily to my overall feeling, and while perhaps none of them alone would have been enough to relax and calm me, they had an additive, cumulative effect. Now if you were doing a scientific experiment to find out whether music alone were enough to produce relaxation in a stressful situation like the dentist's chair right before root canal, you might find that it does in some cases, but more often does not. Same with the dentist's bedside manner. Same with the nitrous oxide. Same with physical position.

Synergy in the Wild: The Mind-Body Connection in Animals

Here's a great example of synergy. It's a dramatic illustration of how mind and body can work together—even in animals—in ways that are frequently missed by experiments that focus on just one variable.

Some time ago, it came to the attention of people who notice these things that frogs were dying at an unprecedented rate, and environmentalists and other concerned citizens were convinced that a prime cause was a particular insecticide called carbaryl that was making its way into the waterways. The folks who manufactured carbaryl said, "No way, José. We've got studies showing carbaryl is not lethal to frogs. It can't be our fault." And indeed, a number of studies showed that if you take, for example, a gray tree frog, and put him in a lab and expose him to the concentration of carbaryl he might normally come in contact with in a natural waterway, he doesn't die.

But here's the thing. Gray tree frogs—and other amphibians—are extremely sensitive to predator cues. They notice when something that's likely to eat them is within a hundred yards. When they sense that they are in danger, they do what every other sentient being does—they secrete large amounts of stress hormones. In the lab, the frogs were pretty unstressed because there were no predators around.

But in the wild, they're constantly surrounded by predators that would like to turn them into a tasty lunch. So in an ingenious experiment (published in the journal *Ecological Applications*), biologist Rick Relyea decided to test what happens when you put frogs in a stressful situation and *then* expose them to carbaryl. Short answer: They become dead frogs.

Carbaryl isn't necessarily lethal to the frogs when they're relaxed. But when the frogs are stressed, something happens to their internal environment and the carbaryl becomes much harder to handle. In two of the six species Relyea tested, carbaryl became much more lethal when combined with predatory stress—up to forty-six times more lethal in some cases.

It wasn't stress that was killing the frogs. And it wasn't carbaryl. It was the *combination*.

But synergy also has a tremendously positive face. In fact, the whole concept of synergy is essential to the paradigm of natural medicine. Acupuncture needles in the ear, for example, won't cure addiction. But when coupled with other treatments, they offer a significant benefit beyond what's accomplished by the other treatments alone, particularly in the area of easing withdrawal symptoms. Quercetin by itself might not completely disable asthma, but couple it with a diet free of trigger foods and a stress-reducing strategy, and you might find yourself without an asthma attack for a long time.

This is how natural medicine works and why so many studies of the effects of a vitamin supplement have been disappointing. The studies are designed like drug studies—"Does this pill cure a headache?" Never mind that there's an enormous disinclination to find benefits for vitamins, minerals, herbs, and other supplements in a research environment largely funded by pharmaceuticals. Even in a "research-neutral" environment, a single vitamin (or other supplement) may not show its full ability to heal and support health if it's asked to work its magic by itself. Vitamins are like basketball players—there are stars, sure, but the real championships are won by teams.

But put them together and—at least in my case—they worked wonderfully.

Unfortunately, Western science uses the "one at a time" model of testing. So, for example, if you want to know the effect of a specific drug, you do your measurements before and after giving it, and then you see whether the drug makes a difference. But the human body responds much more like I did in the dentist's chair. Things work *together* to produce a result— in this case, my complete relaxation. A vitamin might not have a strong effect by itself, but when combined with three other vitamins— and perhaps acupuncture—you may get a powerful effect.

That's why the standard method of testing is not well suited to teasing out the powerful healing effects of vitamins and herbs. And that's why you should be more than suspicious next time you hear an "expert" tell you that the research shows a vitamin doesn't "do" anything. In nature these compounds are found together and often work synergistically, as a team. When tested by themselves—particularly when the research is supported by people who have a vested interest in showing that they don't work, or, who often don't use the right form or dosage to begin with—it's hard to get really solid information. To read another example of what I mean, check out the sidebar on page 20.

How to Lie with Statistics

One of the arguments you will hear repeated endlessly by people who should know better is that there's "no evidence" for nutritional

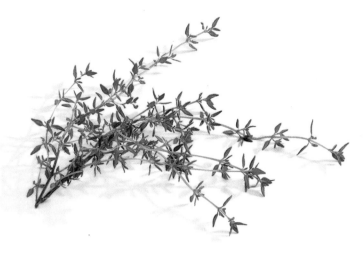

medicine or for natural and integrative approaches to health. With equal certainty, they will tell you about all the evidence that *does* exist for conventional pharmaceutical medicines. A full discussion of the issues this brings up really deserves a book of its own, but it's worth talking about a few examples of how cases can be made with statistics to advance an agenda, or how a built-in bias by researchers (and the media) can distort both findings and the way they're reported.

Just as I was completing the manuscript for this book, a study was published in the *Archives of Internal Medicine* that investigated the effects of vitamin E and vitamin C on women. The study tracked more than 8,000 women who were at high risk for cardiovascular disease over the course of nine years. Here's how the media reported the findings: "Antioxidants do not protect high-risk women from heart disease" (Fox News), "Antioxidants don't lower heart risk" (WebMD), "Vitamins No Magic Bullet for Heart Health" (ABC News), and "Common Vitamins No Help for Women's Hearts" (Reuters).

Hidden Beneath the Headlines

Sounds pretty bad, doesn't it?

Here's what was buried in the data: Vitamin E led to a 22 percent reduction in the risk of heart attack. It also led to a 27 percent reduction in the risk for stroke. And vitamin E, when taken together with vitamin C, lowered the risk of stroke by 31 percent.

Why was it buried? Well, for one thing, lots of people in the study didn't actually *take* the vitamins. (Guess what—you have to take them for them to work!) When the researchers looked at the subgroup of people who actually took their vitamins, the benefits mentioned above were found. When the population as a *whole*—vitamin takers and non-vitamin takers—were mixed together, the results weren't very impressive.

It's interesting that the media reported the negative findings based largely on a press release by—what else—the American Medical Association, not exactly an impartial organization without ties to Big Pharma. Mike Adams—a consumer advocate and investigative health journalist for whom I have enormous respect—launched a grassroots campaign by readers to demand retractions, corrections, or clarifications from major media outlets "all of which," he says, "printed incorrect, incomplete, or misleading statements concerning the results [of the study]."

"If you're going to count the results of all the women who don't take the supplements, why not simply launch the study, give vitamins to no one, then announce the conclusion that vitamins don't work?" asks Adams.

I mention this to drive home the point that the default position of the media and of the medical establishment is pretty much antisupplement and antinatural medicine. Information about natural, nontoxic, nonpharmaceutical interventions (and preventive measures) does not routinely fall on welcoming ears, and how that information is reported and filtered deeply affects what you hear about and learn about natural medicine.

Faulty Studies and the Fine Print

In this book, you'll read a number of stories about studies that were used to debunk the effects of food or supplements. One example comes from an old, poorly designed study on chocolate that was funded by the chocolate manufacturers and used for decades as "proof" that diet has no effect on acne. (You'll read about that on page 203). Another is the phenomenally dishonest reporting on the "ineffectiveness" of St. John's Wort for depression. The study examined subjects with an extraordinarily difficult form of depression that didn't respond to St. John's Wort, but what was left out of the reporting was the fact that these same subjects also didn't respond to prescription antidepressants either! Meanwhile, St. John's Wort is *quite* effective for more moderate or mild depression (but you'd never know that from reading the media reports).

On the other side of the fence, the reporting on the positive effects of prescription drugs can sometimes be as "truthful" as late-night infomercials for hair-growth. Magazine ads for Lipitor leave you with the impression that if your cholesterol is even slightly elevated, taking the popular drug will save your life. But Lipitor is only approved by the Food and Drug Administration to reduce the risk of heart attack *if* you have multiple risk factors for heart disease, and its benefits are based largely on its supposed ability to lower cholesterol, which may *or may not* have anything to do with preventing cardiovascular events and death. In fact, if you read the small print on television ads for Lipitor a couple of years ago, you'd briefly see the following words flash on the screen in tiny letters: "Lipitor has not been shown to prevent heart disease or heart attacks."

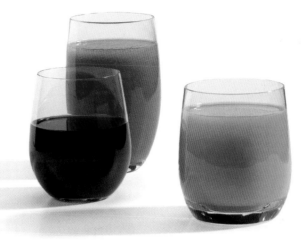

Another example: As of 2004, Fosamax (for osteoporosis) was the third most frequently prescribed drugs for seniors. As my friend John Abramson, M.D., professor of medicine at Harvard and author of the superb book, *Overdosed America*, writes, "One wonders how many of the women taking this drug actually benefit, since … it does not reduce fractures when used to prevent osteoporosis." Abramson also wonders "how many women taking these drugs are aware of the research showing the significant benefits of exercise in preventing fractures and, more important, improving overall health and longevity?"

When Less is Better

Is it "harder" to become a lifelong exerciser than it is to pop Fosamax? Sure it is. But unlike Fosamax, which not only doesn't prevent fractures but also can cause nausea, abdominal cramping, gastrointestinal upset, and in some cases, osteonecrosis (bone loss) of the jaw, exercise pays off with incalculable dividends. And there isn't a single side effect, unless you count losing weight, looking better, and having more energy as side effects!

So am I anti-medicine? Of course not. But my admitted bias is that if you *can* take less of it, you should. And if there are other, more gentle ways that can accomplish the same result for you—diet, lifestyle, nutrition, herbs, natural treatments, or combination of nutrients such as are found in this book—I say try those first. When it comes to powerful pharmaceuticals, less is more. The best goal of all when it comes to drugs is zero. It may not be attainable for everyone, but that doesn't mean it's not worth shooting for.

After all, as my friend Robert Crayhon says, "Depression is not a Prozac deficiency." And you don't get heart disease because you don't have enough Lipitor in your diet.

Conspiracy? No, but ...

A spate of "natural cure" books have looked at some of the marketing practices of the drug companies, the power of the food companies and Big Pharma, and the porous influence of these huge conglomerates on agricultural policy and on the FDA, and these books and authors have concluded that it's all a great big government conspiracy to keep you from knowing what you need to get yourself well and to stay healthy and out of the medical system. That the big evil people in government and in power don't want you to know the truth. Some newsletters capitalize on this sentiment with mail solicitations that lead with lines like *"Doctors' secrets they don't want you to know!"* or *"Why your doctor won't tell you about [fill in the blank]!"*

This sells. I get it. Believe me. And I also understand how easy it is to feel like there is a grand conspiracy whose purpose is to keep you from getting the health info you ought to know about.

The truth, however, is actually more subtle.

There isn't a vast conspiracy out to keep you from knowing about natural cures and treatments. There is, however, a shared and prevalent sensibility—one I've tried to illustrate in the above text—that accomplishes the same thing. It's a sensibility created in part by the paradigm that looks at disease as simply a collection of dysfunctional molecules that can be "cured" or treated by finding a drug to interfere with them. And that discounts any treatment or intervention that can't be tested in the exact same way as you would test a drug. It's a shared, collective prejudice against practices that aren't in the mainstream of Western medicine. It's a subtle, shared distrust of "natural" or non-pharmaceutical interventions (witness the utterly ridiculous website "Quackwatch," which has never encountered a drug treatment it didn't like, or a non-drug treatment that it did). And it's an over-reliance on a particular *form* of scientific investigation that may not always be perfectly suited for uncovering what some of these non-traditional treatments have to offer.

I'm one of the biggest skeptics on the planet, and when possible, I like to see things validated by scientific investigations. That said, I'm *also* not one of these people who needs a double-blind, randomized controlled study published in a peer-review journal before I can believe it. As my friend, nutritionist Robert Crayhon is fond of saying, "there's no double-blind study to prove that water puts out fire, but the entire New York City fire department operates on the presumption that it's a good working hypothesis!"

So What Is Natural Medicine, Anyway?

Try for a minute to come up with your own definition of "natural medicine" and you'll quickly get an idea of the difficulty I was faced with in writing this section of the book. Is it medicine that starts life as a plant? Well, that would include an awful lot of pharmaceuticals (drugs) that are derived from botanicals (plants). Is it medicine that is limited to vitamins and minerals as they occur in nature? That would leave out every supplement mentioned in this book, since

The Stress Connection

One part of natural medicine thankfully does not fall into the "gray" area—it's clearly smack dab in the middle of any definition of *natural* you can come up with. It's unambiguous and essential and occupies a central place in the treatment of almost any disease or condition I can think of.

I'm talking about stress management.

If you do an even cursory glance through this book, you'll notice that the subject of stress comes up time and time again. It's a factor not just in the conditions covered in this book, but in dozens of conditions not even mentioned—fibromyalgia, for example, or the skin condition rosacea. While stress does not *cause* many of the conditions I discuss in this book, it nonetheless makes a major contribution to the way in which the condition plays out. Asthma, allergies, hypertension, acne, insomnia, and obesity are just a few of the many conditions that can be made worse by stress. Stress can trigger symptoms, increase their severity or frequency, and lengthen the time you have to suffer with them. Stress can also compromise recovery. No good holistic or "natural" approach to healing would ignore stress as a critical component of illness.

Specific emotional states like depression, for example, have been linked to "hard-core" diseases like diabetes and heart disease. Conventional medicine continues to obsess over cholesterol as a "risk factor" for heart disease, meanwhile ignoring the very real (and in my opinion, much more serious) risks from trauma, divorce, anger, loneliness, grief, and abusive relationships.

"Evidence is overwhelming that the heart takes a beating after psychic trauma," writes science journalist A.J.S. Rayl in *Psychology Today*.

Natural medicine worthy of the name can never ignore the role of stress, nor of attitude and emotions, in healing the body. That's why you'll see stress management mentioned so frequently in these pages. It's as important to healing as anything you can take in a pill form, even if said pill does come from a plant!

the last time I looked you couldn't pluck vitamin C tablets from a tree.

Applying the term "natural" to medicine (and cures) is just as difficult and imprecise as it is when you apply it to foods, an area in which the term has become virtually meaningless. The very concept of natural cures or natural medicine or natural foods *also* implies that if something is found in nature it's good, and if it's manufactured, it's not. This is patently ridiculous. Poison ivy, crude oil, and toxic mushrooms are all quite "natural," but I wouldn't recommend eating them. And there's nothing natural about a manufactured tablet containing vitamin C, vitamin E, and selenium—but it's pretty darn good for you.

Truth is, the dividing line between what's natural and what's not is both a shifting target and a gray area, without a hint of black or white. There are probably as many definitions of natural medicine as there are authors who have written books on the subject. So let me give you mine, with the caveat that it's a far from "perfect" definition: Natural prescriptions as defined for the purposes of this book include things that are not available by prescription only. For the most part, the natural prescriptions in this book are cobbled together from herbs, vitamins, and minerals, as close as reasonably possible to the way they're found in nature. And the treatments included are more similar to those used by traditional healers than they are to conventional Western medicine.

I can almost hear the objections of the "Quackwatch" contingent, so let me answer them in advance. Sure, in some cases the distinction between what is considered a prescription drug and what isn't is pretty darn arbitrary, and sure, things move in and out of those categories all the time (look at former prescription drugs like Claritin, for example, that are now sold over the counter). And sure, some things that are *not* available by prescription (the hormone DHEA, for example) probably should be. But by and large the substances I've chosen to write about in this book have an overall safety profile that's excellent, have relatively few side effects, and tend *on the whole* to be gentler and more familiar to the body.

Which brings us to Linus Pauling.

Back in 1968, two-time Nobel Prize winner Linus Pauling coined the term *orthomolecular medicine* to refer to the practice of using optimal amounts of substances like vitamins and minerals that are "natural" to the body. (The body, for example, knows quite well what to do with vitamin B12 or with the amino acid tryptophan, both of which it encounters every day of its life. The body does not normally encounter, for example, Prozac or Prevacid.) The concept of orthomolecular medicine has served us well over the years, and while it's been expanded to include many things that we don't necessarily "make" on our own (for example, saw palmetto or green tea), the spirit of the term informs everything that's in these pages—substances that are highly unlikely to hurt us, that our body recognizes for the most part, that are non-toxic, and that come from herbs and plants together with treatments that don't involve drugs.

It's far from a perfect definition, but it's the best I've got, and I hope you'll accept it as a work in progress—if not in every detail, then certainly in spirit. And by the way, if you have a better one, I sure would like to hear it. I'd like nothing more than to be able to "upgrade" the definition of "natural cures" for the next edition of this book.

The Natural Pharmacy Is the Most Powerful

Your brain contains one of the most powerful pharmacies in the world. It has the ability and capacity to secrete neurochemicals that can make you feel ecstatic or horrible. Your food, your lifestyle choices, your relationships— to job, spouse, friends, family, and environment—have the capacity to fine-tune this

A Few Definitions

For purposes of organization, I've divided the book into several sections:

Pure Cures are single nutrients or herbs that have been used by themselves to produce an effect. Vitamin B12, for example, is very effective against aging complications, so it's listed under Pure Cures, as is melatonin for jet lag. This doesn't mean that anything listed as a Pure Cure wouldn't or couldn't be made better by combining it with other nutrients, herbs, or treatments. It's placement under Pure Cures is simply a convenience, reflecting that this particular item has some effect by itself.

Plant Cures are simply cures that come from the plant kingdom—herbal supplements as opposed to vitamins and mineral supplements.

Combo Cures are combinations of nutrients, treatments, and/or foods that, when taken together as a natural prescription, have the best and most dramatic effect. An example is my PMS cure of magnesium, vitamin B6, and evening primrose oil. They too can be used alone or combined with Pure Cures or Natural Treatments (or both). For example: the Combo Cure for PMS (magnesium, B6, and evening primrose oil) goes quite well with the Pure Cure for PMS: krill oil.

Food Cures are simply foods that have medicinal or curative powers on their own. An example: celery for blood pressure. As before, they can be used alone or in combination. (In this case, celery for blood pressure goes very nicely with the Combo Cure for hypertension on page 150.)

Natural Treatments: This category is for actual *healing modalities* as opposed to specific supplements. Acupuncture, chiropractic, image therapy, and other treatments all come under this heading. And, of course, exercise. (By now I hope you realize that any of these treatments can be combined with supplements and healing foods for even more dramatic results.)

Some nutrients have so many uses that I simply could not choose one specific condition to attach them to. Their health benefits are so broad, so helpful for multiple conditions, or so essential for dozens of metabolic processes that I decided to give them their own special category.

Desert Island Cures: These are the supplements I'd like to have with me on a desert island. Choosing which ones belonged in this category was difficult, as you could make a case for dozens more. But if you put a gun to my head, told me I had to join the cast of *Survivor* for a month, and could only take a few pills with me, these would probably be the ones I'd choose.

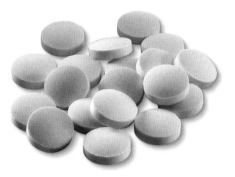

neurochemical mix in ways that can powerfully support your health. The choices you make—and the lifestyle you choose—may be more important determiners of your ultimate health and happiness than any drug on the planet.

A couple of examples. The famous Lyon Diet Heart Study showed that just following a Mediterranean diet (including fish, vegetables, and olive oil), produced a 72 percent decrease in coronary events, a 56 percent decrease in overall mortality, and a 61.7 percent decrease in cancer. Not a drug in the world can get those results. And in the famous ongoing Nurses' Health Study, doing only *five simple things* was associated with an almost unbelievable 83 percent reduction in the incidence of cardiovascular disease. You ready for the five simple things?

- Eat a healthy Mediterranean-type diet
- Exercise regularly
- Don't smoke
- Drink in moderation
- Maintain a reasonable body weight

Did you see drug-taking on that list? I didn't think so. And at the risk of sounding like one of those other "natural cures" guys, I need to point out that there's not a multibillion-dollar industry representing a huge chunk of the American economy that's devoted to telling people to eat fish and vegetables, put down the smokes, and go take a walk.

The Goal of This Book

My goal in this book—and, come to think of it, every book I've ever written—is to empower you. It's to help you become not only an active participant in your own health care, but the leader of your own health-care team. I want you to be captain of Team You. I don't want you to follow me—or any other "'guru'" of health—but rather learn to listen with open heart and mind, try things on, see whether they work, use what does, and throw away what doesn't.

Back in the 1990s when I was working as a personal trainer in New York City, gyms were springing up all over the city. The *New York Times* called the phenomenon "The Gym Wars." There was much discussion about where to go to get the best workout, about who had the best aerobics classes, about which location had the most state-of-the-art equipment, which gym had the best trainers, and so on. I remember being interviewed at the time by one of the magazines, and being asked, "Which gym is best?"

Here was my answer: The best gym is the one you actually *go* to.

I was reminded of this exchange the other day when I was talking to Walter Bortz, M.D., a faculty member at Stanford, the author of *Dare to Be 100*, and the president of a great organization called Fifty-Plus Lifelong Fitness. He's also seventy years old and runs at least one marathon a year. We were talking about exercise and I asked him, as a master's athlete, doctor, and lifelong fitness advocate: What's the best kind of exercise, all things considered?

Here was his answer: *The best exercise in the world is the exercise you actually do.*

I think the germ of truth in both these answers—mine and Bortz's—can be applied to natural cures and healing in general. The best treatment is the one that actually works for you.

In the long run, you are in charge of your health. Listen wisely to those you trust, but ultimately make your own decisions. Remember that your health is both a gift that was given to you and a gift that you give the world. When you are not healthy—when you are less than your best—when you are living, as William James said, "a life inferior to ourselves," you are depriving me and everyone else of the enormous contribution you have to make to the world.

You owe it to yourself and to me and to everyone else around you to be the fullest expression of who you are. That means a healthy body, mind, and spirit.

Don't settle for less.

Enjoy the journey.

PURE CURES

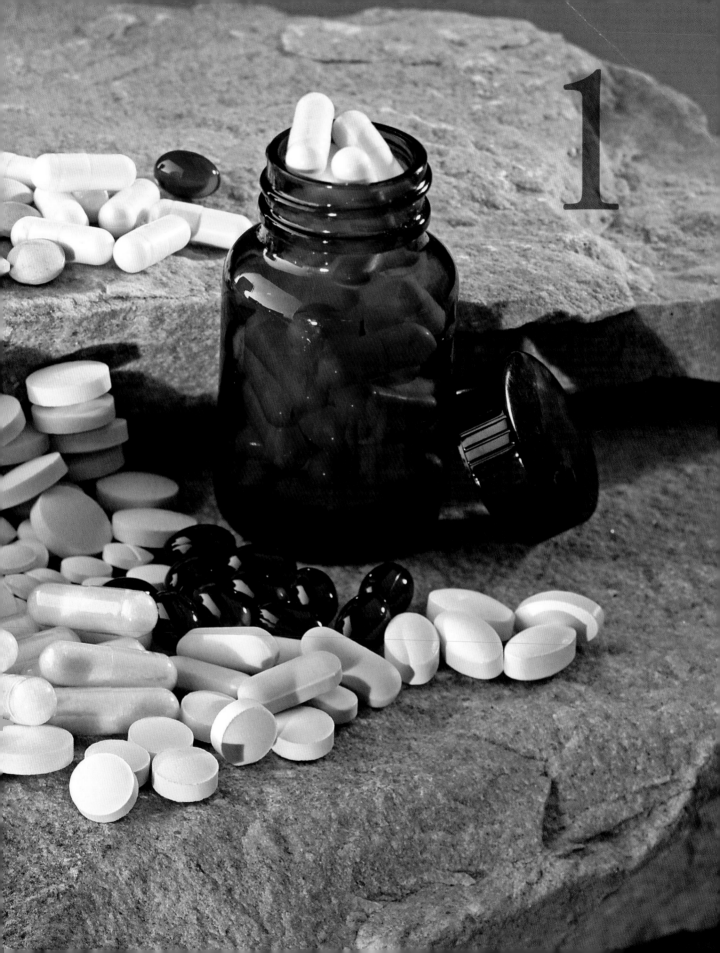

1

Theanine

for Anxiety

EVER WONDER WHY green-tea drinkers never seem to get the "hypers" that coffee drinkers get, even when the green tea is fully caffeinated?

The answer in all likelihood is a nonprotein amino acid found in tea called *theanine*. Theanine is helpful in improving mood and increasing a sense of relaxation. In fact, it's used in Japan for just that purpose. The calming effect of theanine is probably the reason that drinking green tea—even with caffeine—doesn't produce nearly as "jittery" an experience as drinking coffee. If you want to relax, a theanine supplement might be just the thing for you.

Historically, theanine has been used for its ability to reduce anxiety and its overall calming effects. It is known to block the binding of L-glutamic acid—an excitatory neurotransmitter—to glutamate receptors in the brain. If you think of the little glutamic acid molecules as lamps and the receptors as wall outlets, theanine basically closes down some of those wall outlets so fewer lamps get plugged in and there's less bright light; the brain is then less "excited."

A 1999 study measured the brain activity of volunteers after an oral dose of 50 to 200 mg of L-theanine (also known as just *theanine*) and found that the supplement helped generate alpha brain waves, which are usually considered to be associated with relaxation. That may be another way that L-theanine helps promote relaxation. Theanine also seems to promote increased levels of GABA (gamma aminobutyric acid), an inhibitory neurotransmitter that also has significant calming effects in the brain. Some supplements actually combine theanine with GABA. (According to Ray Sahelian, M.D., GABA seems to work better when combined with other stress supplements, so a theanine-GABA supplement like ZEN—available on my website, www.jonnybowden.com—makes a lot of sense.)

Natural Prescription for Anxiety

Theanine: 200 mg

For Added Effectiveness: GABA (200–500 mg) OR inositol (500–1,500 mg)

Note: All dosages are daily dosages and in pill or capsule form unless otherwise noted.

Preliminary evidence shows that theanine might have the potential to reduce blood pressure. (It certainly does in rats—at least rats that are hypertensive.) And it seems to cause a significant increase in dopamine, one of the "feel-good" neurotransmitters. In a 2007 study, it reduced heart rate during an acute experimental stress task. Plus, in animal studies it improves performance on a bunch of tests of memory and learning.

I have a good friend who has one of the highest-pressure jobs in the United States—he's a CIA agent. As you can imagine, his wife has a bit of stress and anxiety in her daily life. (File that under "ya think?") He told me that theanine has been a lifesaver in their home. His wife says that a 200 mg theanine supplement takes the edge off anxiety, without making her the least bit drowsy. Maybe it can do the same for you.

Vitamin B6

and Autism

YEARS AGO, when I was working as a musical director, I had the pleasure of working with Patricia Birch, who was well known at the time for being the director-choreographer of the theatrical version of *Grease*. In addition, she choreographed at least two dozen other Broadway shows, *Saturday Night Live* for six years, music videos for many stars, and earned Emmy Awards during her amazing career. Anyway.

When I first watched her work, I was surprised at how little she seemed to do. She hired amazing dancers and then got out of the way while they did their thing. She pointed, suggested, facilitated, and then seemed to disappear. She was the ultimate catalyst. Broadway legend had it that she didn't really "do" anything, but nothing could be further from the truth. If Pat wasn't there, the good stuff just didn't happen. She was so darn good that she seemed invisible—the dancers got all the credit for the spectacular moves onstage, but there would have been no show without Pat's quiet, behind-the-scenes guidance.

And so it is with vitamin B6.

B6 to the body is like Pat Birch to a Broadway show. Without it, the show just does not go on, and the actors are all headed for the unemployment line. B6 is the quintessential brain food, involved in all different kinds of reactions that affect not only the brain but the colon, heart, kidneys, and lungs. Vitamin B6 is the master vitamin in the processing of amino acids—the building blocks of all proteins and some hormones. It helps make serotonin, melatonin, and dopamine, the happy, sleepy, and peppy neurotransmitters, respectively. It's essential in the regulation of mental processes and mood function.

It's no wonder, then, that studies show that vitamin B6 plays an important role in the management of autism, as this condition has been linked to alterations in normal brain chemistry. Autism, a spectrum of developmental disorders of the brain that appears in early childhood, can be mild to severe and is usually accompanied by symptoms of impaired social interaction and diminished or absent communication skills, as well as unusual behaviors. Though we don't know exactly how, neurotransmitters are undoubtedly involved. Our brains need B6 to perform some of the operations necessary to make those neurotransmitters; if we don't have enough B6, we simply can't make them.

Natural Prescription for Autism

Vitamin B6: For children, start with a dose of 3.5 mg per day per 2.2 lb body weight and work with a doctor if you use a higher dose.

Magnesium: 200 mg

Essential fatty acids: 1,000 mg

Food allergy testing: Try a hypoallergenic diet and remove all food dyes, colorings, and preservatives. Get a food allergy test to identify foods that might cause sensitivities.

Detoxification program: Work with a qualified health-care practitioner.

Note: All dosages are daily dosages and in pill or capsule form unless otherwise noted.

There is currently no agreed-upon cure for autism, but there are a bunch of studies that show B6 can play a helpful role in reducing some of the symptoms, which suggests that our kids are probably also deficient in many nutrients that affect brain function. Some studies suggest that there is a subgroup of autistic children who actually do improve with vitamin B6 supplementation. The children in the studies usually took between 3.5 mg and almost 100 mg of B6 per day (for every 2.2 pounds of body weight). A doctor carefully supervised them throughout the process, as it is thought that high levels of B6 might have a negative effect on the nervous system, although this has never been confirmed. The studies showed that autistic children who took B6 and magnesium combined had significant improvement in their symptoms, including eye contact and verbal (as well as nonverbal) communication.

While adding B6 may not result in a complete turnaround for autistic behavior, there is certainly enough evidence and reason to try supplementing in children.

Other Benefits from This Great Vitamin

Vitamin B6 is one of the most utilized vitamins in the body and plays a vital role in managing such critical conditions as asthma, diabetes (especially diabetic neuropathy), and some forms of heart disease.

In general, people with asthma have a defect in the metabolism of an amino acid called *tryptophan*, which is the raw material from which the body makes serotonin—the happy neurotransmitter. This metabolic difficulty may well be the result of low B6 levels. Some studies show that patients benefit from vitamin B6 supplementation, which seems to correct the blocked tryptophan metabolism. In one study, oral supplementation of 50 mg twice daily resulted in a dramatic decrease in frequency and severity of asthmatic attacks. People with asthma who undergo treatment with the drug theophylline definitely need B6 supplementation, as that medication may significantly suppress levels of *pyridoxal-5-phosphate*, the active form of vitamin B6, which would definitely be bad news. Extra B6 can also reduce the typical side effects of theophylline (headaches, nausea, irritability, and sleep disorders).

WORTH KNOWING

The dose of B6 used in the research mentioned above was pretty high, and as noted, there has been a persistent yet scientifically undocumented worry that high doses of vitamin B6 over time *might* cause problems in the nervous system.

My associate, nutritionist Suzanne Copp, M.S., points out that it's not the high doses of B6 that are a problem, but rather, giving a single B vitamin *without* preparing the body with a foundation dose of all the other B vitamins. According to my friend, the brilliant nutritionist Linda Lizotte, R.D., giving a high dose of one B vitamin (like B6) may create a deficiency in one or more of the other Bs; the "negative effect" you may (or may not!) observe from a high dose of a single B vitamin could actually be a sign of some *other* B vitamin deficiency.

Bottom line: When you take a therapeutic dose of a single B vitamin (B6 or any other), it's important to take a B complex supplement as well. Take it at a different time of day—the B vitamins are like instruments in an orchestra, and they perform best together. But when you want to give one a solo, put it in the spotlight and take it by itself after the orchestra has already laid down the main tracks.

Bone and Brain Disorders

A B6 deficiency is also a common finding in those who suffer from carpal tunnel syndrome, a painful disorder caused by compression of a nerve that passes between the bones and ligaments of the wrist. It can cause weakness and pain when gripping, in addition to burning, tingling, or aching. At 100 to 200 mg a day, B6 has helped to relieve pain. But you must be patient: The average amount of time it takes to feel relief is three or more months.

Because B6 is intimately involved with brain chemistry, it is also beneficial for any type of mood or brain disorder, such as depression, schizophrenia, and epilepsy. Vitamin B6 levels are frequently very low in depressed individuals. They're also frequently low in women taking birth control pills or the hormone replacement drug Premarin. Imagine how many depressed people could be helped just by adding B6 to their diet or supplement regimen—it would help to raise serotonin levels, thus acting as a kind of "natural Prozac."

In this country we're spending upward of $12 billion a year (2004) on antidepressant drugs, and the current thought is that 25 percent of people are misdiagnosed or overdiagnosed as depressed. Imagine what could be done with a little vitamin like B6.

Vitamin B12
for Aging Complications

IN HIS BOOK *Your Nutrition Prescription,* H.L. Newbold, M.D., tells the story of a seventy-six-year-old German woman who came to see him. She had been crying uncontrollably for six months and was unable to function fully because of her state.

Despite her normal blood level of vitamin B12, he still injected her with it. She returned to his office three days later, no longer crying, reporting that she felt stronger than she had in a long time and was even able to sleep through the night for the first time in many nights. Three days after that, she was actually happy again that she could do her housekeeping.

And that, my friends, is the dramatic effect that B12 can have on the elderly.

Know Whether You Are Low in B12

It's been estimated that up to 45 percent of people over the age of sixty-five are deficient in vitamin B12 and, depending on the level you use as a marker, it could be more.

Vitamin B12 is involved in all sorts of things in the human body, including the production of DNA, the making of red blood cells, and the creation of the *myelin sheath*, the insulation that surrounds our nerves. This sheath helps conduct signals in the nervous system. Without enough B12 we start to act and feel old and show more prominent symptoms of aging: ataxia (shaky movements and unsteady gait), muscle weakness, spasticity, incontinence, slowed reactions, memory loss, disorientation, and depression—nothing on the must-have list for any baby boomer I know. Vitamin B12 deficiency is also associated with deafness; supplements have been useful in treating tinnitus and noise-related hearing loss.

To get enough B12 you have to do more than eat it—you have to absorb it. And therein lies the rub. Anyone over 40, especially the elderly, are at risk of B12 deficiency because they

lack enough of a protein that is secreted in the stomach called *intrinsic factor*, which you need to absorb B12.

So even if you're getting plenty of the vitamin in your diet—which, believe me, most people aren't—it won't do you much good if you lack this important protein. To properly absorb (and use) vitamin B12 requires a whole host of chain reactions that involve adequate pancreatic enzymes, calcium, and enough hydrochloric acid (something that many of us don't make enough of, especially as we age). Therefore, many other physiological deficiencies associated with aging can all lead to a B12 deficiency.

Because of this complex absorption process and the risk of many metabolic blocks—from nutrient deficiencies to exposure to toxins to factors in processed foods that cause reduced stomach acid, autoimmune disease, and enzyme disruption—it's perfectly possible to eat adequate amounts of B12 from foods like mollusks (clams, oysters, etc.), liver, beef, fish, and eggs but still develop a deficiency. The real indicator of whether or not B12 supplementation is necessary in the elderly is the symptoms that exist.

Natural Prescription for Aging

Vitamin B12: 10–25 mcg. When vitamin B12 is used for therapeutic purposes (as opposed to correcting a deficiency), injections are usually necessary to achieve results. However, oral vitamin B12 can be used to treat a vitamin B12 deficiency.

Folic acid: 400–800 mcg

Acetyl-L-carnitine: 1,500 mg per day for two to three months

Antioxidants (daily doses):

Vitamin C: 2,000–4,000 mg

Vitamin E: 400–800 IU

Mixed carotenoids (beta-carotene and others): 15,000–40,000 IU

Selenium: 200–300 mcg

CoQ10: 30–150 mg

Lipoic acid: 50–250 mg

Regular aerobic exercise and weight (resistance) training

Note: All dosages are daily dosages and in pill or capsule form unless otherwise noted.

Don't Forget B12 for Memory

Research shows tremendous potential for B12 to reverse mental decline in elderly patients. In one study, 61 percent of patients with mental impairment had complete recovery with supplementation; investigators speculate that those who did not recover had suffered from a deficiency for so long that damage to the nervous system had become irreversible.

Then there's Alzheimer's, a terrible condition for which we currently have no cure. While Alzheimer's undoubtedly has multiple and overlapping causes, there are some interesting areas of investigation involving natural substances like vitamin B12.

In fact, a study in Wales looked at whether Alzheimer's disease was a result of vitamin B12 deficiency. While this subject is still hotly debated among physicians, the study seemed to show very clearly that there is indeed a link. Researchers evaluated members of a family with a genetic predisposition toward Alzheimer's. They found that 67 percent of family members with confirmed Alzheimer's disease also had abnormally low blood levels of vitamin B12, compared to 8 percent who were at equal genetic risk for developing Alzheimer's but had not.

The researchers theorized that the deficiency probably caused impaired central nervous system reactions (specifically a chemical reaction called *methylation*, impairment of which is a characteristic feature of Alzheimer's). They also believe that there might be a genetic predisposition to Alzheimer's, and that some individuals are actually born unable to properly absorb B12.

Keep in mind that supplementation results in less improvement for those who have had full-blown Alzheimer's symptoms for more than six months. So routine early testing for B12 has the potential to prevent mental decline in many of the elderly and to also potentially protect against a condition as devastating as Alzheimer's.

You don't have to be elderly to take B12. Many other reasons support keeping your B12 status at adequate levels. For instance, vitamin B12 can help re-mineralize bones, inhibit the replication of the HIV virus, and fight asthma if the asthma is sulfite-induced. And B12 can greatly improve nervous system function, which also makes it beneficial for those with diabetic neuropathy and multiple sclerosis. It protects against environmental toxins, enhances immunity, and may even help with sleep disorders.

Taurine

for Bloat and Water Retention

IN A MINUTE, I'm going to tell you how good taurine is for the heart (and for arrhythmias). But first let me just pass on a little folk wisdom to you. If you've got PMS—and especially if you feel bloated—think taurine.

One of the most popular products on my website is a product by the wonderful vitamin company Designs for Health called Water Ease. Water Ease is 700 mg of taurine, with a little B6 thrown in for good measure. It's specifically made for easing water retention and bloat, and my clients and Internet customers have found it one of the most useful products on the market for getting rid of that wretched feeling that your tissues are waterlogged. If you've ever tried to fit into jeans during that time of the month, you know exactly what I mean. Obviously, that hasn't happened to me, but it's happened to most of the women that I know, and those who have turned to taurine—one of the most natural diuretics in the world—have been singularly impressed.

The Tale of Taurine

So what is taurine, anyway? And is it a coincidence that it not only works brilliantly for bloat and water retention but is also one of the most important nutrients for heart health, healthy blood pressure, and the prevention of arrhythmias?

Taurine is what's called a nonprotein amino acid. The body makes it from cysteine or methionine (other amino acids), with the help of vitamin B6. The highest concentration is found in the brain, retina, and heart muscle. Taurine represents about 50 percent of the free amino acids in heart cells and the second most abundant amino acid in the muscles.

Taurine is mostly found in high-protein foods. Beans and nuts don't contain it, but they do contain the amino acids from which the body can make taurine. Nevertheless, some integrative medical experts like Steven Lamm, M.D., suggest that vegetarians and those on low-fat diets may have less-than-optimal levels of taurine.

Aiding Arrhythmia

Since 1974, taurine's ability to prevent cardiac arrhythmia has been well documented in research. It's believed that it works by helping potassium (and magnesium) inside the heart muscle cells. Remember that the potassium/sodium balance not only affects blood pressure, but also water retention. When you have too much sodium (and not enough potassium), you retain water. Think of how you feel after you eat a really salty meal (or sometimes Chinese take-out). That's often caused by too much sodium, which translates to increased bloat. By helping tilt the balance in favor of potassium, taurine not only helps lower blood pressure, but acts as a natural diuretic (see above).

Natural Prescription for Bloat and Water Retention

Taurine: 700–1,000 mg, one to two times daily as needed (up to 6 g per day)

Note: All dosages are daily dosages and in pill or capsule form unless otherwise noted.

By helping normalize water via the potassium connection, taurine also helps lower blood pressure, which is one of many reasons why it's so important for the heart. A number of studies have shown just that. My friend Mark Houston, M.D., director of the Hypertension Institute at St. Thomas Hospital in Nashville, points out that animal studies have shown consistent and significant reductions in blood pressure with taurine, and that human studies have shown that many people with hypertension have reduced levels of taurine. Houston's Hypertension Institute program of vitamin supplementation for lowering blood pressure and keeping the heart healthy includes a daily dose of 1,500 mg of taurine. People with diabetes frequently have low levels as well, and stress eats it up, so those under high levels of stress may not have (or make) optimal amounts.

Taurine also helps regulate the levels of calcium inside the cells, protecting the heart muscle from dangerous calcium imbalances that can lead to cell death and heart muscle damage.

Because taurine helps regulate potassium, it may help prevent arrhythmias. Researchers writing in the journal *Medical Hypotheses* searched for nutrient deficiencies that could cause cardiac arrhythmias and found a lot of support for deficiencies of both taurine and L-arginine, another heart-friendly amino acid. The researchers stated that case histories of people with very frequent arrhythmias showed that 10 to 20 g of taurine per day reduced premature atrial contractions (arrhythmias) by 50 percent, and when 4 to 6 g of L-arginine were added, all remaining arrhythmias were terminated. In one of the cases, taurine restored energy and endurance. It has maintained a reputation for being an energy enhancer, leading to its inclusion in a lot of sports and energy drinks. Truth be told, it really doesn't "give" you energy, but it does help balance and restore you if you're burned out. Taurine is seriously depleted under the stress of hard exercise, so a case can be made for including it in drinks if they're truly used by athletes rehydrating during heavy workouts.

Proven Heart Health

Taurine is just a great overall heart nutrient. Nutritionist Susan Mudd, M.S., C.N.S., says "Taurine's cardiovascular functions and protection seem endless: cardiomyopathy, congestive heart failure, and recovery from heart attack, to name a few." Indeed, congestive heart failure is the top use for taurine supplementation listed in the prestigious Natural Medicines Comprehensive Database (www.naturaldatabase.com). In one study of 24 subjects with congestive heart failure, only 2 g of taurine twice a day resulted in clinical improvements for almost 80 percent of patients. In another study, 3 g of taurine outperformed even coenzyme Q10, another superb nutrient with documented results in congestive heart failure.

In 1928, the New York Heart Association published a classification of cardiac patients into four functional classes (I through IV) based on their prognosis and their clinical severity (that publication is now in its ninth edition and still going strong). Some patients with severe heart failure rapidly improve from New York Heart Association functional class IV to functional class II after only four to eight weeks of treatment, and their improvement seems to continue for as long as the taurine treatment is continued. Taking taurine orally improves left ventricular function and symptoms of heart failure.

I recommend taurine for anyone who is having problems with water retention and bloat. But for the same reason that it helps with those annoying conditions, it is also a terrific nutrient for the heart, and should be included in any natural supplement program for heart health, congestive heart failure, recovery from heart attacks, and the prevention of arrhythmias.

5-HTP

for Depression

CONSIDER THIS: You're lying on the couch, unable to motivate yourself enough to get up and get dressed. Everything seems pointless, hopeless, and dark, and all you want to do is stare into space. There's a pill sitting on the coffee table a few feet in front of you that promises to make you feel 100 percent better and take your depression away.

And you can't muster the enthusiasm or energy to get up and get it.

That's the best—and truest—description of severe depression I've ever heard. I don't remember from whom I heard it, but I remember recognizing it instantly as being a perfect description of the hell that is depression.

I know, because it's exactly how I felt for one horrendous year in my life, right after I moved to Los Angeles and promptly got divorced.

Luckily, it didn't last (feeling horrendous, that is—the divorce has gone quite well, thank you). And yes, I did use a pharmaceutical prescription—Lexapro, actually—to help get up off the couch and put some things into motion that actually helped me get rid of the depression. But I haven't used Lexapro for years, and I've seen plenty of other people get off antidepressants—or avoid going on

them in the first place—by using a combination of natural substances from amino acids to St. John's wort.

One of the best of those natural substances is 5-HTP.

Depression Is Not a Prozac Deficiency

The term 5-HTP stands for 5-hydroxytryptophan, and it's the stuff out of which your body makes serotonin, one of the major players in a group of neurotransmitters—chemicals that transmit information in the brain. Though depression is complicated and undoubtedly has many precipitating factors, it's widely accepted that neurotransmitters are deeply involved, especially serotonin. Low levels of serotonin are associated with cravings, anxiety, obsessive-compulsive disorder, aggressive behavior, and depression.

We don't know exactly how all the neurotransmitters work together to cause or affect depression in all its many forms, but we do suspect that low levels of serotonin play a big part in what people experience as depression.

It's not for nothing that serotonin is known as the "feel good" neurotransmitter. Without enough of it we don't do very well. The most popular pharmaceutical antidepressants—Prozac, Zoloft, Lexapro, etc.—belong to a class called serotonin selective reuptake inhibitors (SSRIs). The SSRIs do just what the term says—they inhibit the action of the cleanup crew that "mops up" serotonin from the brain, thus allowing serotonin to hang around longer. The more serotonin, goes the reasoning, the happier the camper.

Enter 5-HTP. Your body makes serotonin from an amino acid known as L-tryptophan. L-tryptophan comes in foods like turkey and seafood. The body then turns it into a metabolite called 5-HTP (5-hydroxytryptophan) and then, with the help of vitamin B6, into 5-HT (5-hydroxytryptamine), better known to all of us as plain old serotonin.

Questionable Safety Concerns

You used to be able to buy L-tryptophan as a separate nutritional supplement, but the Food and Drug Administration—in what I still believe to be an incredible act of bureaucratic stupidity—took it off the market around 1990 after an outbreak of eosinophilia myalgia syndrome (EMS), which was linked to the use of tryptophan.

WORTH KNOWING

There's a lack of info about the effects of taking 5-HTP during pregnancy, so check with your health professional or be on the safe side and don't use it. It can affect prolactin, a hormone necessary for milk production, so it might be a good idea to avoid it while breastfeeding. Because it does increase serotonin, it's wise to check with a knowledgeable health care professional about possible interactions with other drugs or supplements. Really. Though 5-HTP is great stuff, don't start mixing and matching with pharmaceuticals or taking yourself off medications without your doctor's knowledge. It can be done, but do it wisely and with supervision.

EMS is a dangerous and potentially deadly blood disease that is usually associated with parasitic infections or severe allergy. If it was truly caused by tryptophan, the FDA would have been right to get rid of it, but the Centers for Disease Control and Prevention traced the cause of the EMS crisis to a contaminant found only in batches of tryptophan manufactured by a single Japanese company, Showa Denko. Showa Denko, the source of up to 60 percent of all the tryptophan sold in the United States, had used an untested manufacturing process that reduced the amount of activated charcoal used to filter fermented raw tryptophan.

Natural Prescription for Depression

5-HTP: Start with 50 mg three times a day and increase if necessary after two weeks. A common dose for depression and headache is 300 mg daily.

Omega-3 fatty acids: 1–3 g daily

Remove sugar from diet

Exercise daily!

★ FOR ADDED EFFECTIVENESS:

Inositol: 612 g for as long as needed

Note: The above dosages are daily and in pill or capsule form unless otherwise noted.

Taking all tryptophan supplements off the market permanently— which the government did—was akin to permanently banning Tylenol in 1982 because seven people in the Chicago area died after ingesting Extra Strength Tylenol that had been laced with potassium cyanide— which the government did *not* do. I wonder why? It says more about the government's attitude toward supplements than it does about the safety of tryptophan that it acted so unilaterally against this great natural cure, but that's another story.

One Step Away from Serotonin

For years health practitioners had used tryptophan to help people sleep and as a natural aid to relaxation and calm. A lot of people were very upset when it was taken off the market. But lucky for us, 5-HTP is even better. As explained above, it's only one step from 5-HTP to serotonin. In addition, in animal and human studies, 5-HTP, unlike tryptophan, has been demonstrated to increase catecholamine metabolism, specifically working on dopamine and norepinephrine—other "feel good" neurotransmitters that are involved in mood. (It's possible that the antidepressant effect of 5-HTP may be related to a combined effect on serotonin and other neurotransmitters.) Regardless of its effect on other brain chemicals, supplemental 5-HTP surely increases serotonin, and because of that, has a calming, relaxing effect on brain chemistry. It's used for mild and moderate depression and it also may help you sleep better. Why? Because at night, serotonin converts into melatonin (see page 63), which is important for a great night's sleep.

For some people, 5-HTP may perform equally to or better than standard antidepressant drugs and in most cases, without side effects. One study compared 5-HTP to fluvoxamine, an SSRI like Prozac, Paxil, and Zoloft. In the study, subjects received either 5-HTP (100 mg) or fluvoxamine (50 mg) three times daily for six weeks. More patients felt better after using 5-HTP than fluvoxamine, and 5-HTP was quicker acting than the fluvoxamine. And in one other study, patients who were unresponsive to other antidepressant therapy showed significant improvement when using 5-HTP.

Then there are headaches. Because chronic headache sufferers have low levels of serotonin in their tissues, some researchers refer to migraine and chronic headaches as a "low-serotonin syndrome." Evidence from several studies in both children and adults shows that 5-HTP may be effective in reducing both the severity and frequency of headaches, including tension headaches and migraines. (It may be most effective for treating headaches in people with a history of depression or those who experienced severe headaches before the age of twenty.) And fewer pain-relieving medications may be needed when taken with 5-HTP.

There's even some evidence that 5-HTP may be helpful in fibromyalgia. In one study, 300 mg per day of 5-HTP was shown to be effective in reducing many symptoms of fibromyalgia, including pain, morning stiffness, sleep disturbances, and anxiety. A single 100 mg nighttime dose of 5-HTP was shown to be sufficient to improve the duration and depth of sleep.

And 5-HTP may turn out to have a nice role in a weight loss protocol, as it may greatly reduce carbohydrate cravings. By altering serotonin in the brain, it inhibits eating behavior in animals. Studies in humans also suggest that 5-HTP may reduce eating behaviors, lessen caloric intake, and promote weight loss in obese individuals. Appetite reduction and weight loss (averaging eleven pounds in twelve weeks) have occurred with amounts of 600 to 900 mg of 5-HTP daily. In a double-blind, placebo-controlled study of nineteen obese females, those who were given 8 mg per kg of body weight of 5-HTP for five weeks achieved a significant weight loss of about 5 percent. And those findings were confirmed by a second study conducted over a longer period of time.

Listen, I'm the last person to tell you to throw out your pharmaceutical antidepressants. I believe they've helped many people—including me—and probably saved a lot of lives. But if you have mild or moderate depression, or any of the other conditions mentioned above that might respond to a boost in the brain chemical serotonin, you might give 5-HTP a try. And if you're lucky—and many people are—you may find that by using 5-HTP, you may not need the "big guns" at all.

Chromium

A Magical Mineral for People with Diabetes

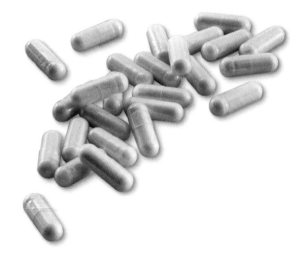

IN 1996, the American Diabetes Association (ADA) stated that "chromium supplementation has no known benefit in patients who are not chromium deficient."

I mention this statement because it's a great object lesson in why you should be careful about swallowing whole—without a spoonful or so of Celtic salt—any statement that comes from an "official" health organization. This statement by the ADA was not the first time—and certainly won't be the last—that an establishment health organization was completely off the mark. (Anyone remember the first edition of the food pyramid?)

One year after the ADA statement, a study published in the journal *Diabetes* divided 180 people with type 2 diabetes into three groups— one group received 200 mcg of chromium picolinate a day, one group received 1,000 mcg, and the third group got a placebo. Supplemental chromium was shown to have dramatic effects on glucose and insulin variables and "significant, sustained reductions in diabetic symptoms were especially noted in those who received 1,000 mcg per day."

Insulin's Little Helper

So what's the deal with chromium? Simply put, chromium is "insulin's little helper."

If you're familiar with the mechanism of diabetes, you probably know something about insulin. In a nutshell, here's what happens: When you eat, your blood sugar goes up, the pancreas secretes insulin, and insulin begins to remove sugar from the bloodstream and escort it into the cells. In at least one in four people (much more by some estimates), this mechanism doesn't work properly. The cells become "resistant" to the effects of insulin, and the person is left with both high blood sugar and high insulin, which often puts you on the fast track to diabetes and metabolic syndrome (itself a risk factor for heart disease; see page 192). It's not a great scenario, and it's increasingly common.

What chromium does is help insulin do its job better. In this way, it works much like certain "insulin-sensitizing" medications, such as glucophage. It literally helps open the doors of the cells so that insulin (and sugar) can get in, thus reducing the burden on the body of having high amounts of both blood sugar and insulin. According to Georgetown University Medical Center professor Harry Preuss, M.D., C.N.S., chromium activates the enzyme tyrosine kinase, which helps insulin attach to insulin receptors. It's like a key to the cell door.

The leading chromium researcher in the world is Richard Anderson, Ph.D., at the U.S. Department of Agriculture. Anderson has done a number of studies on people with diabetes that show positive effects such as lowered blood sugar when people are supplemented with chromium, particularly at the higher doses (800 to 1,000 mcg per day). Chromium has also been shown helpful in the treatment of gestational diabetes and may even be of some help in type 1 diabetes. In one study, even 200 mcg of chromium given to people with type 1 diabetes allowed them to reduce their average insulin dosage by almost one-third.

Dosing the Deficiency

Remember that we don't absorb chromium very well and we don't get a lot of it in our diet (the main source is brewer's yeast, liver, and of course, beer—not the way you'd want to get it if you struggle with blood sugar and weight issues).

Some studies have shown no effect of chromium on blood sugar or other diabetic measures, but Anderson and other experts have

---

Natural Prescription for Diabetes

Chromium: 1,000 mcg*

Cinnamon: 1/2 tsp

Magnesium: 400–800 mg

Biotin: 8–16 mg

Vitamin C: 1–2 g

Omega-3 fatty acids: 2–3 g (balance with 250–500 mg omega-6 fatty acids, like GLA from evening primrose oil, or take a basic essential fatty acid supplement like Omega Synergy (see www.jonnybowden.com for details)

Alpha lipoic acid: 250–1,000 mg

Zinc: 25 mg

Low-carbohydrate and/or high-fiber diet

Exercise: Five days a week

*You can take a higher dosage. At the famed Tacoma Clinic in Washington, noted integrative medicine guru Jonathan Wright, M.D., frequently uses 3,000–4,000 mcg with his diabetic or blood sugar–challenged patients with great results.

Note: All dosages are daily dosages and in pill or capsule form unless otherwise noted.

---

pointed out that this is probably because researchers have not always used the most effective forms of chromium, nor the right dosages. Anderson himself is partial to chromium picolinate, while other experts, like Preuss, favor niacin-bound chromium (chromium polynicotinate or chromium nicotinate, sold under the brand name ChromeMate). There's also GTF chromium (GTF stands for *glucose tolerance factor*), but this is a mislabeling and a misconception; no such substance exists.

Interestingly, a high-sugar and processed-food diet actually drains chromium from the body, so the paradox is that those who need it the most have the least of it. Infection, pregnancy, and stress may also reduce levels. Even those eating a lot of healthy foods like seeds, nuts, and grains may be low in chromium because many of these foods, especially soy, contain phytic acid, which decreases the absorption of chromium (and other minerals).

A Measurement Marker

And don't believe for a second that only people who are chromium deficient will benefit from chromium supplements. There are no good tests for either deficiencies or for body stores and no biochemical marker has ever been able to reliably assess a person's chromium status.

There have been some studies on chromium and fat loss and chromium and muscle gain, but the results are inconsistent. It's possible that the doses used in some studies were less than required to make a difference. Jonathan Wright, M.D., one of the leading lights of integrative

WORTH KNOWING

Don't confuse chromium the supplement with the dangerous form of metal that was poisoning the town in the movie *Erin Brockovich*. That was *hexavalent* chromium, and it is indeed a poison. *Trivalent* chromium, the kind in food and supplements, is amazingly safe. So few adverse effects have been reported that the Institute of Medicine has never established a Tolerable Upper Intake Level for it. According to Georgetown University Medical Center professor Harry Preuss, M.D., C.N.S., rats fed trivalent chromium at levels thousands of times higher than the reference dose for humans, based on body weight, didn't show any toxic effects.

medicine for more than 30 years, routinely uses much higher doses of chromium (3,000 to 4,000 mcg per day, tapering down eventually to 1,000 mcg for "maintenance") with his patients to curb sugar and carbohydrate cravings, and reports great success.

The main thing we can hang our hat on is chromium's ability to help lower blood sugar and make insulin work more effectively. That alone makes it a hugely important addition to the regime of anyone trying to regulate his or her blood sugar and reduce insulin resistance.

Glutamine

for Cravings

NEXT TIME a carbohydrate urge hits, reach for the white stuff. No, not granulated sugar. Glutamine. L-glutamine (also known as glutamine) is the most abundant amino acid in the human body.

The majority of it is stored up in the muscles and used up in really heavy exercise, which is why it's such a popular supplement among bodybuilders and athletes. (It's also critical for the immune system, and since so much is used up during intense exercise, this may be partly why marathoners frequently get sick after the event.) Glutamine's also a very important nutrient for intestinal health and wound healing.

And glutamine can help with cravings. For both sugar *and* alcohol.

The Atkins Connection

I first learned about this from Robert Atkins, M.D., who actually learned about it from Roger Williams, M.D. Williams, a pioneer in nutritional medicine, was the father of the term *biochemical individuality* and the author of several books on nutrition and alcohol. He was one of the first to recognize the deep and intimate connection between cravings for alcohol and cravings for sugar, and he used glutamine for both.

It started back in the 1950s, when Williams did an experiment with alcohol-loving rats.

First he established which rats liked to drink by giving them the opportunity to drink freely from either of two bottles—one filled with tap water and one containing 10 percent alcohol. Then he picked nineteen rats that tended to like the alcohol the most, and divided them into two groups. One group received 100 mg of L-glutamine mixed with their food, the other group didn't. At the end of 17 days, he returned all the rats to a regular diet of Purina rat chow and watched and measured what they drank.

Natural Prescription for Cravings

Take 1 heaping teaspoon of glutamine powder dissolved in water when a craving strikes or as a preventive measure (preferably on an empty stomach).

Alternately, take three or four times a day, in between meals.

Note: The above dosages are daily dosages and in pill or capsule form, unless otherwise noted.

The rats fed the glutamine consumed, on the whole, 35 percent less alcohol over the next 9 days than the rats that were not fed the glutamine. Williams concluded that "glutamine administered orally appears to be a relatively effective agent in decreasing the voluntary consumption of alcohol by rats."

It also seems to work on humans. In a study published in the *Quarterly Journal of Studies on Alcohol* in 1957, Williams found that 1 g of L-glutamine in divided doses with meals significantly reduced both cravings and the anxiety that accompanies alcohol withdrawal. In another experiment, a daily dose of about 3 teaspoons did the trick for about three-quarters of the people studied. Why these studies were never followed up on amazes me, but glutamine continues to be used by many knowledgeable practitioners who work with both alcoholics and sugar addicts, and it's used in many alcoholism programs across the country.

Cure Those Constant Cravings

When you experience a craving, it's because your brain wants sugar. And it wants it now! Glutamine is an alternate source of glucose available to the brain, plus it has the added advantage of getting there quickly! You can open a capsule and put it under your tongue and you'll feel the crave-reducing effect within minutes. Or better yet, put a heaping spoonful in water.

"[Glutamine] provides a ready source of brain fuel for hypoglycemics and helps stave

WORTH KNOWING

You don't have to follow the Atkins recipe, though it does taste good. In fact, I find that sweetening the mix, even with stevia or xylitol, increases my desire for more sweets, but that's just me. (Obviously the folks at the Atkins Center didn't agree!) Most people these days, myself included, just take a heaping teaspoon of glutamine and mix it in plain old filtered or spring water. It works just fine.

off sugar cravings ... that develop when blood sugar levels drop too low," says Joan Mathews-Larson, Ph.D.

Abram Hoffer, M.D., Ph.D., a Canadian psychiatrist and one of the pioneers in the practice of orthomolecular medicine (the practice of using megavitamins and nutrients to treat disease) called L-glutamine "an amino acid that decreases physiological cravings for alcohol" and "one of the two primary energy providers that ... provide fuel to the brain."

Atkins has suggested the following for a sugar urge: Take 1 to 2 g of L-glutamine, preferably with some heavy cream and just a touch of nonsugar sweetener. "The immediate desire to eat something sweet will pass," he said. "For a reference attesting to its efficiency, ask any of the 8,000 Atkins Center patients for whom I have prescribed it!"

Lysine

for Herpes

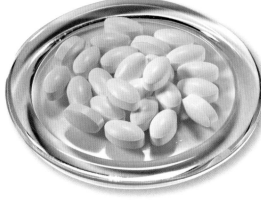

LET'S TALK about herpes. It's probably not your favorite subject, but let's talk about it anyway. I don't know about you, but when I was "coming up," as they say, herpes was the scourge of the sexual revolution.

AIDS was a few years away, and we were still way too naive to know about the dozens of other sexually transmitted diseases like chlamydia or human papilloma virus. If you got herpes back then it was considered the death knell for your sex life. There were herpes support groups, for goodness' sake. (Remember, this was pre-Oprah.) Having herpes was the deepest, darkest secret you could possibly harbor.

Well, times have changed a lot, but herpes is still not something you'd exactly put on your "must-have" list. Herpes simplex virus is a recurrent viral infection that causes outbreaks on any area of the body, particularly the mouth or genitals. (HSV-1 is the cold sore variety, HSV-2 the genital variety.)

More than 60 percent of those infected with herpes virus will have reoccurring outbreaks of herpes. While one person may only have one or two outbreaks per year, and some lucky folks have them only once every few years, others are plagued by this infectious, painful, sometimes dangerous, and always uncomfortable virus several times per month. Chicken pox, shingles, and cold sores—they're all part of the herpes family. And then, of course, there are those familiar outbreaks in the most unwanted of intimate places—always, it seems, just when you have the best chance of getting lucky.

Even if you've been fortunate enough never to have an outbreak of genital herpes, you've probably experienced a plain old garden-variety cold sore. And if you have, you've probably gone on the inevitable quest to find something— anything—that will make it go away: licorice root, homeopathic medicines, vitamin megadoses, avoiding the sun, and any technique that reduces stress. They're all good and can help control an outbreak when it happens. But for true prevention you may want to consider some immune-enhancing strategies, and you might especially want to consider lysine.

Enter the Herpes Slayer

Lysine, an amino acid, has had a reputation as a first-line defense against herpes for a long time. Back in 1978, a multicenter study of lysine therapy in herpes simplex infection was published in the journal *Dermatologica*; the authors found that lysine "appears to suppress the clinical manifestations of the herpes virus."

A number of studies followed over the years—one found that more patients were recurrence-free during lysine treatment (1,000 mg daily) while another found that 1,000 mg of lysine three times a day for six months resulted in fewer infections, less severe symptoms, and significantly less healing time.

In one other study, researchers surveyed 1,543 subjects with a questionnaire after a six-month trial period during which they took an average dose of 936 mg of lysine daily. The study included subjects with cold sores, canker sores, and genital herpes. Eighty-four percent of those surveyed said that lysine supplementation prevented recurrence or decreased the frequency of herpes infection. Whereas 79 percent described their symptoms as severe or intolerable without lysine, only 8 percent used these terms when taking lysine. Without lysine, 90 percent indicated that healing took six to fifteen days, but with lysine 83 percent stated that lesions healed in five or fewer days. Overall, a stunning 88 percent of the people in the study considered supplemental lysine an effective form of treatment for herpes infection! Not bad for a nondrug intervention with no known side effects.

Natural Prescription for Herpes

Lysine: 1,000–3,000 mg (larger doses can be divided into 1,000 mg, three times per day)

Vitamin C and flavonoids: 200 mg of vitamin C plus 200 mg of flavonoids, each taken three to five times per day

Vitamin E: 400 IU, three times per day for three days and then cut back to 400 IU per day. Do not use if you are on anticoagulant drugs.

PLANT STEROLS:

Lemon balm (Melissa officinalis): Lemon balm cream applied two to four times per day for five to ten days

Topical tea tree oil ointment (not the undiluted oil) or

Licorice root gel: Applied to blisters as needed

Diet: Avoid foods that are high in arginine, such as nuts, peanuts, and chocolate. Eat foods high in lysine, such as yogurt and other dairy products.

Note: All dosages are daily and in pill or capsule form unless otherwise noted.

Lysine and Arginine

Lysine is considered an "essential" amino acid, defined as an amino acid that the body can't manufacture and therefore has to be obtained from food (or supplements). It works hand in hand with other essential amino acids to maintain growth, lean body mass, and the body's store of nitrogen, an essential part of all amino and nucleic acids, both of which are necessary to all life. But when it comes to herpes, lysine has a strange relationship with another (very important) amino acid, arginine.

Herpes is less likely to reproduce when the ratio of lysine to arginine favors lysine—when there's too much arginine and not enough lysine, the virus likes to replicate. Therefore, when you're fighting herpes, you want to make sure not to take arginine supplements, great as they may be for other things (like the heart and even sexual performance). Foods that have more lysine than arginine include fish, chicken, beef, lamb, milk, cheese, beans, brewer's yeast, mung bean sprouts, and most fruits and vegetables. Foods that have more arginine than lysine include gelatin, chocolate, carob, coconut, oats, whole wheat and white flour, peanuts, soybeans, and wheat germ. Best to stay away if you're having—or expecting—an outbreak. And if you want the therapeutic benefits of lysine for the prevention or control of herpes, it's best to take supplements. You're just not going to get nearly enough from food alone.

Everyday Prevention

Like many conditions discussed in this book, herpes has a very intimate relationship with stress. Stress makes it worse. A lot worse. Stress can actually bring on an outbreak, and it can certainly make an existing one worse. Reducing stress is one of the best things you can do for yourself if you want to keep outbreaks to a minimum.

And while we're talking about prevention, keep in mind that using lysine as a preventive measure against cold sores without strengthening the overall immune system is a little like rearranging the deck chairs on the Titanic. The stronger your immune system, the less chance that the herpes virus will reemerge to wreak havoc on your social life. If the immune system is working properly, the herpes virus wouldn't find it quite so easy to get inside your cells, replicate, and ruin your chances to get a date Saturday night. Under normal conditions a healthy immune system would destroy the virus before it had a chance to do this. Vitamins like C and E are potent against the virus, and new research points to plant sterols as also playing a role by increasing natural killer cell activity (a good thing) and destroying the virus.

If you're prone to herpes of either variety, you should definitely give lysine a try. But don't stop there. The next time you get a cold sore—or even better, before you get one— think about reducing your stress level and increasing your immune-strengthening vitamins. And don't forget to sleep well. All of these factors will contribute to the prevention of a new herpes attack.

Vitamin D
for Physical Performance

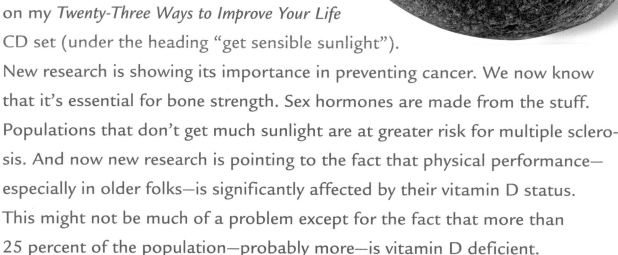

I REALLY CAN'T SAY enough about vitamin D. It's the subject of an entire track on my *Twenty-Three Ways to Improve Your Life* CD set (under the heading "get sensible sunlight"). New research is showing its importance in preventing cancer. We now know that it's essential for bone strength. Sex hormones are made from the stuff. Populations that don't get much sunlight are at greater risk for multiple sclerosis. And now new research is pointing to the fact that physical performance—especially in older folks—is significantly affected by their vitamin D status. This might not be much of a problem except for the fact that more than 25 percent of the population—probably more—is vitamin D deficient.

Let me explain. As of this writing the recommended daily allowance for vitamin D is 400 IU. I—and a growing body of nutritionists and doctors and health professionals—think that's way too low. Oh, I'm being polite. We think it's ridiculous. The current (paltry) levels of vitamin D recommendations are based mostly on vitamin D's effects on bone health.

But as Denise Houston, Ph.D., observes, "higher amounts of vitamin D may be needed for the preservation of muscle strength and physical function as well as other conditions such as cancer prevention." Movement is underfoot to raise the "recommended" level to 1,000 IU, which would be more like it.

But get this: Research from the Institute of Medicine shows that fully 50 percent of women aren't getting even the paltry amount of vitamin D currently recommended, let alone the revised, more optimal level.

Vitamin D and Men's Health

So we know for a fact that women are lacking vitamin D. What about men?

Not long ago, the website *Medical News Today* asked the rhetorical question, "How do we get men more interested in vitamin D?" The site reported that most men could care less. But what if vitamin D were linked to the kinds of things that get guys' attention? Performance? Sex? Hair growth?

Well, vitamin D may not grow hair on bald heads, but new research is showing that it significantly impacts performance and may be especially important for older adults. 2007 research from Wake Forest University School of Medicine shows that older adults who don't get enough vitamin D are at increased risk for both poor physical performance and for disability. More than 900 people over sixty-five years of age from two towns in Italy were tested on their walking speed, their ability to stand from a chair, and their ability to maintain balance in a variety of positions. They were also tested on handgrip strength, which seems to predict future disability very well. The results? Those who had low levels of vitamin D were about 5 to 10 percent lower in most measures of performance. A completely different 2007 study in the *Journal of Clinical Endocrinology and Metabolism* with a randomized Dutch population showed virtually identical results and arrived at a similar conclusion.

When *Medical News Today* continued its discussion of "how do we get guys interested in vitamin D?" they put it to their readers this way: "Actually, what we are asking is: *Does the most potent steroid hormone system in the human body have any effects on balance, muscle strength, muscle mass, reaction time, etc.?*" Well, when you put it that way, fellas…. Interestingly, two studies that looked at physical fitness and athletic performance found that physical fitness peaked in late summer when vitamin D levels are at their highest.

Older adults are especially susceptible to low levels of vitamin D because number one, they get less sun exposure, and two, their skin is less efficient in producing vitamin D from the sun in the first place. And it's not easy to get enough vitamin D from food sources.

New Moms at Risk

The scientist who's done the most research on vitamin D and the one who's been sounding the alarm the loudest about our collective vitamin D deficiency and the need for smart sun exposure is Michael Holick, M.D. He's written a great book called *The UV Advantage*, which I highly recommend. He's looked at the vitamin D levels of pregnant mothers coming into his hospital, and also at the vitamin D levels of their infants once they were born. He found that 76 percent of the mothers were severely vitamin D deficient, and 81 percent of their infants were as well. And the Centers for Disease Control and Prevention reported that 42 percent of African American women were deficient in vitamin D during their childbearing years, especially at the end of winter time. In fact, African Americans are especially at risk for vitamin D deficiency because having dark skin is like wearing a permanent sun protection factor of 15 to 30. Holick says that even 48 percent of Caucasian girls aged 9 to 11 are deficient in vitamin D at the end of the winter, and 17 percent of them remain so at the end of the summer because they're all wearing sunblock.

Natural Prescription for Improved Physical Performance

Vitamin D: 1,000–2,000 IU daily

You can also increase your vitamin D levels by getting unprotected sun exposure for about 10–15 minutes three times a week.

Inositol
for Sleep

LOOK UP "sleep disorder" on Wikipedia and you'll get no fewer than seventeen different entries ranging from *bruxism* (grinding your teeth) to *snoring*. (There's even one called *sexsomnia*. Give up? It means "sleep sex." And no, I did not make that up.) All of the disorders have one thing in common: They interfere with a good night's sleep. And that can spell serious problems indeed.

Many important things happen during sleep. Your brain makes certain hormones (melatonin and human growth hormone, for example) and replenishes vital biochemicals that keep you performing at your best during the day. Lack of sleep has been implicated in everything from obesity to traffic accidents. (It's well known that the day of the year with the greatest number of traffic accidents is the day after Daylight Saving Time ends.)

Sleep disorders are big business. As of this writing, use of sleep medications has grown by more than 60 percent since 2000, and in 2006, makers of sleeping pills spent more than $600 million advertising directly to consumers. Obviously, more than a few people are having some problems catching some good shut-eye.

Inositol might be the answer. This interesting substance is usually considered a member of the B vitamin family, but it's not technically a vitamin (it contains no nitrogen) and it's synthesized by the human body. No matter. This terrific little compound has multiple uses, one of which is that it's absolutely terrific for inducing sleep. What's more, it has none of the side effects of sleep medications. You're not likely to wake up in your kitchen in the middle of an ice cream raid. And you're also not likely to feel drowsy and bleary in the morning.

Inositol is "nature's sleeping pill." Taken before bedtime, it can significantly improve sleep quality. People who take it report a general relaxed feeling akin to having a few calming "sleepy-time" teas.

On "Insomnia Forum," one anonymous Internet poster reported this after adding 1,500 to 2,000 mg of inositol to his bedtime routine: "I'm not sure if it's the inositol, but this is the best sleep I've had in over two years of severe insomnia. It's the refreshing kind too, not the shallow type I've gotten on sleeping pills or other drugs." Normally I wouldn't repeat an anonymous Internet posting, but I've heard this sort of thing from many people over the years and I've experienced it myself.

Natural Prescription for Insomnia

Drink 2 g of powdered inositol in water before bedtime.

Though we don't know exactly why inositol works so well as a sleeping aid, most researchers who are aware of its effects assume it's because inositol is involved in the serotonin pathways. Serotonin, the "relaxing" neurotransmitter, is out of balance in many mental health disturbances, such as depression, panic disorder, and obsessive-compulsive disorder (OCD). Interesting, then, that inositol has been used—albeit in small studies—with good results in treating all three of these disorders. One study in 1996 showed a significant improvement in OCD patients when they were given 18 g of inositol a day. And in a double-blind, controlled crossover test, 12 g of inositol was shown to be as effective in treating panic disorder as the medication Luvox, though without the typical side effects of nausea and tiredness.

Inositol is completely safe. Though you can take it in capsule form (1,500 to 2,000 mg seems to be good for sleep induction), I recommend (and prefer) the powdered form since it mixes easily in water, tastes pretty bland, and makes it way easier to get a significant dose (like 6 or 7 g). Just to get used to it, start with about ¼ to ½ teaspoon (roughly ¾ of a gram to 1½ g) and work up to the dose that makes you feel best and gives you the best night's sleep. A few teaspoons should do it easily. (It's been used safely up to 18 g and is probably safe in amounts even greater than that, though you won't need that much.)

Iodine

for Hypothyroidism

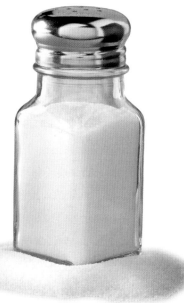

PLEASE PASS THE SALT. And make it iodized. Iodine and the thyroid gland are so closely intertwined that you just can't talk about one without mentioning the other. In essence, iodine is a trace element required for the production of thyroid hormones. The thyroid—a small, butterfly-shaped gland that wraps around the windpipe—uses iodine by attaching it to an amino acid called *tyrosine*. Together they work to make thyroid hormones, which regulate metabolism, or the rate that physiological actions take place in the body. Thyroid hormones stimulate different processes all over the body and play a role in growth, energy, fertility, and immune system support.

Iodine deficiency used to be thought of as rare in the Western part of the world, but there has been a recent and disturbing trend toward decreased iodine intake, which may potentially set us up for an increase in hypothyroidism, a condition in which the thyroid gland fails to function adequately and which results in reduced levels of thyroid hormone in the body; hypothyroidism is already a big problem for a lot of people. At least 20 percent of the world's population is iodine deficient and at risk for the range of iodine deficiency disorders that include goiter (enlargement of the thyroid gland), myxedema, and even cretinism.

In the United States and the Western world in general, the reduction in iodine consumption may be because more people are avoiding dairy, seafood, processed food, and iodized salt, all food substances high in iodine. Vegetarians, depending on the strictness of their practice, are largely deficient in iodine. Symptoms of iodine deficiency include mental fatigue, coordination problems, and stunted growth in children as well as goiter.

The Thyroid Connection

Low iodine levels contribute greatly to hypothyroidism (low thyroid hormones). Approximately 80 percent of the body's iodine pool winds up in the thyroid gland and is used to make thyroid hormones, so if there isn't enough iodine in the diet, the thyroid gland is the first to know it.

The symptoms of hypothyroidism vary from person to person, but commonly include several of the following: fatigue, lethargy, intolerance to

> **WORTH KNOWING**
>
> At a news conference organized by UNICEF, experts said that insufficient consumption of iodine was at once both the most prevailing and most preventable cause of brain damage anywhere around the world. Iodine deficiency is the leading cause of mental retardation, producing typical reductions in IQ of ten to fifteen points.
>
> Interestingly, selenium deficiency can exacerbate the effects of iodine deficiency.
>
> It's okay to supplement with iodine if you are taking thyroid medication like Synthroid or Armour thyroid.

cold, constipation, weight gain, depression, excessive menstruation, dry skin, hair loss, and hoarseness. Hypothyroidism makes one feel like an engine missing a spark plug. The mind and body are sluggish. Digestion becomes poor, cardiovascular function and mental activity slow down, and muscles weaken. The onset of these symptoms may be so gradual that they may go unnoticed for years, and undetected by doctors and patients. There may be several reasons why the thyroid is underacting, but it would be wise to also consider whether you are getting enough iodine in your diet.

Iodine and Your Brain

New and interesting research is also emerging that provides keys to other benefits of adequate amounts of iodine, including brain development.

Natural Prescription for Thyroid Support

Foods: Make sure to include foods in the diet such as seafood, iodized salt, sea vegetables such as kelp, and dairy products, all of which are high in iodine.

Iodine: 150 mcg

Selenium: 200 mcg

Tyrosine: 1–6 g (do not use if you are on an MAO inhibitor)

Note: The above dosages are daily dosages and in pill or capsule form, unless otherwise noted.

For example, iodine deficiency has been called "the world's major cause of preventable mental retardation" by the International Council for the Control of Iodine Deficiency Disorders. Most notably, in 2000, the *American Journal of Clinical Nutrition* published a study that examined 196 iodine-deficient children in Northern Benin. The children were separated into two groups—those whose iodine status was improved after iodized salt was added to the community and those whose status did not change. At the end of the study, the researchers concluded that the children who had iodine increases in diet had a significantly greater increase in performance on the combination of mental tests than did the group with no change in diet.

According to many integrative medicine experts, a simple test can determine whether or not you are iodine deficient: Get a bottle of tincture of iodine from the drugstore and paint a 3-inch patch on your skin. (Arm or belly work well. Be careful not to drop any on your clothes—it stains!) The stain on your skin should last for 48 hours. The sooner it disappears the more profound your iodine deficiency. (There are other tests for iodine deficiency that may be a bit more accurate, but they involve urine analysis; the "at-home" version will do nicely for most people.)

The Iodine Connection

Donald Miller, M.D., a cardiothoracic surgeon at the University of Washington Medical Center and a great practitioner of integrative, holistic medicine, has written eloquently on the importance of iodine in the diet for a number of different conditions. "There is growing evidence that Americans would have better health and a lower incidence of cancer and fibrocystic disease of the breast if they consumed more iodine," he says.

Miller points out that Japanese consumption of iodine through seaweed is many, many times that of the United States, and that the health comparisons between the two countries are disturbing. He suggests that iodine consumption may be one of the many reasons why the incidence of breast cancer is so high in the United States and so low in Japan. Women with goiter—a noncancerous enlargement of the thyroid gland due to iodine deficiency—have three times greater incidence of breast cancer. Interesting.

While Miller's suggestion about the connection between iodine and breast cancer remains an intriguing hypothesis, it's pretty well established that iodine is useful for cyclic mastalgia (cyclic breast pain and unusual breast tenderness and heaviness that often varies with the menstrual cycle). One randomized, double-blind, placebo-controlled, multicenter trial in 2004 found statistically significant improvement in pain for all women treated with 3 mg or 6 mg of molecular iodine, and these were women who were not helped by nonprescription painkillers. And a 1993 study in the *Canadian Journal of Surgery* found that 70 percent of subjects treated with iodine had clinical improvement in their fibrocystic breast disease. The researchers caution that molecular iodine was the most beneficial form.

Seaweed is the best source of organically bound iodine. Try to get the highest-quality noncommercially processed kind you can find. The primary dietary source of iodine is iodized salt, and a lot of people in the United States don't use it. Things that live in the sea—shellfish, white deep-water fish, brown seaweed, dulse, and kelp—are great sources of iodine. So are canned sardines, canned tuna, clams, cod, haddock, halibut, herring, lobster, oyster, perch, salmon, sea bass, and shrimp.

Krill Oil
for PMS

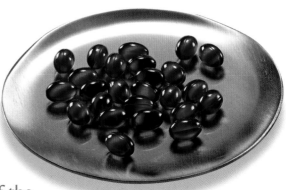

EVER WONDER HOW wild salmon get that nice red color? It comes from a powerful antioxidant called astaxanthin, which just happens to be present in one of the things wild salmon eat: krill. (Farmed salmon don't eat krill, so they get their red color from astaxanthin supplements that may or may not be artificial—plus a nice dose of artificial color chosen from a Salmo-Farm color wheel. But don't get me started.) So what exactly are krill and why do we care?

Krill are little crustaceans that look like shrimp and provide food for everything from salmon to blue whales. And they're one of the most nutritious creatures in the sea. Not only are they loaded with the aforementioned astaxanthin, but they're a great source of valuable omega-3 fatty acids. Krill oil is increasingly being researched for its health benefits (see below), and one of the nicest of those benefits is the effect krill oil has on premenstrual syndrome (PMS).

In a double-blind, randomized clinical trial, seventy patients diagnosed with PMS (by the standards of the *Diagnostic and Statistical Manual of Mental Disorders*, third edition, revised) were treated for three months with either krill oil or plain old omega-3 fish oil. The krill oil group had a statistically significant improvement in dysmenorrhea (painful menstruation) as well as in the emotional symptoms of PMS. The women taking the krill oil also chose to consume significantly less painkillers during the treatment period. JMS Medical Research, the independent research organization responsible for the data analysis, reported that krill oil "significantly improves the overall emotional and physical symptoms of patients suffering from premenstrual syndrome."

This study was particularly interesting because it not only investigated the effect of krill oil on PMS, but it also compared the effect of krill oil to regular omega-3 fish oil. Krill oil won. You'd expect omega-3s in general to have a good effect because of their anti-inflammatory action, but possibly other components in the krill oil work synergistically with the omega-3s.

Ray Sahelian, M.D., a nationally known expert on supplements and the author of *Mind Boosters: A Guide to Natural Supplements That Enhance Your Mind, Memory and Mood*, points out that though fish oil has a higher percentage of the important omega-3 fatty acids EPA and DHA, krill oil has the powerful antioxidant astaxanthin, plus vitamins A and D, and possibly other nutrients (such as small amounts of phospholipids). No matter, in this study, 3 g a day of krill oil was enough to make a big difference in the participants' experience of PMS. It might do the same for you.

Natural Prescription for PMS

Krill oil (Neptune Krill Oil): 3 g daily for 10 days prior to each cycle

★ FOR ADDED EFFECTIVENESS:

PMS Cocktail (see page 162)

Note: The above dosages are daily dosages and in pill or capsule form, unless otherwise noted.

Interestingly, a couple of other studies have since investigated the effects of krill oil on other health issues. One study investigated its effect on cholesterol, triglycerides, and glucose. In this study—a multicenter, three-month, prospective, randomized study followed by a three-month controlled follow-up—patients were given either 1g or 1.5 g of krill oil daily, considerably less than used in the PMS study.

A third group received fish oil. (And a fourth group received a placebo.)

The researchers concluded that krill oil was effective for the management of hyperlipidemia by "significantly reducing total cholesterol, LDL, and triglycerides, and increasing HDL levels." (Note the part about increasing HDL, the "good" cholesterol levels, which is not easy to do. Drugs fail miserably at it.) The researchers stated that "at lower and equal doses, krill oil was significantly more effective than fish oil for the reduction of glucose, triglycerides, and LDL levels."

And right before this book went to press, a study published in the *Journal of the American College of Nutrition* showed that krill oil at a daily dose of only 300 mg "significantly inhibits

inflammation and reduces arthritic symptoms within a short treatment period of 7 to 14 days."

Pretty impressive.

WORTH KNOWING

The Canadian company that sponsored the clinical trials mentioned in this section was Neptune Technologies and Bioresources; the same kind of krill oil used in the studies is often labeled Neptune Krill Oil. In the PMS study, Neptune Krill Oil was given over the course of 90 days. With natural prescriptions for PMS, it's a good idea to give it a try over at least three cycles.

Melatonin
for Jet Lag

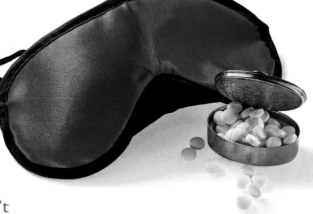

BLIND WOMEN DON'T get breast cancer. Actually, that's not 100 percent true. (It got your attention though, didn't it?) But it is true that their risk for breast cancer is substantially less than sighted women, 50 percent less by some estimates.

And the reason probably has to do with two things—light and a hormone called melatonin. Most people who have heard of melatonin know it as a supplement that can help with sleep (more on that in a moment). And it's great for jet lag. But the melatonin story is a lot more interesting—and complicated—than its ability to serve as a natural cure for insomnia. Melatonin may have a role in protecting you against cancer. It also supports the immune system and is one of the most powerful antioxidants we know of.

Melatonin is produced by the pineal gland, a gland in the brain that helps regulate circadian rhythm. It's actually made along the same metabolic assembly line as serotonin. Both start out as the amino acid tryptophan, which then gets converted into 5-HTP and then to serotonin. Two more steps along the pathway and you've got melatonin.

Natural Prescription for Jet Lag

Melatonin: 3–6 mg at bedtime

Note: The above dosages are daily dosages and in pill or capsule form, unless otherwise noted.

Melatonin is stimulated by darkness and turned off by light. One reason scientists believe that the risk for breast cancer is lower in blind women is that they have less exposure to light and presumably more melatonin. We don't know for sure if that's true, but we do know that in one study, scientists grafted human breast cancer tumors onto rats and then exposed them to blood taken from women during darkness and after exposure to light. The blood taken during darkness slowed the growth of the cancers by a whopping 80 percent; meanwhile, the blood taken after light exposure accelerated it.

The Cancer Connection

Researchers believe that our lights-on-all-the-time, 24/7 lifestyle is one reason that breast cancer is almost five times as high in westernized, industrialized countries as in the developing world. Artificial light (and the subsequent reduction of exposure to darkness) in the words of David Blask, M.D., Ph.D., "turns cancer cells into insomniacs." Night-shift workers are up to 60 percent more likely to get breast cancer.

We can't say for sure that melatonin can help prevent cancer, but it clearly has some relationship to the disease. There's pretty compelling evidence that using melatonin along with conventional cancer treatment like chemotherapy improves the tumor regression rate in breast, lung, kidney, liver, pancreatic, stomach, and colon cancer.

Melatonin plus chemo improved the one-year survival rate by approximately 50 percent compared to chemo alone in one study. Melatonin also seems to help reduce the toxicity of chemotherapy as well as some of the complications from it. One study divided thirty people who had advanced brain tumors into two groups and treated one with radiation therapy and the other with radiation therapy *plus* 20 mg of melatonin. After a year, only one of the sixteen (6 percent) in the radiation-only group was still alive compared to six of the fourteen (43 percent) in the radiation plus melatonin group.

Reboot Your Brain

Then there's melatonin's most famous use—helping to regulate sleep. Melatonin helps sets the brain's internal clock. It's terrific for jet lag and for any time that your sleep cycle is disrupted artificially. A good deal of research shows that melatonin is useful for insomnia, though there's some debate about which is best—regular melatonin or the timed-release kind. The immediate-release kind might be more effective for decreasing the time it takes to fall asleep, but the timed-release kind might be better for improving sleep quality and maintenance.

More Melatonin Benefits

Then there are headaches. In one study, 10 mg of melatonin every evening reduced the frequency of cluster headaches, and some early evidence suggests it might also help with migraines. In one study, 3 mg taken every night before bed significantly reduced migraine frequency, intensity, and duration. The thinking is that melatonin production might be different for people with migraines.

And a single dose of melatonin (.3 mg, less than $1/3$ of a milligram) taken a few hours after nicotine withdrawal seems to reduce both symptoms of irritability and cigarette cravings.

WORTH KNOWING

Melatonin may interact with certain medications, especially benzodiazepines, antidepressants, and central nervous system depressors like alcohol. Those who suffer from depression are advised not to take melatonin. Don't take and drive.

If all this weren't enough, melatonin is one of the most potent antioxidants I know of. It's believed to be many times more effective at protecting cell membranes than vitamin E, and more effective than glutathione (one of the body's antioxidant stars) at neutralizing one of the most dangerous of the free radicals—hydroxyl radicals. And on top of it, melatonin supports immune function in a variety of ways.

Oh, one more thing. In birds at least, melatonin switches on a hormone (gonadatropin inhibitory hormone) that has the *opposite* effect of a hormone (gonadotropin *releasing* hormone) that primes the body for sex. If you're a Japanese quail hoping for a hot sex life, melatonin's probably not the best hormone to take on a regular basis. Switching off gonadatropin releasing hormone shrinks the testes and ovaries as part of the bird's yearly cycle. What that has to do with humans we have no idea, but I thought you'd like to know.

Though some claims have been made for melatonin as an "antiaging" hormone supplement, these claims are bogus. They were based on the idea that you have significantly less melatonin (and serotonin) as you age, but that's turned out to be a questionable assumption, even though melatonin production is greatest when you're one to three years old.

MSM

for Pain and Inflammation

A FEW YEARS AGO I used to regularly hike in Runyon Canyon in the Hollywood Hills with a friend of mine who used to be a big television star. (Now he does reality shows, but that's another story.) This guy is in great shape, but his years as a professional dancer and athlete had taken a toll on his knee and he was beginning to have some real difficulties with our usual hike. He was beginning to limp a little. In fact, he had been talking to his doc about a knee replacement, which as you can imagine, didn't exactly make him feel good, particularly since he's in a profession where you're constantly being reminded about your age and anyone over thirty better have a really good relationship with at least one Beverly Hills plastic surgeon.

I suggested to my friend that he try MSM. He promptly told me some Hollywood version of "been there done that."

"That stuff doesn't work," he told me. "I tried it for a while and nothing happened." When I questioned him more closely, I found out he had been taking one or two capsules a day. "Like the bottle says to," he added. And how much was in each capsule? He had no idea, but I checked. Each capsule was 500 mg.

Fuggedaboudit!

I put him on 8 to 10 grams a day of MSM. Since that comes to about 16 to 20 capsules, I put him on the powdered form (available on my website, www.jonnybowden.com), which comes in either raspberry or lemon flavors, isn't too bad tasting, and makes it really easy to get about 10 grams into your system by simply adding a couple of spoonfuls to either water or a smoothie.

Within a month, he was hiking again. With no limp. And markedly reduced pain and irritation.

MSM for Arthritis

Arthritis sufferers are one of the largest groups of individuals suffering from chronic disease. In fact, as of this writing, more than forty million Americans are affected by some form of arthritis, and many have chronic pain that limits daily activity. Osteoarthritis affects more than twenty million Americans and there are more than a hundred other forms of the disease, which makes arthritis the most common chronic condition in the United States.

Accompanying symptoms include pain, inflammation, and reduced mobility. Add to that the increased knee replacement surgeries (more than 300,000 each year), visits to orthopedists for generalized back and muscle discomfort, and you're looking at a rapidly growing epidemic of the stiff, the sore, and the achy. And baby boomers, like my hiking buddy, are not only living longer, they're not going to take a life of inactivity sitting down (pun intended).

So how do we help alleviate the discomfort that comes with our weekend warrior lives and our rapidly degenerating joints?

Enter MSM.

Natural Prescription for Pain and Inflammation

MSM: Start with 1,000 mg per day and gradually work up to 4,000 mg per day. Because MSM helps to detox the body of heavy metals, watch for signs of rash, sweating, or headaches. (Nutritionist Suzanne Copp, M.S., frequently sees acne breakouts on the back, so be prepared!) It may just mean that you are detoxing too quickly. If this happens, reduce the dose and wait one week before increasing it again.

Boswellia: 150 mg, three times daily, for two to three months. It has been used effectively in combination with ginger, turmeric, and ashwagandha and proved beneficial for inflammation and pain associated with osteoarthritis and rheumatoid arthritis.

Turmeric: 400 mg in capsules, taken three times a day.

SAMe: It should be taken with folic acid at 800 mg and vitamin B12 at 1,000 mcg.

*Glucosamine: 1,500 mg per day for three months, at which point you should see improvement. Then reduce to 500–1,000 mg per day.

*See also glucosamine for arthritis on page 96.

Note: The above dosages are daily dosages and in pill or capsule form, unless otherwise noted.

MSM, which stands for methyl sulfonyl-methane, is actually a naturally occurring compound found in trace amounts in fruits and vegetables. It's long had the reputation of being great for joint health and the pain of arthritis. The key to MSM's abilities as a miracle worker is its high sulfur content, which makes sense when you realize that for centuries people have visited sulfur-rich hot springs for muscle aches and pains.

"From a structural point of view, sulfur is extremely important for maintaining connective tissues and joints," says Jacqueline Jacques, N.D. The biochemical precursor to MSM—dimethyl sulfoxide—has been studied extensively for pain and reduction of inflammation for years. In our bodies, sulfur is present in the muscle, skin, and bones and is necessary for making collagen, the primary component of cartilage, skin, and connective tissue. It's the fourth most abundant mineral in the body, which means that we need a lot of it. MSM is present in small amounts in foods, including milk, garlic, onion, and green vegetables. But heat and processing can destroy the MSM content, leaving us with suboptimal levels. In fact, borderline deficiency of MSM is common among Americans.

MSM can reduce pain. It's an effective natural analgesic and anti-inflammatory. It blocks the transmission of impulses in nerve fibers that carry pain signals, and it decreases pain by changing collagen linkages, which reduces scar tissue. Studies in laboratory animals showed less degenerative change of knee joints in those whose diet included MSM. MSM also increases

WORTH KNOWING

It has been estimated that 20 to 60 percent of patients with arthritis may also be affected by food sensitivities and could benefit from food elimination trials (see Rotation Diet, page 210).

the effectiveness, but not the amount, of cortisol, the body's anti-inflammatory hormone, and inhibits the production of fibroblasts, compounds which cause swelling. And finally, MSM also binds to fluid in swollen tissue and helps to remove it.

In animal and human studies, MSM has been shown to help arthritis, either alone or in combination with another popular nutrient, glucosamine sulfate. In one randomized, double-blind, placebo-controlled study published in the journal *Clinical Drug Investigation*, the addition of only 500 mg of MSM to 500 mg of glucosamine resulted in greater reduction of pain and swelling, improvement of functional ability of joints, and better and more rapid improvement, all without major adverse effects. (And in my opinion, the results are way better with higher doses—as happened with my hiking buddy.)

In another recent study involving fifty individuals with knee osteoarthritis pain, short-term supplementation with 6 g a day (3 g, twice daily) of MSM improved symptoms of pain and physical function, again without any major adverse effects. The researchers, while careful not to draw a definitive conclusion from this one study, nevertheless stated that "MSM … produced improvement in performing activities of daily living."

The Benefits Don't Stop with Pain Relief

MSM is useful is easing a number of other health issues. MSM's ability to reduce inflammation has significance for allergy sufferers as well. Inflammation is common in allergic reactions, and MSM can help with both environmental allergens like hay fever and food allergies.

A 2002 study in the *Journal of Alternative and Complementary Medicine* posted impressive results—upper and total respiratory symptoms were reduced significantly with the use of MSM. Lower respiratory symptoms were also significantly improved. And as a bonus, energy levels increased.

Sulfur is also a constituent of glutathione, arguably the most important and abundant intracellular antioxidant in the body. This makes MSM a great detoxifier. Because many individuals' sulfur stores are depleted, the ability to detox the body of heavy metals becomes diminished. MSM is helpful as it supplies the sulfur needed to chelate, or bind up, metals so they can be excreted by the body. This is especially true for mercury, which in excess in the body can contribute to or in some cases even cause such conditions as Alzheimer's disease, kidney dysfunction, infertility, multiple sclerosis, thyroid problems, and an impaired immune system.

While there isn't a ton of research supporting MSM for arthritis, there's a lot of what we call anecdotal evidence, meaning people report being helped a lot. Considering the many benefits of sulfur in the diet, there's no real downside to trying MSM. Just be sure to use enough to make a difference, and give it a trial of at least a month.

Niacin

for High Cholesterol

OKAY, FULL DISCLOSURE. I am a cholesterol skeptic. Obviously that doesn't mean I think cholesterol doesn't exist. I just think it's been way oversold as a health risk and that the emphasis on that single number has caused us to take our eye off the ball when it comes to a dozen far more significant risks for heart disease. Fully half the people who have heart attacks have normal cholesterol, and half the people who have elevated cholesterol have perfectly healthy hearts.

There's more. While total cholesterol used to be neatly divided into "good" cholesterol (HDL) and "bad" cholesterol (LDL), the truth turns out to be a far more complicated affair. LDL has at least six types, and one of them (LDL a) isn't very harmful at all while another (LDL b) is quite atherogenic. And some very impressive research shows that you can reduce the risk for cardiovascular disease significantly and dramatically without having a single thing happen to your cholesterol (the Lyon Diet Heart Study). Add to that the fact that "reducing cholesterol" has become a multi-, multibillion dollar business (Lipitor and Zocor, the number-one and number-five, respectively, top-selling drugs of 2005, did a combined total of more than $18 billion in sales)—there are some pretty serious

stakes in keeping the idea that cholesterol "causes" heart disease alive.

This is not the place to debate the cholesterol issue. (Those wanting to look into it further should Google *Uffe Ravnskov, M.D., Ph.D.*, check out his website, www.thincs.com (the society for cholesterol skeptics), read his book *The Cholesterol Myths*, or read another excellent book, *The Great Cholesterol Con* by Anthony Colpo.

But I digress.

Though I have my doubts about the *emphasis* on cholesterol, I respect my colleagues who, while agreeing that it is overemphasized, still believe it's something to keep an eye on. When there's too much of it in the arteries, there's a greater chance of some of it becoming oxidized or inflamed, which is the only time it becomes a problem. So in deference to those who want to do something about high cholesterol "naturally," I give you ... niacin.

The One-Two Punch of Niacin

Vitamin B3, or niacin, is found mostly in enriched foods such as flour, rice, and cereal, as well as peanuts, fish, and red meat. And it has a long and impressive résumé when it comes to heart health largely for its role in managing blood lipid profiles, a key strategy for the maintenance of cardiovascular health.

As of this writing, mainstream medicine still sees the cholesterol story this way: Excess amounts of LDL, or "bad cholesterol," cling to the walls of arteries. Over time, a buildup of these deposits, called plaque, will narrow the arteries and restrict blood flow to the heart. Heart disease and heart attacks are often a result of the restricted blood flow caused by the plaque. HDL is considered "good cholesterol" because it reverses the action of LDL by removing the plaque. Enter niacin. What niacin does that medications can't do is both lower the LDL cholesterol and raise the HDL cholesterol. This one-two punch can't really be done with medications, most of which lower either total cholesterol or LDL cholesterol but don't do anything to raise the "good" stuff. In numerous human studies, niacin has consistently shown increases in HDL by up to 45 percent and decreases in LDL by as much as 54 percent. And no matter where you stand on the cholesterol controversy, raising HDL cholesterol is a good thing.

Natural Prescription for High Cholesterol

For high cholesterol, high triglycerides, and low HDL:

Niacin as inositol hexanicotinate: 400 mg, three or four times daily OR

Niacin: 300 mg, three times daily

Essential fatty acids: At least 1 g of omega-3s, balanced with 200 mg omega-6s

Vitamin C: 1–3 g

Vitamin E: 400–800 IU

L-carnitine: 2–3 g

Pantethine: 300 mg, three times a day

Exercise

Low-carb diet: Make sure to include plenty of important fats like omega-3s (fish and fish oil), omega-9s (olive and macademia nut oil), and garlic.

Note: All dosages are daily dosages and in pill or capsule form unless otherwise noted.

The beauty of taking niacin is that it's even complementary when used in conjunction with statin drugs, like Lipitor. A study in the 2002 *American Heart Journal* showed that a relatively small amount of niacin added to a statin drug regimen led to significant improvements in HDL cholesterol. (Remember, statin drugs are usually good at reducing the "bad" LDL cholesterol but do not have a significant impact on raising the "good" HDL cholesterol.) Niacin did not cause any major side effects, and only 20 percent of the patients experienced the typical "niacin flush," an annoying but completely harmless sensation of itching and burning of the skin that often accompanies high-dose niacin therapy. This study is noteworthy in that a comparatively small amount of niacin produced a beneficial effect when combined with a prescription cholesterol-lowering drug. The change in HDL, though small, may have a dramatic effect on heart disease incidence. One study found that a 6 percent increase in HDL led to a 22 percent reduction in the incidence of fatal and nonfatal heart attacks.

Which Types of Niacin Are Best?

You may have heard the names of different forms of niacin, and keeping them straight is like taking chemistry all over again, but this time with fewer brain cells. Because they all work fairly differently (and some, by the way, don't work at all), it's best to understand the different forms and names so that you can find an effective form and one that delivers the least amount of side effects.

Vitamin B3 comes as two basic types—niacin (also called nicotinic acid) and niacinamide (also called nicotinamide). Got that straight? Don't worry about it. Doctors generally recommend inositol hexaniacinate (a form of the nicotinic acid) for individuals who need large amounts of niacin, as it has not been shown to be toxic in larger amounts. While possibly not as effective as plain niacin, it does appear to lower cholesterol.

> ## WORTH KNOWING
>
> Niacin can be irritating to the liver, and I never recommend it for anyone who has liver problems like hepatitis. If you do have liver issues or diabetes, check your liver enzymes regularly when using niacin and use it only under a doctor's supervision. Vitamin B3 in any form should not be taken in amounts greater than 1,000 mg per day, unless supervised by a doctor.
>
> According to my good friend Shari Lieberman, Ph.D, C.N.S., vitamin B3 may be lost in cooking water, so steam, bake, or stir-fry vegetables to spare as much of it as possible.

Niacinamide, the alternative source of vitamin B3, offers no benefit in cholesterol management.

Some products are promoted or labeled as "no-flush niacin" but are really only niacin-like compounds, which may have nutritional value or improve circulation but have not been tested exhaustively in humans like niacin has for its cholesterol benefit. The ingredient section on supplement packaging will indicate the source of the raw ingredient. Make sure the label shows "niacin or nicotinic acid."

Because niacin is a vasodilator—it causes blood vessels to dilate—it may cause temporary flushing in some individuals with doses as low as 50 mg to 100 mg. Flushing is the physical sensation of warmth, tingling, and redness of the skin and is a direct result of increased blood circulation. It's harmless, but it's a pain in the neck. For this reason, the extended-release instead of the immediate-release niacin may be a better option.

To reduce the likelihood of flushing, try these steps: 1) take niacin with food, such asa low-fat snack; 2) take 325 mg of aspirin approximately 45 to 60 minutes before the first dose of niacin; and 3) avoid alcohol, hot showers, spicy foods, and hot beverages soon after taking the medication.

Wobenzym N
for Arthritis and Pain

MARC KROON IS A baseball pitcher who was drafted by the New York Mets in 1991. He pitched for a bunch of teams, including the triple-A Albuquerque, while honing his skills and perfecting his fastball, which looked to be the stuff of which sports legends are made.

Then in 2000, he exploded his elbow. Doctors told him that the ligament and nerve damage he had suffered pretty much ended his pitching career. That could have been the end of the story. Kroon couldn't even flex his elbow comfortably let alone play catch with his kids. But in 2004, after missing three seasons, he walked out on the field as a member of the Colorado Rockies. Pitching, I might add, 97-mile-per hour fastballs. Alan Schwartz in *Baseball America* called it the "best comeback story of 2004."

If you ask him how he did it, he'd probably tell you one word: enzymes.

First Kroon tried acupuncture, which he didn't feel helped. As he was leaving his last appointment, he remembers the acupuncturist saying, "Hey, I've got these enzymes that athletes from Germany take. They're pretty good stuff. Why don't you try 'em out?" Kroon recalls laughing at the $100 per bottle price, but at his mother's insistence, decided to give it a shot.

Good thing he did.

In 2003, after an amazing season as a relief pitcher, he joined the Rockies as a Major League pitcher. And in 2005, he joined the Yokohama Bay Stars in Japan and set the record for the fastest pitch ever in Japanese baseball at 100 miles per hour. "I think it was all the enzymes," Kroon has said.

The Power of Enzymes

Enzymes are biochemical catalysts. They're the body's little "dealmakers," joining with one molecule and converting it into another molecule. An enzyme fits into its target molecule like a key fitting into a lock, does its little magic, and then jumps out to live on and do its work somewhere else, leaving a changed (catalyzed) molecule in its wake. Almost everything that happens in a cell requires enzymes—by some accounts about 4,000 biochemical reactions are catalyzed by them.

Truth be told, enzymes are needed for each and every chemical reaction that makes life possible. No vitamin, mineral, or hormone can perform effectively in the human body without the involvement of enzymes. Because of this, enzymes play a key role in the functioning of a strong immune and cardiovascular system, a healthy central nervous system, and optimal hormonal balance in the body. But as we age, increase our medications, and continue to eat a crummy diet, our enzymes get depleted. This can ultimately leave you with a variety of health issues.

You may be most familiar with the kind of enzymes known as digestive enzymes. Digestive enzymes work on the food you eat and help the body break it down into smaller units (like fatty acids, glucose, and the like) that your body can use. But there are other enzymes in the body as well, known as systemic enzymes. While digestive enzymes are responsible for breaking down food and aiding digestion, systemic enzymes are something different.

Systemic enzymes break down a number of biochemicals that are intimately involved in pain and inflammation. These systemic enzymes are what allowed pitcher Marc Kroon to pitch again.

Natural Prescription for Pain

Wobenzym: *500–1,000 mg between meals.

Calcium: 1,000 mg

Magnesium: 400–800 mg

Glucosamine: 1,500 mg per day in divided doses

Chondroitin: 1,200 mg per day in divided doses

Omega-3 fatty acids: 1,000 mg

Gamma-linolenic acid: 300 mg

*Only Wobenzym N needs to be taken on an empty stomach. The dose can be considerably higher, especially for difficult cases. There are no side effects, and it is completely safe at much higher doses.

Note: The above dosages are daily and in pill or capsule form unless otherwise specified.

"Systemic enzymes exert their beneficial effects at a cellular level, replenishing, in advanced years, the declining reservoir of naturally occurring enzymes in cells," says Aftab J. Ahmed, Ph.D.

The Athlete's Secret Weapon

Wobenzym N is a proprietary enzyme product from Germany and one of the oldest and most respected of the systemic enzyme formulas. It contains such plant ingredients as bromelain (from pineapple), papain (from papaya), the systemic enzymes chymotrypsin and trypsin, and the flavonoid *rutin*. It has a long history of being used successfully against the pain of arthritis and inflammation.

"Wobenzym N has the ability to turn off the switch that produces inflammatory compounds," says Gary Gordon, M.D., who has been using the product in his medical practice for decades.

You don't take Wobenzym N or any systemic enzymes the way you take digestive enzymes. You actually take it *away* from meals (on an empty stomach). Why? Because proteolytic enzymes digest something very different from food—they "digest" little pain-causing compounds called *circulating immune complexes*. Here's how it works: When your gut is functioning optimally, it keeps everything out of the bloodstream that doesn't belong. The gut digests and breaks down your food and sends the nutrients extracted into the bloodstream, where they can deliver nourishment to the cells, organs, and tissues. But when the gut walls become somewhat permeable—a condition we call "leaky gut"—stuff gets through that doesn't belong.

Little, incompletely broken down particles get through the barrier and enter the bloodstream. The immune system sees them and puts up a red flag, essentially saying, *Hey, this stuff doesn't belong here! Alert!* It sends out antibodies to deal with what it sees as invaders, and these antibodies attach to the offending particles, forming what's called a circulating immune complex (CIC). These CICs are the cause of all sorts of problems and mischief, starting, but not ending with, achy joints and general joint pain.

Systemic enzymes like Wobenzym N go after these particles. You don't need Wobenzym N to digest your food—you need it to go after the food that escaped undigested that joined with the immune system antibodies, created CICs, and generally wreaked havoc throughout the body.

The Drugs of the Future

A number of studies done in Europe and Russia have shown Wobenzym N to be effective in producing relief from arthritic symptoms, including pain. It's also used to maintain healthy joints and for sports injury recuperation (just ask Marc Kroon). And it may even help protect cartilage from destruction.

"I've seen people able to give up their crutches within three days of going on Wobenzym N," says Gary Gordon, M.D. He cautions, though, that not everyone will get that result and that if you don't, you should adjust your dose and be very patient. "But remember," he says, "if you're using drugs, you're only suppressing the symptom and allowing the joint to continue to deteriorate."

In arthritis, certain kinds of immune system cells penetrate the joint and attack the cartilage. These invaders—activated immune cells— produce a whole bunch of inflammatory chemicals known collectively as *cytokines*. The cytokines in turn trigger more inflammation. The destructive process continues and eventually you're left with pain, swelling, and loss of joint movement. Systemic enzymes actually help reduce the production of the inflammatory cytokines and may prevent further destruction of the cartilage.

"Systemic enzymes help to reduce local pain and regional swelling and gradually improve joint function," Ahmed says. "They empower the body to heal itself."

The claims for Wobenzym N go way beyond its ability to help relieve pain and prevent further deterioration in arthritis. Because proteolytic enzymes have such power to modulate both inflammation and the activity of the immune system, they've been used for everything from heart disease to autoimmune disease.

And, although it's way beyond the scope of this book, it's worth noting that the brilliant maverick researcher Nicholas Gonzalez, M.D., is currently in the midst of a groundbreaking clinical trial (supported by a $1.4 million grant from the National Cancer Institute) testing a combination of enzymes and nutrition as an alternative to chemotherapy.

"Wobenzym N gives you the same effects as aspirin, ibuprofen, and NSAIDs without any of the side effects," Gordon says. "When you take NSAIDs [nonsteroidal anti-inflammatory drugs such as Advil], you're suppressing key parts of your body that could have helped you heal. With Wobenzym N you're getting at causes, not merely the suppression of the pain. The differences are dramatic."

Enzymes allow you to work with your body to suppress inflammation without allowing the damage and joint destruction to proceed. Drugs, on the other hand, frequently suppress the symptoms while allowing the joint to continue to deteriorate.

"Enzymes are truly the drug of the future," Gordon says. "Our problem now is to get doctors to learn this."

Nattokinase
for Prevention of Stroke

WHEN I WROTE *The 150 Healthiest Foods On Earth,* I not only included the food natto, I gave it a star. And it deserves it, largely because it is rich in a remarkable enzyme called *nattokinase,* a "natural cure" if there ever was one. But I also wrote that—unfortunately—natto has a few cosmetic and olfactory obstacles to overcome before it makes it into most people's diet.

Natto is kind of sticky and not too appealing to Western palates. It doesn't help that it has an odor reminiscent of eau de New Jersey Turnpike. Back in 1945 when the United States occupied Japan, it prohibited the sale of natto because it thought that cholera and typhoid were likely caused by "such a rotten food." And yes, folks, it sure does smell like rotten eggs. But natto is a rich healing food, and the enzyme nattokinase may be your best (natural) weapon against stroke and a tremendous weapon against heart disease. Read on.

Natto has been a traditional Japanese food for more than 1,000 years; ancient Samurai consumed natto on a daily basis and even fed it to their horses to increase their speed and strength. Natto was also given to pregnant women to ensure healthy newborns. To this day, the people of Japan consume natto regularly, and it may be one of the reasons why they live longer. In his excellent book *Reversing Heart Disease*, Stephen

Sinatra, M.D., suggests eating natto two or three times a week for both prevention and as part of a therapeutic program.

Supplementing with Soy

What's so amazing about a bunch of boiled, fermented soybeans? In a word, nattokinase. Beneficial bacteria known as *Bacillus natto* are added to boiled soybeans, producing a fermented food rich in this healing, health-giving enzyme. Note well: You don't get this enzyme from soy chips, soy milk, or any other commercial soy product. Unfermented soy products such as soy milk or even tofu don't have a drop of nattokinase.

If eating natto is out of the question for you, nattokinase is now beginning to be offered as a supplement by high-end supplement companies that deal mainly with health professionals. And for good reason: It's a natural clot buster. To understand how it works, you need to

Natural Prescription for Thrombosis/Blood Clots/Strokes

Nattokinase: 25–100 mg. Make sure the fibrin units (FU) value is more than 20,000 FU/g

Multivitamin: Take one with high levels of vitamins B6, B12, C, and folic acid to guard against high homocysteine levels (Note: Homocysteine is an inflammatory marker in the blood that has been linked to higher levels of heart attack and stroke)

Magnesium: 400–800 mg

Vitamin E: 400–1,000 IU

Essential fatty acids: 1,000 mg of omega-3s, and 250 mg of omega-6s

Note: All dosages are daily dosages and in pill or capsule form unless otherwise noted.

understand the wonderful system of checks and balances the body has to keep blood flowing with just the right thickness. Our bodies naturally produce clotting compounds like fibrin and fibrinogen, which form a kind of weblike mesh that acts as a blood thickener so that you don't bleed to death from a minor injury. But too much fibrin would result in dangerous blood clots every time you cut yourself shaving! To guard against this, the body also produces an enzyme called plasmin, which breaks down excess fibrin. The result? Not too much bleeding, not too much clotting. This system of checks and balances is part of nature's great design.

But sometimes the system doesn't work so well. The plasmin (anticlotting enzyme) can be overwhelmed, and you're left with too much clotting ability and not enough clot-dissolving ability. (That's when conventional docs will frequently prescribe blood thinners like Coumadin.) Nattokinase works by helping to dissolve fibrin, thus acting as a natural clotting agent. According to Ralph E. Holsworth Jr., D.O., who introduced it in the United States, nattokinase "provides a unique, powerful, and safe way to eliminate clots or reduce the tendency to form clots, and thus decrease the risk of heart attacks and stroke."

Breaking up Blood Clots

Thrombosis is the formation of a clot (or thrombus) inside a blood vessel that winds up obstructing the flow of blood. Some people have a genetic condition called thrombophilia, which is a predisposition to form clots. Sinatra reports that an estimated 5 to 7 percent of Caucasians of European descent in the United States have an increased tendency for thrombosis. In *Reversing Heart Disease*, Sinatra says that abnormal clot formation contributes to more than 600,000 deaths per year in the United States alone. For anyone at risk for clots, nattokinase can literally be a lifesaver.

Hiroyuki Sumi, M.D., discovered nattokinase in 1980 while working as a researcher at the University of Chicago. Being Japanese himself he actually enjoyed the taste of natto and frequently had it for lunch. As curious scientists are prone to occasionally try something just for the hell of it, Sumi one day decided to drop some of his lunch into a petri dish of thrombus (a blood clot). Bingo! The natto started breaking up and destroying a significant amount of the clot, which dissolved in record-breaking time. Sumi stated: "I studied more than 200 foods from all over the world, but none surpassed natto in terms of fibrinolytic activity."

There's quite a bit more research on natto-kinase since. In one study, six men and six women were each fed 200 g (7 oz) of natto and then had their thrombinolytic (clotting) activities measured. Researchers found that eating natto literally cut in half the time needed to completely dissolve a clot. Another study recently published in the medical journal *Angiology* demonstrated that nattokinase can protect against deep vein thrombosis during long airline flights. Maybe Japan Airlines was on to something when it started using dried natto—which was developed about ten years ago—for in-flight meals and as a snack with beer.

Natto is also highly antibacterial, in part because it has a high nutritive value and is easy for the body to absorb. In years past in Japan, food poisoning was very common, and people used natto to prevent cholera, typhoid, and dysentery. Natto accomplishes this by suppressing the growth of harmful bacteria that are found in food, while at the same time supporting the growth of the beneficial bacteria like lactobacillus.

Natto contains another useful component, namely vitamin K2. Vitamin K2 helps to prevent osteoporosis, which it is estimated will affect

WORTH KNOWING

If you're already on blood-thinning medications, be sure to work with your health practitioner if you're eating natto or taking nattokinase. Nattokinase will affect your clotting factors. As discussed above, natto itself contains vitamin K2, which while great for healthy bones, can also interfere with blood-clotting medications. Work with someone knowledgeable in both medications and natural substances if you're going to either get off blood clotting meds or use them with natural substances that work similarly.

Also keep in mind that as natto becomes more popular it will probably be embraced, coopted, and therefore ruined by the food industry. Since it's not very palatable in its natural, sticky state, it's inevitable that food companies will attempt to make it taste better. If history is any guide, it will wind up losing much of its effectiveness in the process. Either develop a taste for the real thing—highly recommended—or go for high-quality supplements of nattokinase.

more than 52 percent of women and men aged fifty and older by the year 2010. Nattokinase helps to make vitamin K2, which in turn helps to make a protein called *osteocalcin;* osteocalcin helps get calcium into the bones where you need it. Research has also shown that those who already have osteoporosis also have a lower level of vitamin K2.

Zinc

Your Key to Infection Protection

IF MINERALS WERE ancient gods, zinc would be Zeus: superhero mineral, protector of the immune system, defender of bodily invaders, and involved in virtually every aspect of infection prevention. If you've got a cold, an infection, or a cold sore, zinc may just be your best friend.

Critical for more than 300 enzymatic functions in the body, zinc is found in every one of our eighty trillion cells. Without it we wouldn't survive. Zinc helps us grow and develop, breathe, and digest our food. One of its primary functions is in wound healing and tissue repair. In the language of the twenty-first century, it is a "healing" nutrient. Because our bodies are constantly being subjected to little injuries (and big ones), we need zinc for the rebuilding process (healing). Without it, we'd simply break down.

If you're like millions of people in America, you're likely to reach for zinc lozenges at the first sign of a cold. That would be smart. A study at the famous Cleveland Clinic showed that zinc lozenges decreased the duration of colds by an impressive 50 percent.

The Natural Standard database, one of the most respected sources of supplement and medical data I know of, rates the evidence of a positive effect for zinc on the immune system a very respectable B, meaning "strong scientific

evidence." Considering that getting a B from the Natural Standard is like getting a B at Harvard, I'd say that's pretty good.

Zinc possesses antiviral activity and will attack viruses that may cause the common cold. The *American Journal of Clinical Nutrition* reported a recent study demonstrating that after one year of either zinc supplementation or no supplementation, those taking zinc experienced far fewer colds than those who took a placebo. In addition, 88 percent of participants in a study of the elderly developed colds when they didn't take 45 mg of zinc regularly. Note that these participants ranged in age from 55 to 87—could there be a need for higher levels of zinc as we age? Zinc lozenges became popular after a well-publicized 2000 study done at Wayne State University showed that they significantly reduced the duration of the common cold. They work because they bathe the throat tissues where viruses multiply. So reach for zinc lozenges during cold and flu season.

Nixing the Naysayers

Of course, like most natural treatments, zinc has its naysayers. One study in particular is widely touted by the antisupplement brigade as evidence that zinc has no effect on the common cold. But let's go to the videotape. Three dosages of zinc were given to subjects with colds—5 mg, 11.5 mg, and 13.3 mg. These amounts are pretty paltry; 5 mg isn't even 65 percent of the recommended daily allowance (RDA) for women, and it's less than *half* of what's recommended for healthy men. (It could reasonably be assumed that sick folks might need *more* than the RDA.) When the researchers "averaged" the results for all three groups, sure enough these little bitty doses of zinc didn't make a difference.

However, for the group getting the 13.3 mg dose, the duration of the cold was about 30 percent shorter. I don't know about you, but if a tiny drop of zinc cuts my cold length by a day—which happened in this study—I'm taking it.

This study also used two different types of zinc—zinc acetate and zinc gluconate, and only one was effective (the gluconate). The lesson here *isn't* that zinc has no effect on the common cold, it's that you've got to use the right *amount* and the right *type* of zinc. Note: To alleviate cold symptoms, for several days try lozenges providing 13 to 23 mg of zinc gluconate or zinc gluconate-glycine every two hours while awake. The best effect is obtained when lozenges are used at the first sign of a cold.

Natural Prescription for Immune Support

Zinc: 30–50 mg*

Vitamin C: 1–2 g

Selenium: 200 mcg

Probiotics: 10 billion bacteria

Multivitamin/mineral: Do not exceed 35–40 mg of zinc per day unless you are working with a health-care provider.

Echinacea: 300 mg

Diet/lifestyle: Reduce sugar, consider a detox program

*Because taking more than 50 mg of zinc daily over a long period of time can lower copper levels, it's advisable to also take a low dose of copper during this time.

Note: The above dosages are daily and refer to pill or capsule form unless otherwise noted.

Zinc: The Missing Link for Superimmunity

Studies have shown that severe zinc deficiency significantly depresses immune function because zinc is needed for both the development and the activation of a very important class of white blood cells (lymphocytes) called T cells. When people with low zinc are given zinc supplements, their T-cell count goes up and they're better able to fight off disease.

There's a fair amount of research showing that malnourished children given zinc supplements have shorter courses of infectious diarrhea. Zinc supplements also can help heal skin ulcers and bedsores for people who are low in zinc to begin with. (When zinc levels are normal, however, supplements don't seem to make the wounds heal any faster.)

Problem is, how do you know when your levels are normal? You don't. There's no single laboratory test that consistently and accurately measures zinc status. (Nutritionists have been using the simple *zinc taste test* for years, but not everyone knows about it and it's somewhat subjective. See the box for more information.) Test or no test, one thing we know for sure is this: Most of us don't get nearly enough zinc. According to the U.S. Department of Agriculture's 1996 Continuing Survey of Food Intakes, more than 70 percent of Americans don't consume the recommended daily allowance, which is only 8 mg a day for women and 11 mg a day for men. (Ten percent of individuals don't even consume half the RDA!)

Emily Ho, Ph.D., a research scientist at Linus Pauling Institute of Oregon State University, estimates that zinc deficiency affects more than two billion people worldwide, about one-third of the entire planet. Liping Huang, a geneticist at the ARS Western Human Nutrition Research Center at Davis, California, notes that "mild zinc deficiency may exist in the United States among otherwise healthy infants, toddlers, preschool children, pregnant and lactating women, and seniors." Vegetarians who avoid meat and dairy are also at risk for mild zinc deficiencies.

Not Just a Man's Mineral

Zinc has something of a reputation in the men's health magazines as a "guy's" nutrient, largely because it is critical for the production of both sperm and the male hormone testosterone. (Little fun fact: The reasons oysters are thought to be such a "sexy" food—even an aphrodisiac—is that they're loaded with zinc.) And the normal human prostate gland has a higher level of zinc than any other soft tissue in the body, compared to cancerous prostates, which have a lot less zinc than normal ones.

Then there's the infertility connection. Infertility affects 20 percent of all couples in the United States, and the main culprit (35 percent of couples) is sperm abnormalities. Since zinc is needed for pretty much every aspect of male reproduction, including hormone development, healthy and numerous sperm, and sperm motility, it makes sense—especially if you're a guy—to get enough zinc in your diet. Zinc levels are usually much lower in infertile men with low sperm counts. One study showed that increasing zinc and folic acid levels helped increase sperm counts in infertile men.

But zinc is hardly just a man's mineral. It has been shown in studies to aid children with attention deficit hyperactivity disorder (ADHD) and help prevent or retard the progression of macular degeneration, the leading cause of adult blindness. It fights fatigue for both sexes, diminishes white spots in fingernails, reduces brittle hair and nails, and it can help with menstrual problems, impotence, and painful knee and hip joints. And whether you're a man or a woman, if strengthening your immune system is high on your list of priorities, zinc needs to be an important part of your diet (or supplement program).

Finally, we need zinc to help decode the instructions in our DNA, the genetic version of a user's guide for how to keep our body functioning. Our bodies use these instructions to make the proteins that keep muscles, bones, hormones, enzymes, and dozens of other biochemicals in our complex internal systems running smoothly. Zinc is an essential component of about 400 of these proteins.

A Little Goes a Long Way

And zinc isn't one of those nutrients you need to "oversupplement" with. (Quite the contrary: Too much zinc interferes with copper absorption, and the two minerals need to be in balance.) For example, while prostate health depends on adequate zinc levels, one study indicated that men who supplement with 100 mg of zinc or more a day have more than twice the risk of developing prostate cancer. We don't know why, though some nutritionists, like my associate Suzanne Copp, M.S., think that it might have to do with a copper deficiency that can be created by taking too much zinc.

Point is, you can do really well with supplementing in the 15 to 50 mg range, although for some situations (like macular degeneration or fighting off a cold or healing a wound) it's perfectly okay to use a higher dose for a short time. In general, a basic 15 mg a day seems to help fend off most common problems. Certain seafoods, notably oysters, along with milk, whole grain breads, dark meat poultry, and nuts like cashews also provide plenty of the mineral.

WORTH KNOWING

A study done a couple of years ago showed the benefits of zinc supplementation in the treatment of children with attention deficit hyperactivity disorder (ADHD). Four hundred healthy children diagnosed with ADHD were randomly assigned to receive either 40 mg of zinc (as zinc sulfate) per day or a placebo for twelve weeks. At the four-week evaluation, the average total ADHD score had improved significantly more in the children given zinc compared with the children given a placebo. Specifically, the zinc-treated children had significantly greater improvement in scores on hyperactivity, impulsiveness, and impaired socialization scales than the children given the placebo. At the twelve-week evaluation, the improvement in the zinc group was even more pronounced.

Let's stop overmedicating our kids and start looking for the root causes of conditions like ADHD. Maybe then—with a little help from zinc and other nutrients—we can start to reduce the number of school-age children in the United States who are currently diagnosed with this disorder.

But a number of factors can interfere with zinc absorption—phytates in cereals and soy foods, for example are compounds that bind to minerals and keep them from being absorbed. Even fiber may decrease zinc's availability. Stress definitely depletes it, and very easily!

The Zinc Taste Test

Nutritionists have used a test for years called the *zinc taste test*. Here's how to do it at home: First you get some liquid zinc. (Liquid zinc is available at better health food stores or through health practitioners. You can't use a flavored kind—it has to be pure, clear, and tasteless, like Zinc Talley by Metagenics.) The test is simple: You just hold a capful or two of the liquid zinc in your mouth for about a minute. If it tastes like metal, you're not zinc deficient. But if it tastes like water, you are.

Many anorexics see some improvement when they start taking zinc as part of an overall treatment program. (It's better for them to take it in liquid form so they can test their levels through the taste test; at the same time, they'll get better absorption.) It's possible that because it helps with taste perception, it may help them get better in touch with their experience of food and hunger ("When am I hungry, when am I full?").

Both my associates, nutritionists Suzanne Copp, M.S., and Susan Mudd, M.S., C.N.S., routinely use zinc in their private practice when working with clients who have eating disorders. "Invariably, the zinc tastes like water to them," Copp says, "meaning their levels are pretty depleted."

Zinc Carnosine
for Stomach Ulcers

WHAT DO YOU GET when you cross the mineral *zinc* with the amino acid *carnosine*? The answer may be your ticket to the end of stomach worries.

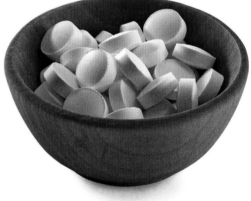

Zinc carnosine is fairly new in the dietary supplement category. It's showing great promise in the treatment of ulcers. And that's good news for the twenty million ulcer sufferers in the United States, most of them over the age of sixty and female. Zinc carnosine may not necessarily be for everyone, but if you suffer from stomach or intestinal ulcers, it may be for you.

Ulcers start as an irritation in the lining of the stomach wall, which if left untreated, can cause perforations and the all-too-familiar symptoms of heartburn, stomach pain, nausea, or even vomiting.

And what do you normally do when this happens?

Plop, Plop, Fizz, Fizz

Well, if you're like millions of Americans, you turn to drugs. Prevacid and Nexium are among the five top-selling prescription drugs in the country, and millions of people use such over-the-counter acid-suppressing drugs as Tums, Maalox, Rolaids, and Mylanta on a daily basis. This is a really bad idea. Over time those antacids do more harm than good.

The only way to get nutrients that our bodies need to function is through digestion, and without the right amount of stomach acid, trying to digest your food and absorb your nutrients is like trying to box with one hand tied behind your back. The major enzyme in the stomach responsible for much of the work of digestion is called pepsin. It's the stomach's principle protein-digesting enzyme, and it requires acid to get "turned on" so it can do its work. Turn off the acid with pills, and pepsin is incapacitated, along with your digestive process.

"Chronic use of antacids may permanently impair normal stomach function," says my friend, naturopathic physician Andrew Rubman,

Natural Prescription for Ulcers

Zinc carnosine: 75 mg in divided doses. Use for eight weeks to see results

Probiotics: 1–10 billion bacteria

Glutamine: 1–20 g per day in divided doses

Aloe vera juice: 5–30 ml, two or three times per day

Deglycyrrhizinated licorice (DGL) powder: 200–400 mg dissolved in 200 ml warm water

Cabbage juice: One quart fresh juice per day. Start slowly and work up to that amount gradually to avoid stomach upset.

Note: All dosages are daily dosages and in pill or capsule form unless otherwise noted.

N.D. Some antacids will cause your stomach to produce more acid, a condition called *acid rebound* (or reflux), which worsens your gastrointestinal problem. And some health practitioners believe that overuse of antacids will change the acid-alkaline balance in the gut, upsetting the balance between "good" and "bad" bacteria and setting the stage for infection with *Helicobacter pylori (H. pylori)*, a common stomach bacterial infection that is a major cause of stomach ulcers.

So antacids are not the answer, not to heartburn and certainly not to ulcers. But zinc carnosine might be. Zinc carnosine dissolves in the stomach and adheres to the ulceration (or wound) on the stomach lining, and it does this more effectively than any other form of zinc.

Once dissolved, zinc carnosine goes to work stabilizing membranes, healing wounds, and repairing tissues, all in an effort to support the mucosal barrier—the defensive wall of the stomach.

The Japanese have been using zinc carnosine since 1994 and, in a number of studies, have produced "remarkable improvement" of ulcer symptoms, including heartburn, belching, and abdominal distention.

Gut Science

But the goal here is not just to suppress symptoms—it's to get to the cause of the ulcer in the first place. And that's where zinc carnosine really shines.

The two major causes of ulcers are *H. pylori* and nonsteroidal anti-inflammatory drugs (NSAIDs). *H. pylori* affects about 20 percent of adults in the United States. It's found in 70 to 75 percent of gastric ulcer patients and 90 to 100 percent of duodenal ulcer patients. A new study in *Alimentary Pharmacology & Therapeutics* showed that taking antibiotics to kill *H. pylori*, along with medication to control stomach acid, has an 86 percent success rate, but when zinc carnosine is added to the mix, the success rate climbs to a perfect 100 percent.

NSAIDs, which also include pain relievers such as aspirin and aspirin-like compounds like ibuprofen and naproxen sodium, aren't as innocuous as they seem. They come with their own set of potential side effects, one of which is that they can increase what's called *gut permeability*—essentially a weakening of the lining in the gut that serves as a protective barrier for the bloodstream, keeping out things that don't belong. When those "borders" are weakened, i.e., when the gut becomes more permeable, all manner of digestive "riffraff" can get in, causing myriad health problems. (This is known as *leaky gut* in integrative medicine.)

NSAIDs can complicate the issue. And they've also been linked directly to ulcers. While NSAIDS don't "cause" ulcers, it has been reported that 50 percent of patients who regularly take NSAIDs have some level of gastric erosion and as many as 15 to 30 percent have ulcers.

In early 2007, researchers at the Queen Mary's School of Medicine and Dentistry conducted a series of studies to determine whether zinc carnosine would help protect against the gut-eroding effects of the NSAID drug indomethacin. They treated volunteers with 150 mg of indomethacin every day for five days. But along with their NSAID, half the volunteers also received 75 mg of zinc carnosine a day. The other half of the volunteers received a placebo. Here's what happened: In the NSAID/placebo group, there was a threefold rise in gut permeability. But in the NSAID group that also received the zinc carnosine, there was virtually none.

The researchers were convinced that zinc carnosine protected the gut against the damages that would have been done by NSAIDs alone, meaning that if you are going to use NSAIDs, taking zinc carnosine at the same time is a really good idea. (An even better idea would be to try zinc carnosine as part of a natural prescription for healing and dump NSAIDs altogether, at least the regular and extended use of them.)

In addition to protecting the intestines, zinc carnosine may help with wound healing in general. In the above-mentioned study, zinc carnosine was found to decrease gastric and small intestinal injury in addition to protecting against gut permeability. Researchers have also found that zinc carnosine encourages cells to travel to a simulated wound area and trigger increased cell proliferation, suggesting that zinc carnosine improves wound healing.

Satiatrim
for Appetite Control

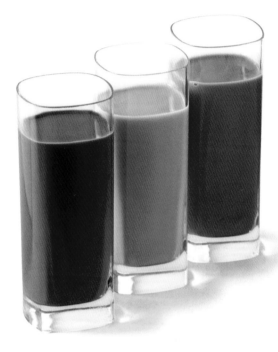

A FEW YEARS AGO, when I was writing *Living the Low Carb Life: Choosing the Diet that's Right for You from Atkins to Zone,* I was researching the chapter on drugs and supplements for weight loss and I came across a product that I had never heard of called Satiatrim.

It sounded good, and the thinking behind it was solid—design a low-calorie drink that would naturally stimulate the release of a hormone in the gut called cholecystokinin or CCK. The job of CCK is to signal your brain that you've had enough to eat. The scientists working on the product reasoned that if you could trick your body into releasing CCK before a meal, you'd have a natural appetite suppressant.

While there have certainly been other "appetite suppressants" on the market, many have worked by using stimulants (like ephedra), which simply speed you up and make you jittery. Satiatrim is based on the concept of using real food to stimulate the body's natural appetite control pathways—a concept that makes sense to me.

Most of us eat way too fast to allow CCK to travel to the brain in time to shout "Hey, put down the fork!" By the time it reaches its destination, you've overeaten by hundreds of calories. To complicate matters further, CCK really responds best to protein and fat, which are not your typical binge foods. A carb feast slows CCK down, making it even tougher to put down the fork (or the spoon buried in that pint of Ben and Jerry's). Satiatrim stimulates CCK before you eat, so you're less likely to binge and be hungry in the first place.

I was intrigued with Satiatrim because I liked the principle behind it and because the people working on it were serious, smart, and had good scientific credentials.

Only trouble was, it wasn't on the market. Now it is.

How Satiatrim Works

I got a hold of a case of the stuff as I was writing this book and I can tell you it works quite well. It's effective at curbing appetite. Why? Because it really makes you less hungry, and does that by cleverly manipulating your body's "satiety" signals. You simply drink it a half hour or so before eating, and let nature do its work. You eat less because you want less.

Robert Portman, Ph.D., is the chief scientific officer of the company that makes Satiatrim. "When we eat, our stomach expands," he explains, "causing the release of CCK. A principal action of CCK is to close the valve between the stomach and intestine, thereby slowing the movement of food. By slowing the movement of food, Satiatrim acts as a gastric pacemaker, helping us to feel full while eating less. And because food stays in the stomach longer, we feel full for an extended period of time."

One reason I like Satiatrim is because Pacific Health—the company that makes it—isn't trying to sell it as a magic cure that will help you look like a fitness model in ten days. Satiatrim won't melt pounds off while you sit back and gorge on fast food, and no one claims it will. But it *will* help you to eat less food without going hungry. One of the primary reasons diets fail is hunger.

"Satiatrim is like a glass of willpower," says Portman. "It can help overweight individuals stay on their diet until they achieve their weight goal." Having used it myself when fighting those last ten pounds that somehow keep sneaking up from time to time, I can tell you that it really helps stave off hunger pains when you're dieting so that you feel less like overeating and are genuinely satisfied with less food.

Extending Satiety

A number of studies have been conducted on Satiatrim, one of which, as of this writing, is scheduled to be presented at a meeting of the North American Association for the Study of Obesity. Tanya Little, Ph.D., at the Department of Medicine at Hope Hospital in Manchester, United Kingdom, summarized the findings: "Our studies have demonstrated that Satiatrim dramatically slows the movement of food through the stomach. We have also been able to demonstrate that Satiatrim achieves this important effect by stimulating the release of a number of gut peptides [proteins], including cholecystokinin. The end result is that Satiatrim enhances and extends satiety [a feeling of fullness] and reduces the amount of food consumed in a subsequent meal." Little concluded that Satiatrim is potentially beneficial for anyone trying to lose weight.

I think so, too. Satiatrim comes in little single-serving containers that look like juice boxes, and is available in three flavors. While it won't fool you into thinking you're drinking a chocolate milk shake, the taste really isn't bad. Each serving is only 45 to 50 calories, but regular use before meals may wind up saving you hundreds of calories a day. A typical serving has a couple of grams of protein, a couple of grams of fiber, very few carbs (2 g), and a few grams of fat.

Full disclosure to those who have read everything I've written with eagle eyes (thank you for that, by the way). There is a tiny bit of milk, soy, sunflower oil, and safflower oil in this product—four ingredients I haven't been a huge fan of over the years for various reasons. But my feeling here is this: We have to choose our battles in the food arena, and obesity is way more of a problem for health than a couple of grams of an omega-6 oil or a drop of soy. On balance, this is a really well-designed product that works—not by magic, but by taking into account the body's own inherent wisdom.

That makes sense to me.

COMBO CURES

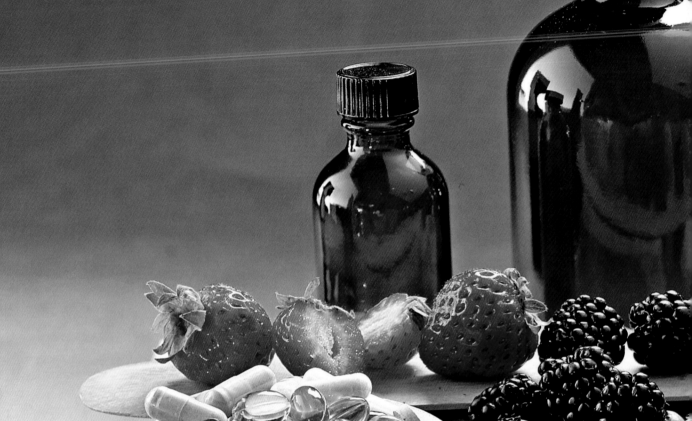

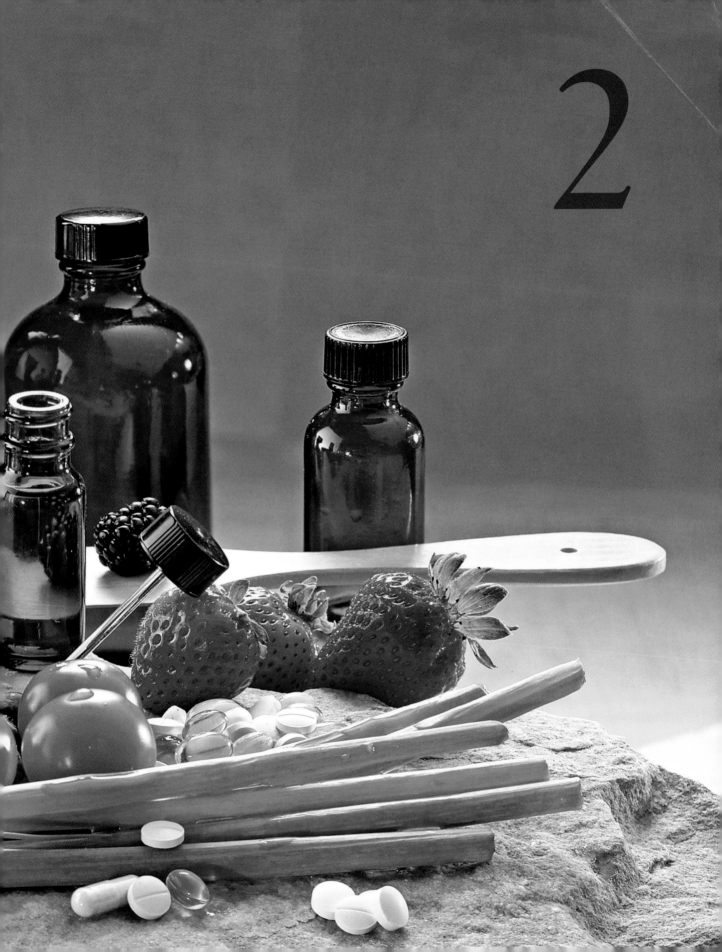

2

Health Recovery Center Treatment
for Alcoholism

WHAT CAUSES ALCOHOLISM? Is it a character flaw? Do people drink to avoid deeper complex psychological issues? Or are they driven to drink by their genes and biology? Is it some combination of all of the above? And most important—how can you treat it?

"Most alcoholism treatment in the United States today is a version of the Minnesota Model developed in the 1940s and 1950s by the Hazelden Foundation of Center City, Minnesota," says Joan Mathews-Larson, Ph.D. "This form of treatment is based on the presumption that drinking is a way of dealing with painful emotional or psychological problems and that once those problems are identified and confronted, the alcoholic will no longer be driven to drink irresponsibly." The self-knowledge gained through group meetings, support, and counseling is believed to lower the need for compulsive drinking.

The most famous of these peer counseling groups is Alcoholics Anonymous (AA). But AA is not actually a treatment for alcoholism—it's a support group. AA members would bristle at the idea that alcoholism can be "cured" and consider themselves alcoholics for life, "in recovery" even if they haven't had a drink for twenty-five years.

AA is a self-described *fellowship* that allows alcoholics to become and remain abstinent, with the help and support of other members. In that regard it's firmly in the mainstream of traditional views on alcoholism. That it is a wonderful program and has saved lives is not in question. But it has never addressed the biochemical underpinnings of alcoholism.

The Sugar Connection
Some people feel the time to do just that is long overdue. They argue that our view of alcoholism as a "character defect" that can be treated exclusively by talking and support is out of date.

According to Mathews-Larson and others in the forefront of this movement, trying to "treat" alcoholism by talking is akin to using a support group to treat inborn errors of insulin metabolism in diabetics. While not taking anything away from AA, these maverick innovators are using vitamins, minerals, amino acids, and other nutritional protocols to treat alcoholism by addressing underlying biochemical causes. By correcting what they feel are the driving mechanisms of alcohol cravings, they believe they can offer alcoholics more than just the ability to learn to coexist with their symptoms.

"Scratch an alcoholic and you will find a hypoglycemic," says Mathews-Larson, whose Health Recovery Center in Minneapolis has treated alcoholics with vitamins, minerals, and amino acids for several decades. She believes addicts don't metabolize sugar properly, which is responsible for a good deal of the cravings and addictive behavior and that without correcting this situation, no treatment of alcoholism can be entirely successful, even if it does lead to abstinence.

"Alcoholics die twenty years before the rest of us, whether they stop drinking or not," she told me, "because there's no repair of this mechanism."

Testing Tolerance

In one in-house study done at the Health Recovery Center, Mathews-Larson performed a glucose tolerance test on 100 alcoholics. The glucose tolerance exam is a five-hour medical test that determines how well the body deals with sugar and is conventionally used to screen for diabetes, insulin resistance, and hypoglycemia— a condition of low blood sugar that can cause symptoms ranging from lightheadedness to irritability to anxiety or even violence.

"Eighty-eight of them tested hypoglycemic," Mathews-Larson told me.

She's not alone in making this connection. Nutritional medicine pioneer Emanuel Cheraskin, M.D., believed that between 75 and 95 percent of alcoholics he studied were hypoglycemic.

"Too much therapeutic emphasis has been placed on psychological factors while more basic biochemical deficiencies and defects in body chemistry have received relatively little attention," he says. Douglas Baird, D.O., medical director of the Hypoglycemia Support Foundation, goes one step further, saying: "I have never, ever seen an alcoholic who wasn't hypoglycemic. It just doesn't occur, it's the same problem."

Indeed, studies dating back to the 1970s have suggested a connection between alcoholism and impaired sugar metabolism or hypoglycemia, which, as noted above, is linked to violent symptoms. (The Quolla Indians of Central America, for example, were known for their violence, including unpremeditated murder. Anthropological studies in the 1970s showed that every single one of the tribesmen tested turned out to be hypoglycemic.)

"When you're hypoglycemic and your blood sugar is very low, your brain is craving sugar," explained Mathews-Larson. "Alcohol goes right to the brain and gives the brain its fuel."

First Things First: Sugar, Nutrients, and the Yeast Connection

The first order of business at the Health Recovery Center is a multilevel assessment that includes the glucose tolerance test as well as tests for thyroid function, serum zinc, and copper levels.

"Alcohol destroys zinc, which can in turn cause an increase in copper levels leading to a number of 'psychological' disorders, including paranoia," explains Mathews-Larson. She also tests for the presence of *Candida-albicans* (yeast). "Three-quarters of the people we treat are filled with candida," she told me. "In the brain, candida can cause depression, spaciness, and tremendous fatigue. And all candida lives on is sugar."

The Health Recovery Center addresses the sugar addiction with a combination of diet and natural nutrients including glutamine. "This amino acid has a truly amazing ability to reduce cravings for alcohol," says Matthews-Larson (see glutamine for cravings, page 49). Indeed, in a 1957 study in the *Quarterly Journal of Studies on Alcohol*, glutamine was shown to significantly diminish the desire to drink, and many nutritionists use it to this day for its ability to reduce sugar cravings.

"You can quench a sudden desire for alcohol by opening a 500 mg glutamine capsule and letting it dissolve in your mouth," said Mathews-Larson. Glutamine is also available in powder form, and a tablespoon dissolved in water seems to reduce cravings considerably for many people I spoke with.

"Glutamine is used directly as fuel for the brain," Hyla Cass, M.D., told me, "and it has been shown to decrease addictive tendencies." Cass, an assistant clinical professor of psychiatry at UCLA and author of *Natural Highs*, recom-

Acupuncture for Withdrawal

Acupuncture needles in the ear are widely used to calm down cravings of all sorts and have been well documented as being helpful in the treatment of withdrawal. Both the Lincoln Hospital in New York and the Haight-Ashbury Free Clinic have had very positive results incorporating some form of acupuncture in their drug and alcohol treatment programs, especially when used for the pain and anxiety of withdrawal and cravings.

"Ear needles can be a valuable adjunct in helping people get through the difficult phases of withdrawal," says Robert Duggan, M.A., founder and president of the Tai Sophia Institute, whose center uses a variety of methods to treat addicts and alcoholics, including twelve-step programs and ear needles.

mends taking 2 to 5 g of glutamine a day for curbing cravings (the equivalent of a teaspoon of powder). It's best taken between meals for maximum absorption.

Next: Individualized Treatment

Other components of the natural nutritional treatment for alcoholism include amino acids, the building blocks of protein. Amino acids are converted into brain chemicals (neurotransmitters) that control mood. "Alcoholics and drug addicts are often so depleted of amino acids that they can't create these neurotransmitters, leading to depression, hostile and aggressive behavior, confusion, anxiety, and paranoia," says Mathews-Larson.

The formulas given at the Health Recovery Center vary and are based on an individual's needs, but most include a multivitamin, multi-mineral, B-complex supplement, gamma-linolenic acid, which reduces withdrawal symptoms and improves mental processes, and melatonin for better sleep, according to Mathews-Larson. Some alcoholics receive vitamin and mineral infusions intravenously as well. Depression, anxiety, and sleep disorders—which frequently accompany alcoholism and remain even after a person has stopped drinking—are treated in a similar fashion, by providing the nutritional building blocks of the neurotransmitters that are low in these conditions.

Because the Health Recovery Center believes, as I do, that every addict needs to be treated as an individual and there is no one perfect "formula" for treating something as complicated as addiction, there is no "Natural Prescription" for addiction. However, Mathews-Larson does strongly recommend three nutrients for just about everyone: glutamine, for its ability to help with cravings; chromium (see page 46) for its ability to help with controlling blood sugar and hypoglycemia; and the amino acid taurine (see page 39).

"Everyone is low in taurine," she told me, a statement I tend to agree with. "Without taurine, they can't absorb their magnesium, or most other minerals." She recommends 2,000 to 4,000 mg a day.

Support in Various Forms

Finally, let me be clear that the Health Recovery Center does not discount or dismiss the power of twelve-step groups. They just believe that correcting and treating the underlying biochemistry of addiction (and blood sugar abnormalities) with diet and supplements helps an alcoholic or addict get the most value from support and spiritual programs of their choosing.

Speaking of Alcoholics Anonymous and Women for Sobriety (another support group), Mathews-Larson says this: "I cannot overemphasize the importance of these invaluable human resources. Nowhere else can you find others who have a gut-level understanding and appreciation of what you have been through."

Glucosamine and Chondroitin

for Arthritis

I'VE ALWAYS BEEN impressed by how far ahead of the curve veterinarians are. You go to your vet and you don't hear a whole bunch of political drug-company propaganda about the "unproven" effect of supplements. They just tell you what works. If a dog has a skin rash, for example, and the vet gives it a vitamin supplement and soon the skin rash is gone, the vet will recommend the supplement. Done deal.

MSM

Glucosamine
Chondroitin
Sulfate

Vets worry less about whether there are seventy-five randomized, controlled, double-blind studies on skin rashes. If the vitamin supplement works—and does no harm—the vets use it.

I was hearing about glucosamine from vets long before the medical establishment decided to get on board. It helps dogs—and people—with the pain, stiffness, and infirmity of arthritis. Since almost all dogs eventually suffer from arthritis, and larger dogs frequently suffer with a painful joint condition called hip dysplasia, the use of glucosamine is of more than theoretical use in veterinary practice. And there are no "placebo effects" with dogs. They don't get better because they think they're "supposed" to— they either feel (and act) better or they don't.

And if their behavior is any indication (and what other indication do we have—the last time

I checked, they couldn't really communicate in English), their joints seem to feel a lot better when they're given a hefty dose of glucosamine.

A Vital Building Block

Glucosamine is actually classified as an amino sugar (technically an amino-monosaccharide). It's naturally synthesized in the human body (and in the bodies of vertebrates and marine creatures as well) and is a basic building block of connective tissue, like the cartilage in your knee, for example. While we have an ample amount of the stuff when we're young, we lose some of it as we age, leading to the thinning of cartilage, which frequently progresses to the common condition known as *osteoarthritis*.

Osteoarthritis is one of the most common of the chronic health conditions. About two-thirds of all people over the age of sixty-five have physical signs of it that would be visible on an x-ray, but many don't know it because they have no symptoms. For others, the symptoms range from mildly annoying (a pain in the joint when it rains) to downright debilitating. After all, when cartilage in the joints wears down, eventually you're left with little or no shock absorbers—just bone rubbing on bone. That's got to hurt. And over time, this rubbing will permanently damage the joint. Any joint can be affected; though it's very common in the knees, arthritis can also affect the hips, neck, lower spine, hands, and feet.

A Joint Partnership

Glucosamine—and its partner chondroitin—can help.

Many studies have shown that glucosamine and/or chondroitin are beneficial in helping to repair damage to the joints caused by osteoarthritis (more on chondroitin in a minute). While it can't bring cartilage back, it can prevent further loss as well as reduce symptoms of pain, swelling, and stiffness or noise in the joints.

This is important, especially for post-menopausal women, who have a greater propensity toward osteoarthritis than men. In two independent, three-year, randomized, placebo-controlled studies, glucosamine sulfate was shown to slow the progression of osteoarthritis symptoms. After three years, postmenopausal participants in the groups given the glucosamine sulfate showed no joint space narrowing

whatsoever, while those given a placebo did. Not only that, the glucosamine sulfate group showed a significant improvement in their WOMAC Index (a standardized measure of pain) while there was a trend for worsening of pain in the placebo group.

Let's face it: Joint pain is uncomfortable and frustrating, especially for those who are used to living an active life. For relief from the pain, many reach for remedies like the prescription drugs in the category known as COX-2 inhibitors (Celebrex and Vioxx are famous examples), or pain relievers such as acetaminophen (Tylenol) and nonsteroidal anti-inflammatory drugs (Aleve). These drugs do offer immediate relief, but they're hardly without problems (witness the class-action suits over Vioxx).

Keep in mind that none of them address the underlying cause of the joint pain. Natural supplements like glucosamine not only help with pain—albeit a bit more slowly—but have the potential to stop the progression of the condition that's causing it. Best of all, they do so without any serious side effects.

The Role of Chondroitin

You'll often hear glucosamine mentioned together with another supplement called chondroitin. There's a reason for that. Chondroitin sulfate is another building block of connective tissue. It actually stimulates the cartilage cells (called chondrocytes), and therefore works beautifully when paired with glucosamine to speed the regeneration and recovery of bone tissues. While chondroitin taken alone doesn't seem to

Natural Prescription for Arthritis

Glucosamine from glucosamine sulfate (glucosamine hydrochloride if you're allergic to sulfate or shellfish): 1,500 mg per day in divided doses (okay to take 3,000 mg a day for the first month)

Chondroitin sulfate: 1,200–1,500 mg (okay to reduce to 500 mg per day if you like, after the first few months)

MSM: 1,000–4,000 mg

Omega-3 fish oil (or essential fatty acids): 1–5 g (1,000–5,000 mg)

Bromelain: 100–400 mg

DL-phenylalanine: 500 mg

Sea cucumber: 400 mg

CMO: 100 mg

Exercise: Water aerobics or tai chi

Note: The above dosages are daily and in pill or capsule form unless otherwise noted.

do very much, when taken together with glucosamine it offers significantly greater improvement of osteoarthritis than when either is used separately.

Well-absorbed and associated with only minor side effects, chondroitin sulfate can also decrease pain and slow the rate of cartilage loss in people with osteoarthritis. The Annual Scientific Meeting of the American College of Rheumatology in 2005 reported that the combination of glucosamine and chondroitin sulfate is at least as effective as the prescription drug celecoxib (brand name Celebrex) in treating pain caused by moderate to severe osteoarthritis of the knee. So for best results, use them together.

Glucosamine/chondroitin therapy requires patience: You may have to wait anywhere from eight to twelve weeks to see results. Some studies suggest that about two-thirds of adults who use glucosamine and chondroitin will experience benefits but that one-third will experience nothing.

To increase the odds that you'll be in the majority of people who reap the benefits of this terrific natural combination, use it properly. There are different "versions" (called salts) of glucosamine, including glucosamine sulfate, glucosamine hydrochloride, and glucosamine hydroiodide. (Glucosamine hydrochloride actually provides more glucosamine than the glucosamine sulfate, but this may not matter if your supplement is standardized for the amount of glucosamine it contains.)

Most studies have used glucosamine *sulfate*, so unless you're allergic to sulfates, that's probably your safest bet. The best studies used 1,500 mg of glucosamine sulfate a day, though I've heard some health practitioners swear by the idea of "loading up" with 3,000 mg a day for the first month and then dropping down to the recommended 1,500 mg. Some evidence suggests the dose has to be adjusted for obesity. Chondrotin seems to work well at around 800 to 1,500 mg daily.

Adding to the Arsenal

In addition to glucosamine sulfate and chondroitin sulfate, other nutrients have been shown to have benefit and may work synergistically with glucosamine and chondroitin.

Methyl sulfonylmethane (MSM) (see page 66) is terrific for joint pain, largely because of its high sulfur content. (There's a reason people all over the world flock to hot sulfur baths for pain relief.) MSM blocks the transmission of impulses in nerve fibers that carry pain signals. Studies in laboratory animals whose diet included MSM showed less degenerative change of the articular joint compared to the control group. In the June 2004 journal *Clinical Drug Investigations*, scientists reported that glucosamine and MSM individually improved pain and swelling in arthritic joints; the combination of the two was more effective in reducing symptoms and improving the function of joints.

And speaking of sulfur-containing natural compounds, there's bromelain, the general name for a group of sulfur-containing enzymes that digest protein. Derived from pineapple, bromelain's usefulness in osteoarthritis comes from its anti-inflammatory properties. Bromelain also stimulates the production of plasmin, an enzyme that helps to break down clots, which in turn prevents swelling. Plasmin also blocks the formation of pro-inflammatory compounds.

Phenylalanine is an amino acid that is a primary building block for pain control. (The DL form of the amino acid, known also as DLPA, is especially potent in this respect.) Research supports the use of DLPA in relief of back pain,

arthritis, aches, pains, and menstrual cramps. Phenylalanine slows the body's breakdown of endorphins, the body's internal painkillers. The more endorphins you have hanging around, the less pain you have.

Note: If you have a condition known as phenylketonurea (PKU) *do not* use this nutrient. PKU is a rare genetic disorder characterized by the inability to break down phenylalanine. Aspartame is made from phenylalanine, which is the reason Equal comes with a warning label for

WORTH KNOWING

In those patients who are obese, have peptic ulcers, or are taking diuretics, the effectiveness of glucosamine sulfate is reduced. So if this applies to you, work with a health-care provider to increase the doses shown here.

Those who are allergic to sulfates may take glucosamine hydrochloride and not glucosamine sulfate, and they should avoid chondroitin sulfate. Glucosamine is derived from shrimp, oyster, and crab shells, and chondroitin is derived from cartilage of cows, pigs, and sharks. There is no synthetically made glucosamine on the market.

Glucosamine and chondroitin help regrow cartilage. However, if you have no cartilage left, these nutrients will not do any good to artificial knees. They may help, though, with your other joints. The best option is to prevent the joint from getting to a stage of destruction by using nutrients that help keep cartilage tissue healthy.

people with PKU. If you don't have PKU, DL-phenylalanine is perfectly safe.

Oil Those Joints

Cetyl myristoleate or CMO is less known than glucosamine or chondroitin, but is also worth knowing about if you have arthritis pain. Clinical studies have shown that it increases joint mobility for up to 60 percent of the people who take it.

CMO is an all-natural oil found in certain animals like cows, whales, mice, and beavers. Harry W. Diehl, Ph.D., a researcher at the National Institutes of Health, first discovered it in 1972. It has been used in a lot of arthritis research over the last 25 years. It works by inhibiting the production of certain inflammatory compounds in the body. Studies have shown that the effectiveness of CMO is actually superior to over-the-counter prescriptions such as nonsteroidal anti-inflammatory drugs.

In treating any inflammatory condition like arthritis, we never want to overlook the king of the natural anti-inflammatories, omega-3 fatty acids (fish oil). Fish oil works by reducing the number of inflammatory messenger molecules made by the body's immune system. The Arthritis Foundation recommends eating at least two fish meals a week—particularly in fatty fish such as salmon, mackerel, and sardines.

High-quality fish oil supplements are an excellent way to get the many health benefits of the omega-3 fatty acids (see page 299).

Other ingredients you may see on the ingredients list in a glucosamine-chondroitin formula may include sea cucumber (*Cucumaria frondosa*), grape seed extract, boswellia, and turmeric, all of which have varying degrees of anti-inflammatory action.

Exercise for Arthritis

You may feel like exercise is out of the question if you have arthritis. Not so. Moderate exercise can be your best friend—building strong muscles around the joints can go a long way toward relieving joint pain, not to mention the benefits exercise provides to overall endurance, well-being, and mood. Two exercise modalities worth checking out are tai chi, a very gentle form of martial arts that involves soft, flowing movements and no stress on the joints, and water aerobics, which can be done at different levels of difficulty without putting any stress on the joints. For more ideas, the www.about.com website has an excellent introduction to exercise with arthritis. And if you or someone you love is truly unable to get out of a chair, there's still hope—the Sit and Be Fit program is a wonderful resource. Check it out at www.sitandbefit.com.

Quercetin/Magnesium/ Vitamin B6

for Asthma

CONVENTIONAL MEDICATIONS ARE often helpful for treating acute asthma attacks and for preventing recurrences. However, despite the best that modern medicine has to offer, many patients continue to experience acute attacks and/or chronic, low-level breathing difficulties. Moreover, most of the medications used to treat asthma can cause side effects. New ideas are needed if we are to win the battle against asthma.

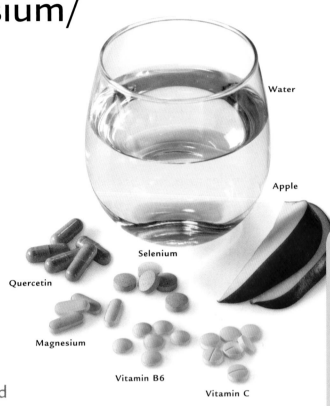

Water

Apple

Selenium

Quercetin

Magnesium

Vitamin B6

Vitamin C

—Jonathan Wright, M.D., co-author of *Natural Medicine, Optimal Wellness*

If you've ever seen someone having an asthma attack, you know it's not pretty.

And according to those who suffer from them, an attack can be one of the scariest experiences in life. Muscles around the sufferer's airways tighten up, less and less air can get in, inflammation increases, the airways become even more swollen and narrow, and it becomes harder and harder to breathe. During a bad attack, the person with asthma may literally feel like he's suffocating and can't breathe. In severe cases, the airways can close so much that not enough oxygen gets to the vital organs—at which point it's a full-blown medical emergency.

You can die from that kind of attack, and approximately 4,000 to 5,000 people a year do just that. And asthma is a contributing factor to 7,000 other deaths each year.

What Is Asthma?

Asthma comes from Greek words meaning either "panting" or "sharp breath." It's a chronic disease affecting the pathways that carry air in and out of the lungs. Those airways become inflamed and very sensitive to any of a variety of substances (in air, food, or the environment) that are irritating or allergenic. That's one reason asthma is so often linked to allergies.

Sharp-eyed readers may notice that the words *inflamed* or *inflammation* have shown up in both of the above paragraphs. Keep an eye out—they're going to come up again. Remember that when we start to talk about quercetin.

Asthma is widely understood by almost everyone to be an immunological problem. The immune system mistakenly identifies substances—pollens, dust, dander, foods, etc.—as being dangerous and overreacts, setting up a cascade of events that leads to inflammation in the lungs and a narrowing of the air passages.

If that overreaction of the immune system to everyday stimuli sounds somewhat like the description of an allergy, it's because they're not entirely dissimilar. Allergic asthma is a specific type of asthma that can be triggered by an allergy to, for example, pollen or mold. And it's common: In the United States, it's estimated that about half of asthma sufferers have allergic asthma.

Because allergies (and asthma) are inflammatory disorders, it makes sense that a diet high in natural anti-inflammatories (e.g., vegetables and some fruits) is going to be a good idea for sufferers. And for asthma—and allergies—one of the best and most powerful of the natural anti-inflammatories is a substance called quercetin.

The Most Important Flavonoid

In the coloring of fruits and vegetables there are thousands of molecules known collectively as polyphenols. One particular class of these polyphenols is called *flavonoids*. And the most abundant, most bioavailable, and most studied of these flavonoids is a compound called *quercetin*. Apples are a significant source of quercetin, which has quite a résumé of health benefits.

Quercetin—which was called "the most important flavonoid" by the peer-reviewed journal *Nutrition in Cancer*—is highly anti-inflammatory, making it very useful in helping to calm the symptoms of asthma (and allergies). It's found in onions, apples, berries, tea, red wine, and supplements. In one study published in 2002 in the *American Journal of Clinical*

Nutrition, higher quercetin intakes were associated with a lower incidence of asthma.

"Quercetin has a very unique molecular structure," says David Nieman, Ph.D., author of *Nutritional Assessment* and head of the Appalachian State University Human Performance Lab. "It has many effects in humans. It impacts the immune system, it reacts against cancer cells, and it's a powerful anti-inflammatory."

In the voluminous literature linking dietary habits and disease, quercetin has an impressive history of being linked to a reduction in heart disease as well as to a reduction in lung cancer. Epidemiological studies have suggested that high consumption of apples may protect against asthma, and quercetin may be the main reason why.

The quercetin in the apple is, interestingly enough, in the peel. "The peel prevents the harmful effects of the UV rays of the sun from hurting the fruit," Nieman says. "It also prevents microbes from getting in. So quercetin is the first line of defense for the apple. It appears to have many of these same protective effects on human cells."

One of the reasons quercetin is so helpful with asthma (and with allergies) has to do with cells in the body known as *mast cells*. Mast cells are responsible for a lot of the crummy symptoms you have when you get an allergy attack or experience asthmatic wheezing. The mast cells, which are actually part of the immune system, carry around all sorts of granules, the most famous of which is histamine. During an attack—of allergies or asthma—the mast cells release histamine and other chemicals like cytokines and leukotrines, causing the characteristic symptoms that drive everyone, especially the sufferer, crazy. Quercetin stabilizes the mast cells, calming them down. When you put quercetin in a test tube with mast cells, they relax. And that's exactly what you want, whether you're suffering from an allergy attack, asthmatic wheezing, or both.

But quercetin's ability to help with asthma doesn't stop with the mast cells. It also inhibits two enzymes—tyrosine kinase and nitric oxide synthase—that turn the volume up on inflammatory reactions. These enzymes essentially act as cheerleaders for the inflammatory response, urging it on and making things worse. Quercetin inhibits both of them. It also turns down the volume on another inflammatory chemical in the body called NF-kappa B. All of these anti-inflammatory actions make quercetin a powerful natural weapon against both allergies and allergic asthma.

Asthma and Allergies: Overlapping Components

Asthma and allergies share a number of overlapping components. Take bacterial infections, for example. At least two studies suggest that *Candida albicans*—the bacteria more commonly known as yeast—may be an important agent in the cause of both asthma and allergy. Let's not forget that those little "yeasty-beasties" are actually living organisms that produce waste products of their own, which can cause an attack.

One study found that 8 to 10 percent of chronic asthma and rhinitis patients are likely sensitive to one of three yeasts (one of which was candida). For about 5 percent of candida-allergic patients studied, bronchial asthma was the major symptom of their yeast problem. (See page 179 for suggested treatments for candida.)

Asthma and allergies share a relationship to emotional stress. Even conventional doctors, especially the younger ones, now know that asthma has significant emotional triggers in addition to its physical components. Anxiety and stress are common asthma triggers—just as they are for so many other conditions and symptoms. It's not that emotions cause asthma, but they can make symptoms a lot worse. Strong emotions can even trigger an attack.

Stress management may be one of the best "natural cures," or "adjuncts," for managing asthma severity. Learn to recognize both thought patterns and behavior patterns that are stressful for you and develop some techniques for cutting them off at the pass. Image therapy (see page 278) is a great tool to use. It can help prevent you from panicking or stressing out at the first sign of an asthma event, which only makes everything worse. Buteyko therapy, which teaches a different way of breathing, is also worth looking into (see page 331).

Food Allergies and Sensitivities

Though some asthma is triggered by external environmental substances (like pollen), some is triggered—or exacerbated—by food. According to Alan Gaby, M.D., unrecognized food allergy (and/or food intolerance) is a contributing factor in at least 75 percent of people with childhood asthma and about 40 percent of those with adult asthma.

"As early as 1959, Albert H. Rowe, M.D., a pioneer in the field of food allergy, successfully treated 95 asthmatic patients with dietary changes alone," Gaby says. At the top of the list of foods most likely to provoke asthma? Dairy products. Other usual suspects include eggs, chocolate, wheat, corn, citrus fruits, and fish. Tartrazine (yellow dye #5) is believed to be a trigger for thousands of people.

A rotation diet (see page 210) is a good way to identify any food triggers, but it is a tad labor intensive. Even easier is the shotgun approach called an elimination diet, whereby you simply get rid of all the dietary "usual suspects" that cause most of the problems in most other people with asthma—then see whether there's an improvement (there almost always is). You can always add foods back one at a time to zero in on just what's causing the most symptoms—or you can just stop eating all of them and call it a day, though after looking at the list of "usual suspects" you may not think that's a great option. Most important to eliminate: dairy, wheat (or even better, grains), and sugar. Start by eating a diet free of dairy products, refined carbohydrates (e.g., sugar and flour), hydrogenated fats (partially hydrogenated oils or trans fats), and as many additives, preservatives, and chemicals as possible. The more whole organic foods that don't have bar codes, the better. A "clean" whole foods diet like this should clear up symptoms for many people, since it basically eliminates everything that's likely to be a problem.

The Stomach Acid Connection

One reason why food sensitivities and asthma show up together so often can be found in a study done decades ago by George Bray, M.D., and it has to do with stomach acid. In 1931, Bray compared children with and without asthma and found that while only one out of five nonasthmatic children were deficient in hydrochloric acid (HCl), four out of five of the asthmatic kids were. Low levels of HCl can significantly impair digestion and can increase allergies—or sensitivities—to foods.

In Bray's study, when the low-acid kids were given HCl before or during meals and when they continued to avoid trigger foods, they had noticeable improvements in asthmatic attacks, and the attacks became shorter and less severe.

Natural Prescription for Allergies and Asthma

Quercetin: 500 mg, twice a day (preferably taken with bromelain)

Magnesium: 300–600 mg

Vitamin B6: 50–200 mg

Vitamin C: 1,000–3,000 mg

Selenium: 200 mcg

Note: All dosages are daily dosages and in pill or capsule form unless otherwise noted.

This is not the only time you'll hear about the connection between low stomach acid and symptoms and diseases. Many of the best people in the field of complementary medicine, including Jonathan Wright, M.D., believe that low acid is endemic in our society and can cause a host of problems that clear up or improve noticeably once the low acid level is corrected.

Selenium: The Powerhouse Antioxidant

People with asthma are subjected to increased oxidative stress, the damage done to cells by free radicals of oxygen molecules. One super antioxidant that has special importance to people with asthma is selenium (see Desert Island Cures, page 313). A number of studies have reported low selenium levels in people with asthma, and one study—in the *American Journal of Respiratory and Critical Care Medicine*—reported that study participants with the highest intakes of selenium were only about half as likely to have asthma as those who consumed the least. (Not much selenium was needed for the positive effect—under 100 mcg.) The researchers suggested that part of the blame for Britain's rising asthma rate might be the nation's declining selenium intake.

Selenium is also part of an important enzyme called *glutathione peroxidase*, which is critical in protecting against free-radical and oxidative damage associated with asthma and is especially important in reducing the production of inflammatory compounds like leukotrines. What's more, asthma drugs significantly decrease the body's glutathione levels, and glutathione is arguably the most important antioxidant in the body. For all those reasons, selenium supplementation for asthma is an important part of any natural prescription. Even the extremely cautious and conservative *Cochrane Reviews* stated "there is some indication that selenium supplementation may be a useful adjunct to medication for patients with chronic asthma."

I'm way less cautious: I say take selenium every day for its myriad of benefits, not the least of which is that it may help your asthma.

Other supplements that may help with asthma include magnesium, vitamin B6, and vitamin C. Low levels of B6 and magnesium are frequently found together with asthma, and some research has shown improvement in the frequency and severity of asthma symptoms with supplementation. B6 and magnesium tend to be at the top of everyone's list for supplementation when it comes to nutrition and asthma. Vitamin C is included in the natural prescription for its powerful action as an overall antioxidant.

Digestive Enzymes and Probiotics

for Bad Breath

BAD BREATH IS another fine example of how the body has a limited number of ways to respond to an infinite number of "insults" or problems. The conventional wisdom is that it's caused by some-thing in the mouth—poor oral hygiene, for example. But just as skin blemishes are only sometimes a surface issue and more commonly stem from something systemic, bad breath only sometimes comes from the mouth.

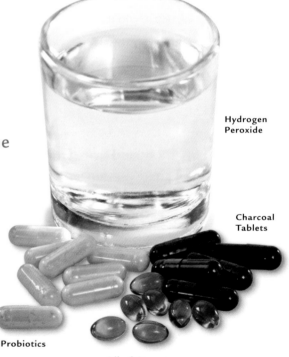

Hydrogen Peroxide

Charcoal Tablets

Probiotics

Oil of Oregano

A great deal of bad breath actually originates in the gut. Poor digestion is a frequent culprit. Enter digestive enzymes. Digestive enzymes that contain hydrochloric acid (HCl) would probably benefit most people over forty regardless of whether they have bad breath. Not only do they address some of the causes of bad breath at the root, they also help us break down and use protein, which can become a lot more difficult for people over forty. Many folks don't make sufficient HCl to adequately break down protein and other foods, so a capsule that combines digestive enzymes and HCl is highly recommended.

Many holistic physicians and health practitioners have recently written about the myriad health problems associated with low stomach acid. Bad breath, bloating, gas, and even fatigue are among the many symptoms of low stomach acid, which HCl can help.

A great way to determine how much HCl you need is this: Take one HCl capsule before a big meal. At the next big meal, take two capsules, and at the third big meal take three capsules, and so on. Continue to do this until you feel a warming sensation in your stomach. Then back off one capsule, and that is the dosage you need to help you with digestion.

Gut health depends on the proper balance of bacteria, so if you suspect digestive problems are at the root of bad breath, a good probiotic supplement—acidophilus and/or bifidus—is a great idea. Fructoogliosaccharides (FOS)—a particularly healthy form of nondigestible carbohydrates—are sometimes included in such formulations because they act as food for the "good bugs."

A Diet for Bad Breath

When gut ecology is properly balanced between the "good" and the "bad" bacteria, it's like having a garden that's overgrown with weeds. The weeds in this case are bacteria like *Candida albicans* (yeast), which can cause all sorts of health problems, not the least of which is really bad breath. Oil of oregano capsules are a great way to kill the little buggers. You also want to starve them. Since they live on sugar, an "anti-yeast" diet—something like the early stages of the Atkins Diet, with no sugar, bread, pasta, rice, cereal, or even fruit for a couple of weeks—is just the ticket. Protein, vegetables, and good fat are the way to go.

Activated charcoal is another great supplement that can help with odors and even toxins originating in the gut. It may also sweeten your breath.

Chlorophyll is nature's deodorizer and, according to some naturopaths, a great blood purifier, meaning it helps support detoxification. The popular breath-freshening gum Clorets capitalized on this connection between chlorophyll and deodorizing, but truth be told, chlorophyll packs a powerful wallop. Some practitioners recommend taking a few capsules or tablets on an empty stomach to support gut health and detoxification. And more fiber in your diet—always a good idea—promotes the elimination of toxins from the body.

Since highly processed foods loaded with bad fats and sugar can contribute to digestive problems (and to bad breath), the more whole foods you can incorporate into your diet the

Natural Prescription for Bad Breath

Digestive enzymes: 1 or 2 with every meal

Probiotics: 1 or 2, three times a day or as directed. You can also take the powdered form with water.

Charcoal tablets in between meals: Activated charcoal absorbs toxins and is a natural purifier. (Take it with plenty of water, and not at the same time as nutritional supplements or medications, as it may theoretically interfere with absorption.)

Hydrogen peroxide: Gargling and rinsing with hydrogen peroxide has been found to be terrific for many people.

Oil of oregano: 2 capsules, three times a day

Green drinks: Daily

Note: All dosages are daily dosages and in pill or capsule form unless otherwise noted.

better. I've long been an advocate of daily, fresh-made vegetable and fruit juice (see *The 150 Healthiest Foods on Earth*). Vegetables and fruits also help balance the system by providing a nice alkaline balance to our highly acidic, overly processed standard American diet. Alternately, some of the "green drinks" now found in health food supermarkets are a great choice

and accomplish some of the same things. These drinks frequently contain nice doses of chlorophyll-containing grasses.

Natural Breath Mints

In addition to the above recommendations, herbs and spices can sweeten your breath. Try the following.

Parsley and mint. Chewing parsley or mint leaves has been a natural remedy for thousands of years. These herbs are especially good if garlic and onions are the source of your bad breath. Parsley is very high in chlorophyll. Try chewing a few parsley sprigs dipped in vinegar for immediate relief. If you swallow the leaves after chewing them they will be digested and continue to provide fresh breath for a while. These plants seem to reduce the production of intestinal gas by promoting better digestion.

Peelu is a natural twig fortified with minerals that help clean the teeth and other inhibitors that prevent gums from bleeding. It also has cleaning agents that kill microbes and germs and a scent that makes breath naturally fresh. Peelu is an ideal brush that has been naturally endowed with more breath-freshening, mouth-cleaning compounds than any artificially made toothpaste.

Finally, herbs like coriander, ginger, cumin, and fennel are helpful. Indian restaurants usually provide a little bowl of fennel seeds for customers. Chewing on them freshens the breath in the nicest and most natural way.

Combo Cure

for Aging Brains

IF YOU'RE A baby boomer, at some point in your life you've undoubtedly heard yourself say the following words: "Senior moment!" And if you aren't a baby boomer, chances are you still know what your boomer friends mean when they say them. (If you don't, let me translate from boomer-ese. A "senior moment" means "I can't remember where I put my keys. Oh my God, is this the beginning of Alzheimer's?") Well, the good news is ... not necessarily. Not *necessarily* because some degree of memory loss—or what's clinically called *cognitive decline*—is expected as we grow older. It happens to many people, if not to everyone.

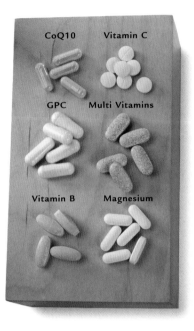

But there's good news. First, some amount of memory loss or cognitive decline doesn't necessarily translate to any meaningful impairment of your brain power or ability to function. Second, cognitive impairment doesn't always progress to Alzheimer's. And third, just like there are things you can do right now to protect your heart, your muscles, your liver, and other organs, there are things you can do right now to protect your brain.

"The brain is like every other organ in the body, only more so. It's more delicate, more metabolically active, more easily damaged, requires more energy, and is in more need of serious nutritional and lifestyle support if it's to stay fit longer," says brain surgeon Larry McCleary, M.D., author of *The Brain Trust Program*.

The Cost of Aging

Keeping your aging brain fit is what this entry is all about. As of 2006, the youngest members of the group of more than seventy-eight million people in the United States known as baby boomers will have passed their fortieth birthday. The older members of the group, which include George W. Bush and Bill Clinton (and me), turned sixty in this same year.

About thirty million of us will suffer some form of dementia, according to *New York Times* columnist David Brooks. A somewhat greater degree of decline, clinically known as *mild cognitive impairment* or MCI, will affect 10 percent of the over-65 population—about 15 percent of that group will go on to develop full-blown Alzheimer's. There are now more than five million people in the United States living with Alzheimer's, estimates the Alzheimer's Association. Someone develops Alzheimer's every seventy-two seconds, and, for what it's worth, the direct and indirect financial cost of Alzheimer's and other dementias have a price tag of more than $148 billion a year.

I'm sure I don't need to tell you that Alzheimer's disease and dementia are no laughing matters. Nor is the overall health of your brain. It's a major concern of many people in this country, particularly baby boomers or those of us who have had to care for aging parents with some form of dementia. It's not fun—not for them, not for us, and it's a fate every one of us would do anything to avoid. I can't promise you that the supplements in this combo cure will prevent Alzheimer's. But I can promise you that every one of them—separately or in combination—has been shown to produce some improvements in mild cognitive impairment and/or in full-blown Alzheimer's.

(Brain) Size May Not Matter

You're born with roughly 100 billion neurons (brain cells), and the brain increases its mass about threefold until you reach your early twenties. (Which is why my friend Janet, when exasperated, frequently says to her teenage daughter, Molly, "I'll have this conversation with you in ten years when your brain is finished developing!")

The rate at which neurons die off is very individual, and, contrary to conventional wisdom, you do continue to grow new ones all your life—it's just that the rate of growth slows down, while the rate of dying continues, leaving you with a somewhat smaller brain. By the age of eighty, your brain is about 10 percent smaller than it was when you were a quick-witted smart alec at age twenty. (Part of this is due to neurons shrinking as well as dying.)

But the good news is that brain size may not matter that much. While you do lose neurons, your brilliantly resilient brain is able to continue to form new neural connections and pathways, meaning that the loss in size can easily be compensated by an increase in versatility and new learning. Your functional capacity needn't be deeply affected at all. That, of course, assumes you keep your brain healthy so it can maintain its ability to "retrain" itself, and to continue to function sharply until the day you die.

And you do that in three ways—with the foods you eat, the lifestyle choices you make, and the supplements you take.

Basic Brain Nutrition 101

Back in 2003, reports from the Chicago Health and Aging Project started documenting the powerful effects that nutrients can have on cognitive decline and Alzheimer's disease. The project was a study of common chronic health problems of older persons, and especially of risk factors for

> *"The sad realities of dementia being epidemic and treatments for dementia still so limited make it a moral imperative to explore all possibilities for relief."*
>
> —Parris Kidd, Ph.D.,
> *biochemist and nutritionist*

Alzheimer's disease. These studies were conducted in a biracial neighborhood of the south side of Chicago. The researchers looked at more than 3,000 participants over the age of sixty-five and with a racial mix of 60 percent African American and 40 percent white. The simple executive summary of what they found is this: Nutrient deficiencies can increase the rate of cognitive decline. And adopting a few simple healthy eating habits—like including fish and vegetables in your regular diet—can slow down cognitive decline by the equivalent of up to nineteen years. Pretty impressive for a nondrug intervention—especially since that same dietary strategy (fish and vegetables) has been shown to reduce heart disease as well.

Food aside, certain nutrients continue to be mentioned, studied, and verified on the subject of preserving brain power. Used in combination, they are a powerhouse for mental protection.

Acetyl-L-Carnitine: The Memory Keeper

The mitochondria are tiny little two-membraned structures in the cytoplasm of the cell that are known as the cells' power source—they're little energy production factories where most of the chemical energy needed for life is generated. When your mitochondria are in trouble, so are you. The term for that—*mitochondrial dysfunction*—contributes to all sorts of human pathologies from neurodegenerative disease to stroke, heart attack, and diabetes. Neurosurgeon Russell Baylock, M.D., says acetyl-L-carnitine improves the function of the mitochondria, "returning them to the way they were when you were twenty."

Sign me up!

Acetyl-L-carnitine is a kind of supercharged version of carnitine that has a particularly positive effect in the brain. Carnitine acts as a shuttle, transporting fatty acids into the mitochondria where they can be "burned" for energy—one reason it's so important for the heart (see the awesome foursome for heart disease on page 141). Neurologist David Perlmutter, M.D., author of *The Better Brain Book*, describes acetyl-L-carnitine as a "neuronal energizer." He also points out that it helps remove waste products from the mitochondria energy production factory, enabling them to be eliminated from the body.

"This is a very important job," he says. "If toxins are not removed from mitochondria, they can damage the mitochondria, which will slow down energy production even more."

Several clinical trials have suggested that acetyl-L-carnitine may delay the onset of age-related cognitive decline and improve overall cognitive function in the elderly. It also protects the brain from damage due to poor circulation and helps to repair injured nerve cells. After three months using recommended doses of acetyl-L-carnitine, there is marked improvement in general cognitive function. One study found that a dose of 1,500 mg of acetyl-L-carnitine taken once a day for ninety days substantially improved reactions to stress, memory function, and mood.

Acetyl-L-carnitine helps the brain form *acetylcholine*, a neurotransmitter needed for memory and thinking. A number of studies have demonstrated positive effects of acetyl-L-carnitine supplementation in Alzheimer's patients, especially with regard to tasks that involve concentration and attention. One study done in 1991 and published in *Neurology* divided 130 Alzheimer's patients into two groups. One was treated with acetyl-L-carnitine while the other received a placebo. In thirteen of the fourteen outcome measures (including long-term verbal memory, selective attention, and logical intelligence), the acetyl-L-carnitine group had better scores. Those patients who had "good treatment compliance"—meaning they actually listened to the doctor and took their supplements on a regular basis—showed even greater benefit. More

recent studies continue to show positive effects, but younger patients seem to benefit even more.

Perlmutter believes that carnitine is one of the few substances that can help slow down the progression of Alzheimer's, pointing out that people with Alzheimer's disease have "strikingly low levels of carnitine." According to the *Physician's Desk Reference*, preliminary evidence shows that acetyl-L-carnitine can slow mental decline in the elderly who are not afflicted with dementia. Perlmutter suggests that "supplementing with this vital amino acid in midlife, when levels begin to decline, may help prevent this brain degenerative disease in the first place."

Membranes Matter

Phosphatidylserine (PS) is a member of a class of biochemicals called phospholipids. It's a naturally occurring nutrient that's found in the cell membranes, but it's most concentrated in the brain. As neurologist Jay Lombard, M.D., author of *The Brain Wellness Plan* says, "The first step in treating patients with Alzheimer's disease is to rebuild defective membranes."

Membranes matter.

PS has been available as a supplement for decades and has been shown in well-documented studies to restore brain function. It helps improve learning and name recall, concentration, face recognition, the ability to remember telephone numbers, and the ability to find misplaced objects. One of its primary functions is to regulate the release of various neurotransmitters.

"Our brain health depends on … phosphatidylserine for a number of important metabolic effects," Lombard says, "including making it possible for nutrients to move freely in and out of neurons."

In one large trial, over the course of three months, 142 subjects aged forty to eighty were given 200 mg of PS a day or a placebo. On the scales normally used to assess Alzheimer's, those treated with the PS showed a small but statistically significant benefit. A large study in Italy titled *Cognitive decline in the elderly: A double-blind, placebo-controlled multi-centered study on efficacy of phosphatidylserine administration* followed 494 elderly subjects over six months, all of whom had moderate to severe mental decline. One group received 300 mg a day of PS, the other received a placebo. The PS group performed significantly better in both mental function and measures of behavior. Interestingly, symptoms of depression also improved, a finding that has been suggested by another study on elderly women.

Steven Bratman, M.D., author of *The Natural Health Encylcopedia*, a database on herbs and supplements that's used by many hospitals, says that "… it is not a great leap to suspect that [PS might be] useful for much less severe problems with memory and mental function, such as those that seem to occur in nearly all of us who are older than forty." And my good friend, biochemist and nutritional supplement expert Parris Kidd, writes: "The findings from …. clinical trial(s) are unequivocal: dietary supplementation with PS can alleviate, ameliorate, and sometimes reverse age-related decline of memory, learning, concentration, word skills, and mood."

But there's a controversy.

Nearly all of the good studies on phosphatidylserine used PS from the brains of cows. For obvious reasons—like concerns with viruses like mad cow disease—no one is using or selling PS from bovine sources anymore. The PS now on the market as a supplement comes from soy, and there is a huge controversy over whether it's as effective.

Phosphatidylserine is basically a serine molecule attached to some fat, and the fat in a cow's brain is 7 percent omega-3, which is what the serine molecule likes to bind to. There's no omega-3 in the soy. But Kidd, a renowned authority on nutritional supplements, explains that while the two phosphatidylserines are indeed different, if you have plenty of omega-3 in your body it shouldn't make a difference. The serine molecule will simply bind to the omega-3 (assuming you've got enough) and that will be that. Though that's theoretical, it makes sense. One product—PS Synergy by Crayhon Research—even combines PS with omega-3 fatty acids for you (it's available on my website at www.jonnybowden.com). If you take a plain PS product without built-in omegas, be sure to also take some omega-3s (or essential fatty acids) at the same time.

The Miracle Antiaging Nutrient for Your Brain

Glycerophosphocholine (GPC) is a supplement that has been extensively researched for its effect on mental performance, attention, concentration, and memory formation. Like PS, it's a member of the class of biochemicals known as phospholipids, which are important in making healthy cell membranes. GPC is found in abundant quantities in mother's milk, which ought to tell us something about its importance in human life. There are only tiny amounts in food, so to get the full therapeutic value of this wonderful substance, supplements are the way to go.

A large body of scientific research has demonstrated GPC's importance for the brain. "I continue to be fascinated by GPC's capacities to salvage function in the damaged brain, to sharpen mental performance even in people who are healthy, and to give new vitality to the aging brain," Kidd says.

I'll tell you one of many examples that demonstrate the scientific validation of this remarkable nutrient. One set of trials involved a fascinating phenomenon called *scopolamine amnesia*. It seems that if you administer a chemical called scopolamine (by injection or by mouth) to people, they will very quickly experience near-total amnesia. They just forget everything. It's remarkable—all information skills, including memory, attention, and learning, just seem to disappear. The chemical is harmless, the effect is only temporary, and it wears off in a few hours, but it allows researchers to do all sorts of clever studies.

In two of these studies, researchers first gave healthy young volunteers GPC or a placebo over the course of a week to ten days. Then they gave them the scopamine injection and watched them carefully for the next six hours. They wanted to determine the degree to which GPC could protect their minds against the (inevitable) amnesia brought on by the drug.

The researchers had the subjects perform a test called free recall (twenty words are read

Natural Prescription for Alzheimer's and Cognitive Decline

Phosphatidylserine: 100–300 mg

Acetyl-L-carnitine: Start with 250 mg per day and increase up to 4,000 mg per day in divided doses

GPC: 300–1,200 mg in the morning

Alpha lipoic acid: 100 mg

Omega-3 fatty acids (either in capsules or liquid fish oil): 1,000–3,000 mg

B-complex vitamin: Include extra B12 (1,000 mcg may be best for older people)

CoQ10: 100 mg

Vitamin C: 1–2 g

Multiple vitamin and/or antioxidant formula: 1 per day or as directed

Magnesium: 800 IU

Diet: Increase vegetables (especially spinach), fish, and berries (especially blueberries)

Exercise: Mild to moderate exercise at least three days a week

OPTIONAL:

Vinpocentine: 10 mg, three times a day

Huperzine A: (see page 247)

Note: The above dosages are daily and in pill or capsule form, unless otherwise noted.

aloud three times and subjects have two minutes to write down as many as they can remember), and a test of attention called the *cancellation test* (subjects are given a matrix of 1,200 randomly generated numbers and told to find three that are identified as "targets" and eliminate them from the matrix within three minutes).

The results were pretty amazing. In the free recall test, the GPC held off the amnesia all the way through the six-hour trial. In the cancellation test, it held off the amnesia for three hours (a partial but very real effect on attention). The researchers concluded that GPC protected the brain's attention and memory capacity. Even more interestingly, the GPC group scored higher in a baseline test of word recall—given to all subjects before they were given the scopolamine, meaning the seven to ten days of treatment with GPC had had a positive effect on their brains even before the experiment began!

Kidd sums it up best when he says, "Along with its sister phospholipid PS, GPC has a proven track record against age-related decline and other brain damage. These are the two most clinically proven brain nutrients, and both are widely needed, especially since there are no pharmaceuticals available that provide lasting benefit against cognitive decline." If you use this supplement, take it in the morning, as it's possible that taking it late in the day may keep you up well after you're ready for bed.

Other Cognitive Defenders

Alpha lipoic acid, discussed elsewhere in this book (see page 148) for its terrific effect on blood sugar (page 148) as well as the liver (page 148 [Hep C cure]), first gained attention as a potential brain nutrient through the work of one of the most respected researchers in nutrition and biochemistry, Bruce Ames, Ph.D. Ames, a professor of the graduate school division of biochemistry and molecular biology at the University of California, performed a series of experiments in which he gave aging rats a combination of acetyl-L-carnitine and lipoic acid. Animals taking the mix performed better on memory tests and also showed general signs of vitality.

"With these two supplements together, these old rats got up and did the Macarena," Ames says. "The brain looks better, they are full of energy—everything we looked at looks more like a young animal." Indeed, analysis of the rats' brain tissue showed that they had less damage to the mitochondria—the power centers of the cells—and less oxidative damage to the memory center of the brain (the hippocampus).

Some researchers—notably neurologist Perlmutter—suggest that alpha lipoic acid's usefulness as a brain nutrient may be due to its powerful effect as an antioxidant, including its ability to significantly boost what Perlmutter considers the brain's most important antioxidant, glutathione. As an antioxidant, alpha lipoic acid helps protect against devastating damage from rogue molecules called *free radicals*. "If your brain is being devoured by free radicals, you will not be able to think clearly, stay focused, or retrieve information when you need it," he says.

But don't stop there!

Vinpocentine is a chemical substance synthesized from vincamine, a natural constituent found in the leaves of a plant in the periwinkle family (*Vinca minor*). While it's not a superstar nutrient in the cognitive arsenal, it does seem to have some effect. In one multicenter, double-blind, placebo-controlled sixteen-week study, patients with "mild to moderate" cognitive impairment problems were treated with vinpocetine. They were then tested on cognitive performance tests and on measures of "global improvement." Their results were compared with the results of a similar group that received placebo, and those treated with vinpocentine did significantly better. Another study tested vinpocentine against a placebo in elderly patients with cerebrovascular (circulation in the brain) and central nervous system degenerative disorders, and similarly good results were found. Vinpocentine so far has not been shown to be helpful with Alzheimer's, but it may improve blood flow in the brain.

Then there's vitamin B12, which is essential for the proper functioning of the brain. B12 plays an important role in creating and maintaining the protective coating around neurons, called the *myelin sheath*. Because B12 is necessary for proper nerve conduction, if and when you have less of it, the nerve impulses or messages are less effective at getting to their destinations, so B12 is essential for the proper functioning of the brain. A deficiency of B12 may lead to mental disorders including confusion, depression, memory loss, and impaired coordination.

Vitamin B12 is also protective against the toxic buildup of another substance called *homocysteine*. In an article in the prestigious *New England Journal of Medicine*, researchers from the department of neurology at Boston University School of Medicine found that a high level of homocysteine in the blood "is a strong, independent risk factor for the development of dementia and Alzheimer's disease." Homocysteine levels are easily brought back down by vitamin B12, vitamin B6, and folic acid. It is quite common for the elderly to be deficient in B12. In one study reported in *The Archives of Internal Medicine* in 2006, researchers gave subjects B12 injections once per day for a week, then weekly for a month, then monthly thereafter for six to twelve months. "Striking improvements" in cognitive function and anemia were noted.

Vitamin B12 doesn't work alone, however. Having adequate amounts of all the B vitamins, especially folic acid and vitamin B6, is also critical for protection against homocysteine and cognitive decline. All work together nicely to reduce homocysteine levels and protect against anemias as well as mental disorders.

In 2004 the *Nutrition Research Newsletter* reported a "memory" study done in Switzerland, where participants were divided into groups with varying stages of cognitive problems. The researchers not only discovered that a high homocysteine level may be an early risk factor for dementia, but that a low folic acid level may precede the onset of Alzheimer's disease. The

Veterans Affairs Normative Aging Study confirmed similar results in 2005. The trio of vitamin B6, vitamin B12, and folic acid is the best remedy for eliminating the risk factor of homocysteine.

The Fountain of Youth

Genetic makeup is partly responsible for determining the rate at which people lose cognitive function and whether or not they will develop dementia, but lifestyle choices play a huge role as well. So does diet. Just ask James Joseph.

James Joseph, Ph.D., a scientist at the Laboratory of Neuroscience at the U.S. Department of Agriculture's Human Nutrition Research Center on Aging at Tufts University, has a special interest in what we should eat if we want to keep our marbles intact as we grow older. In Jospeh's lab, he's got something he calls the rat olympics. He tests motor function and memory function with mazes and assorted tests for muscle strength and coordination. Around middle age, rats start showing the same kinds of decline in performance that humans do. But Joseph's studies show that when you feed lab animals extracts of blueberries, wonderful things start happening—or, more accurately, bad things don't happen.

Such as mental deterioration.

Rats that chow down on blueberries in the Joseph lab act like they've found the Rat Fountain of Youth. Blueberries actually help neurons in the brain communicate with one another more effectively.

"Old neurons are kind of like old married couples," Joseph says. "They don't talk to each other so much anymore." Memory goes down and the "processing" necessary for coordination and balance tends to decline. The technical term for this communication is *signaling*, and special compounds in blueberries called *polyphenols* actually "turn on" the signals. "Not only can you get one neuron to talk to another more efficiently, but you can actually enable the brain to grow new neurons," Joseph explains in an interview. "Call the blueberry the brain berry."

While blueberries have emerged as a superfood for the brain, they're not the only food that has an effect. Researchers writing in the *Journal of Neuroscience* reported that rats that consumed an extract of blueberries, strawberries, and spinach every day showed improvements in short-term memory.

And let's not forget the value of fish and fish oil. Inflammation is a big component of every degenerative disease, including Alzheimer's, and fish oil is one of the most anti-inflammatory substances on the planet. Your grandma was right when she told you fish was brain food. About 60 percent of your brain is fat, and most of that is an omega-3 fatty acid known as docosahexaenoic acid or DHA. Where is it found, you ask? In fish. I consider omega-3s one of the most protective supplements you can take for many reasons (see page 299 [desert island cure]), not the least of which that they go a long way toward protecting your brain.

Niacin intake from foods has also been shown to be inversely associated with Alzheimer's disease. Higher intake of niacin from food has been shown in some research to be associated with a slower annual rate of cognitive decline. Foods like eggs, liver, fish, and broccoli are great sources. Bottom line: Eat your fruits and vegetables, but don't forget your fats and protein.

The Power of the Crossword Puzzle

Much has been written about mental aerobics, brain teasers, and other ways of keeping your brain young. Obviously all that good press for mental gymnastics has had an impact (what other possible reason could there be for the popularity of Sudoku?).

Recent research at the National Institutes of Health showed that seniors who practiced certain thinking skills maintained their ability to perform those skills better than those who didn't practice them. I've often believed one of the reasons symphonic conductors live so long and conduct well into their seventies and eighties and beyond is because they're constantly studying new scores.

They're also throwing their arms around a lot—and don't think for a minute that mild aerobic exercise doesn't have an effect on your brain. It does. Women who exercise regularly have a 20 percent risk decrease for cognitive impairment. Additionally, physical activity can improve reaction time, memory span, and overall well-being. One study reports that going for walks may be enough to stem the age-related decline in physical reaction time.

Recent research shows that regular exercise can not only increase the ability of the brain to function, but it can actually increase its size. This was demonstrated recently in an intriguing study by Arthur Kramer, Ph.D., professor of neuroscience and psychology and director of the biomedical imaging center at the University of Illinois, and his colleagues. They put a group of sixty volunteers in an MRI machine—a very sophisticated kind of x-ray machine that can pinpoint changes and abnormalities in body tissues.

"These folks were basically couch potatoes," Kramer told me, "healthy but sedentary, and ranging in age from sixty to eighty." The researchers then divided them into two groups. One group went into an aerobics program, the other into a "toning and stretching" program.

"The aerobics group started at fifteen minutes a day, at a pretty slow pace," Kramer says, "but after two months they were up to forty-five to sixty minutes, three days a week." This continued for six months, after which the subjects went back into the MRI machine, and the researchers examined their gray and white matter. (The gray matter of the brain is composed of neurons or *computational units*, while the white matter is the axons, or interconnections—"telephone wires between the neurons," says Kramer.)

Both the gray matter and the white matter showed increased volume, showing that exercise can literally build up your brain. And the best part is that it doesn't take much. A pretty moderate level can do the trick, in this case just walking forty-five to sixty minutes, three times a week.

And even if you don't much care about the physical size of your brain, exercise has also been shown to reduce the risk of Alzheimer's disease and other forms of dementia. One theory is that it does so by increasing blood flow to the brain. A study in the *Archives of Internal Medicine* evaluated the cognitive functioning of seniors over the age of sixty-five for almost six years and found that the less they exercised, the quicker the rate of cognitive decline and the higher the risk for dementia, including Alzheimer's disease. In a sobering finding, those who didn't exercise were three times more likely to develop dementia.

Avoid the Number-One Brain Shrinker

I've written elsewhere about the effect of stress hormones on weight. Executive summary: Stress makes you fat. And now I'm going to give you more bad news: It also shrinks your brain.

No kidding.

An important structure in the brain essential to memory called the hippocampus actually shrinks as a result of stress. The total number of cells decreases, and if that weren't bad enough, the existing cells shrink. (The hippocampus is also one of the first regions to suffer damage in Alzheimer's disease.) A ton of research has validated this shrinkage, and this chapter is long enough as it is, so I'm going to give you the bottom line: If you don't handle your stress, very bad things will happen.

Stress aggravates virtually every disease and condition we've talked about in this book, and in some cases, it makes the difference between really bad symptoms and mild ones you can easily live with. The effect of chronic levels of stress hormones on the brain are incalculable. If you think you can't afford to take the time to do some stress-reducing activities, rethink that.

You can't afford not to.

Ways to reduce stress are as easy to find as your own bathroom. A soak in a warm bath works wonders, especially when you add some epsom salts (loaded with relaxing magnesium). Ditto lying in bed by candlelight reading a book that doesn't have anything to do with work. Making love works great, plus it raises both your serotonin and the bonding hormone oxytocin. Try spending time with an animal. Or in the sunshine. (Better yet—spend time with an animal in the sunshine!) Meditation is probably the most reliable and proven way to bring down stress hormones, but if that's not your cup of tea try some simple breathing exercises. (There's a reason they tell you to take a deep breath when you're boiling mad—deep breathing and stress are incompatable.) If you want a really easy, structured way to reduce stress, try the Relaxation Response (see page 291).

Whatever you choose, do something.

Ultimately the health of your brain depends on it.

Healthy Bacteria Plus a Healthy Oil

for Eczema

ASKED TO NAME a bunch of organs, most people would go right to the obvious—heart, lungs, kidneys, and liver. You might not immediately think of skin. But skin is an organ, and it's actually the largest organ of the human body. That's why when it bellows in rage, you should listen to it.

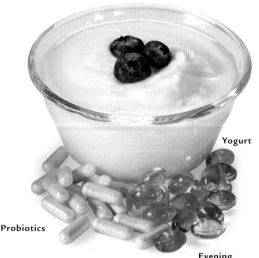

Yogurt

Probiotics

Evening Primrose Oil

Okay, I know, the skin doesn't bellow. Not really. But it does have multiple ways of letting you know that it's unhappy with something that's going on. It can itch uncontrollably. It can form big nasty cysts. It can break out in acne. It can get red and irritable and swollen. It can get dry and flaky. All of these are symptoms that something's going on inside, and it's time to pay attention.

Technically, eczema is not exactly a disease, but rather the general name given for a host of skin irritations and symptoms ranging from mild to very annoying. The two main types are contact dermatitis, which is aggravated when the skin comes in direct contact with an allergen such as household detergents and chemicals, or even cosmetics; and atopic dermatitis, which is aggravated by ingested or inhaled allergens such as certain foods, pollen, dust, or animal dander.

These external triggers ultimately irritate and strip away the outermost layer of skin—called the stratum corneum—causing moisture to escape. From there, it's a vicious cycle: The moisture escapes, which lets in more allergens, which triggers another drying reaction, and so on. The result is what we commonly call eczema. It affects 15 million Americans and nearly 10 percent of all infants and children.

Atopic dermatitis, the kind of eczema we're talking about in this entry, is one of the first signs of allergy during infancy and is believed to be due to delayed development of the immune system. It affects between 10 and 20 percent of all infants, but almost half of these kids will "grow out" of eczema between the ages of five and fifteen, according to the American Academy of Dermatologists.

But many won't.

Two wonderful supplements—evening primrose oil and probiotics—may help.

Scratching Beneath the Surface for Causes

First understand this: Eczema can be difficult to treat partly because you have to do some detective work to figure out just which stressors may be triggering the dry, scaly skin in the first place. Meanwhile, you're fighting the overwhelming urge to scratch and rub the dry, irritated skin, which only makes it more prone to soreness and infection. The arsenal of conventional medical treatments pretty much consists of symptom-treating steroids, antihistamines, and even antibiotics. These treatments will most definitely provide short-term relief, but they in no way address the root cause of the eczema. Moreover, and especially in the case of antibiotics, they will probably do more damage to your health in the long term.

If you want to heal eczema naturally, a great place to start is by examining possible food triggers. There's a connection between atopic dermatitis and food sensitivities or allergies, and believe it or not, your food triggers can be programmed as early as in the womb. A recent study in the *American Journal of Clinical Nutrition* showed that eating certain foods during the last four weeks of pregnancy increases the risk of eczema for the infant. High intakes of vegetable oil and margarine, for example, were associated with an almost 50 percent risk. (Celery—believe it or not—was associated with an 85 percent risk.) And it doesn't end in the womb.

A 1990 study in the journal *Pediatrics* found that there were clear and consistent associations between eczema and the diversity of a child's diet during the first four months of life. The more variety of solid foods that a mother introduced to her baby before the age of four months old, the greater were the odds of the baby developing atopic eczema. Kids who were exposed to four or more different types of solid foods before the age of four months had almost three times the risk of recurrent or chronic eczema than those who weren't exposed to solid feeding (one more strong argument for breast milk, but that's another story).

Adding plenty of the right essential fatty acids to your diet while you're pregnant may seriously decrease the risk of your child getting eczema, not to mention all the other benefits that both you and your baby receive from a high intake of essential fatty acids during pregnancy (more on that in a moment).

Regardless of what your mother ate during pregnancy, remember this: Eczema is treatable, even more successfully if you take a little time to find out what triggers it. Once you identify those triggers in your diet or your child's, you can begin to eliminate or reduce them. Add in the combo cures we're about to discuss, and you're on the way to relief.

Eliminating the Triggers

Many studies have linked food allergies to eczema, so a good place to start in your detective work is with an elimination diet. (If after using this approach you are still stumped, it's time to move on to food allergy/food sensitivity testing, but you may not have to.)

An elimination diet is a nice, easy, low-tech way to help yourself identify which foods can be causing you problems. (Though we're discussing eczema here, it's worth pointing out that the elimination diet is a great tool for identifying problem foods in any condition where foods may be a trigger, for example, asthma or headaches.)

Natural Prescription for Eczema

Omega-6 fatty acids (found in evening primrose oil): Start with 2 g and work up to 6 g. Use for at least four weeks. Balance with 1 g of omega-3 fish oils.

Probiotics: At least 10 billion bacteria

Food allergy testing: IgG allergy tests are best. (Many doctors who practice integrative or complementary medicine will perform these.)

Zinc: 25 mg

Selenium: 200 mcg

Chamomile: A natural anti-itch treatment. Boil up tea and pat on affected areas with cotton. (Let the tea cool first, lest you replace itching with burning.)

Witch hazel: A soothing anti-itch remedy. Apply on eczema as needed.

Colloidal oatmeal bath: Lukewarm, before bed, whenever necessary

Note: All dosages are daily and come in pill or capsule form unless otherwise noted.

All you do is select a "potential offender" and then eliminate it completely from your diet for a minimum of four or five days—three weeks is even better. Then you just notice whether you feel better or your symptoms improve.

Obviously, this can be a long process if you go through every single food on the planet, but the fact is that most people eat about thirteen foods all the time. It might seem counterintuitive, but start with the foods you consume most frequently, even those you're "sure" couldn't be a problem because you eat them all the time.

The most common foods that exacerbate eczema are cow's milk, eggs, wheat, soy, peanuts, fish, cheese, chocolate, coloring agents, and tomatoes. When these foods are removed, eczema has been shown to go into remission. Keep in mind that we are all biochemically unique—everyone reacts differently to foods, and even though the usual suspects such as wheat, dairy, and the like may be triggers for a large number of people, there are always people who will be allergic to weirdly improbable, and sometimes extremely healthy, foods like asparagus.

My associate, Maryland nutritionist Sue Mudd, M.S., C.N.S., once did a food sensitivity test (known as an ALCAT test) on an eight-year-old boy with a severe case of eczema and found that he tested positive for blueberries, apples, and broccoli. (Huh?) Once these seemingly innocuous (and healthy!) foods were removed from his diet, the eczema cleared up. His mother still can't believe it: Gone are the nights she spent with him, up at 3 a.m. because his back was unbearably itchy. Go figure.

With any luck you'll be one of the fortunate ones who solve the food allergy connection on the first try using an elimination diet (a variation of which is called the *Rotation Diet*—see page 210). If you're still stumped, it may be worth the money to invest in a test that identifies food and environmental irritants to effectively solve the eczema dilemma. A good, qualified health-care practitioner can help you with the right test. (Two tests that my associates, Mudd and Susan Copp, M.S., think very highly of are the ALCAT test and the LEAP test. The ALCAT test is provided by Cell Science Systems Corporation in Florida and is available in more than eighteen countries as of this writing. The LEAP test (Lifestyle, Eating and Performance) is administered by Signet Diagnostic Corporation in Florida and has an outstanding medical advisory board. To find out more about the ALCAT test, call (800) 872-5228 or go to www.alcat.com. For more information on the LEAP test, call (888) 669-5327 or go to www.nowleap.com.

If you want the really simplified version of what to do—the eczema version of those "quick start" instruction sheets that come with your electronic devices—simply do this:

- Eliminate grains, especially wheat, dairy, and sugar.
- Read about the rotation diet (see page 210). If necessary, try it.
- If you're still stumped, talk to your health-care practitioner about the ALCAT or the LEAP tests.

Now it's time to include the natural cures.

Adding in the Combos: Fats and Bugs

A common school of thought holds that eczema may be caused by the lack of—or blocking of—an important enzyme called delta-6-desaturase. Here's how it works: Fatty acids go through a number of metabolic transformations in the body and are the "building blocks" for both other fatty acids and compounds known as prostaglandins (or eicosanoids), which can be inflammatory or anti-inflammatory. (That's one reason you want the right balance of fatty acids in your diet.)

Delta-6-desaturase is one of the important enzymes that works on this fatty acid assembly line. Your body needs this enzyme to create a very important omega-6 fatty acid called gamma-linolenic acid (GLA). Too little delta-6-desaturase, too little GLA. And GLA has been shown to be highly beneficial in the treatment of eczema, leading many to believe that not having enough of it could aggravate eczema. The solution? Take it in supplement form.

(Little fun fact: GLA is actually a member of a class of fatty acids called omega-6s, and generally speaking, omega-6s tend to increase the level of inflammatory compounds in the body, especially when they're not balanced with enough omega-3s. Not GLA, however. Research supports the idea that reducing omega-6 fatty acids in the diet can lead to a reduction in inflammatory skin conditions, but actually adding GLA to the diet—through supplements, for example—offers significant improvement! GLA is found in evening primrose oil, black currant seed oil, and borage oil. You can also get it as a supplement called GLA.)

If you've got a picky toddler and you're panicked about how to get him to take evening primrose oil, try rubbing the oil on the affected areas at night (see box on page 123 for other oiling suggestions). Symptoms will improve gradually, and you'll very likely see a decreased need to use antihistamines.

Bugs That Make You Well

Now for the bugs. Probiotics is the name for a general class of "good" bacteria that are absolutely essential for the proper functioning of the digestive system. If digestion isn't working properly, the body is more prone to allergies and skin disturbances.

A 2007 Swedish study published in the *American Journal of Allergy and Clinical Immunology* reported that probiotic-supplemented children of mothers with allergies experienced significant reductions in eczema. "Treated infants had less … eczema at two years of age and therefore possibly run a reduced risk to develop later respiratory allergic disease," wrote lead researcher Thomas Abrahamsson from Linkoping University Hospital. And that research is in line with a previous study from Finland that reported that children who received a particular kind of probiotic—the Lactobacillus rhamnosus GG bacteria—were a whopping 40 percent less likely to develop atopic eczema at four years of age than children who received a placebo.

Your digestive system is like a large garden with flowers and weeds. The flowers are the good bacteria (probiotics), and the weeds are things like *Candida albicans*, bacteria that can result in local or systemic yeast infections. Antibiotics are like powerful weed killers that wind up killing your rosebushes along with the pests. People who are given antibiotics a lot tend to have a much greater tendency to have an imbalance in their gut ecology—it's easier to grow more weeds than it is roses. Probiotics will help offset that unhealthy balance.

Probiotic supplementation is especially critical if a lot of yeast is present, and will help restore a healthy balance of microbes in the digestive tract. Since a healthy digestive tract is critical for prevention of allergies, working with a health-care provider who can eliminate yeast and replenish some of the good bacteria through probiotics use will help to diminish eczema flare-ups.

Folic Acid and NAC

for Hearing Loss

IF YOU'RE A woman and you're at an age when it's even possible that you can get pregnant, you've probably heard that you should be taking folic acid on a daily basis. What you may *not* have heard is that folic acid can also help with hearing loss.

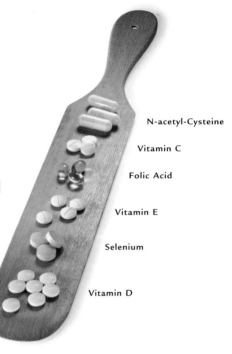

N-acetyl-Cysteine

Vitamin C

Folic Acid

Vitamin E

Selenium

Vitamin D

First let's get the pregnancy issue out of the way. If you're pregnant, folic acid supplements can significantly reduce the baby's chance of having one of a particularly nasty form of birth defects called neural tube defects. Neural tube defects are deformities and abnormalities of the baby's brain and spine, such as spinal bifida (an incompletely formed spinal cord) and anencephaly (born without part of the brain). The American Academy of Pediatrics and the U.S. public health service both recommend that all women capable of becoming pregnant consume 400 mcg of folic acid daily.

Why "capable of becoming pregnant"? Because neural tube defects start to develop in the first trimester, often even in the first month, and usually before a woman is aware she's pregnant. If you wait until you know you're already pregnant, you may have missed the boat.

Folic Acid for Life

Here are three things to know right off the bat: Folic acid does a heck of a lot more than just preventing birth defects, the recommended daily minimum is too low, and folic acid supplementation is just as important for men as it is for women.

Oh, and one more thing—if you're a woman, your need for it doesn't start and end with your childbearing years. It goes on for life.

Every single one of our 100 trillion cells relies on folic acid. What you look like and what traits you pass on to your offspring are dependent in part on how well folic acid functions in your body. So in large measure, whether you look like Marilyn Monroe or Cruella De Vil is going to be influenced by folic acid.

That's because folic acid (also known as folacin, folate, or even vitamin B9) is necessary for the constant, faultless replication of our DNA, the body's genetic blueprint. It also is needed for the building blocks of RNA, which is important for protein synthesis in every cell.

Natural Prescription for Hearing Loss

Folic acid: 800 mcg

ANTIOXIDANTS:

N-acetyl-cysteine: 1,000 mg

Vitamin C: 1–2 g

Vitamin E: 400–800 IU

Selenium: 200–400 mcg

Test for food sensitivities: Especially cow's milk, which was shown in a 1994 study in the *American Journal of Nutrition* to be associated with hearing loss.

Vitamin D: 800 IU

Note: The above dosages are daily dosages and in pill or capsule form, unless otherwise noted.

Folic acid deficiency has been implicated in a wide variety of disorders from Alzheimer's disease to atherosclerosis, heart attack, stroke, osteoporosis, cervical and colon cancer, dementia, and cleft lip. Nutritionists have long known that high doses (I'm talking 5 to 20 mg, not mcg) of folic acid can have a nice brightening effect on mood. That's not surprising because over the past thirty-five years, many studies have shown a high incidence of folate deficiency associated with depression (as well as other mental symptoms like cognitive decline). And depression is more common in patients with folate deficiency.

Folic Acid and Hearing

That folic acid has a positive effect on mood, aging, cognition, and pregnancy is fairly well known. What's not as well known is its effect on your hearing.

To understand why folic acid might help your hearing, it helps to understand the workings of a substance in your blood called *homocysteine*. Homocysteine is an amino acid (a building block of protein) and is a natural product of metabolism. But it's an inflammatory biochemical that—when it builds up in the body—puts you at increased risk for heart disease and stroke. What does this have to do with folic acid?

Everything. The tried, true, and foolproof way to bring down blood levels of homocysteine is with—you guessed it—folic acid (in conjunction with its relatives in the B vitamin family, B6 and B12). And if you're feeling a little like Sherlock Holmes (or Columbo) right now and trying to connect the dots between lowering homocysteine and improving your hearing, let me help you out: High levels of homocysteine contribute to hearing loss.

A recent study from the Netherlands published in the *Annals of Internal Medicine* reported that both homocysteine and folic acid play a role in age-related hearing loss. The Netherlands was chosen as a good test location because foods there are not currently fortified with folic acid. The participants of the study were fifty to seventy years old and had moderately high levels of homocysteine to begin with. The researchers gave them either 800 mcg of folic acid per day or a placebo. At the end of the three-year study,

Regarding folic acid: The recommended daily allowance for adults is 400 mcg and 600 mcg for pregnant women. I say nonsense. I'd like to see 800 mcg as the minimum, and I routinely use amounts in the *milli*gram (not the smaller *micro*gram) level. In fact, one of my favorite folic acid supplements (Super Folate Supreme) comes in an eyedropper—one single drop of the fluid gives you 800 mcg. I routinely put at least four or five drops (4 mg to 5 mg) in a smoothie or fresh vegetable and fruit juice (the folic acid is tasteless!).

One more thing: Government agencies don't recommend high levels of folic acid supplementation, but the reason has nothing to do with the safety of folic acid. Doses of up to 20 mg (20,000 mcg!) have been used safely with humans, plus it's a water-soluble vitamin, which means you'll get rid of any you don't need.

So the problem isn't with taking a lot of folic acid. The problem is that folic acid can mask the symptoms of B12 deficiency. With folic acid supplementation, you'll get rid of the symptoms of B12 anemia, but not the nerve damage that might ensue. (This is especially important for older adults because they're at greater risk for a B12 deficiency.) The government doesn't want you walking around with B12 deficiency and thinking you're fine, so it warns against taking too much folic acid. Makes sense, but there's a much better solution—take some B12 with your folic acid and there's no more problem! The Super Folate Supreme I like has 6 mcg of B12 (100 percent of the recommended daily allowance) in every drop. (Super Folate Supreme is available through my website, www.jonnybowden.com) If you use another brand, no problem, just make sure you're getting B12 every day as well.

the folic acid group had significantly less hearing loss than the placebo group. This difference was even more pronounced in people who had particularly low folic acid levels prior to the study. (Incidentally, there was also a not-too-surprising 26 percent drop in homocysteine levels in the folic acid–supplemented group.)

And who's low in folic acid? Probably you. It's been estimated that 88 percent of North Americans suffer from a folic acid deficiency. Both the National Health and Nutrition Examination Survey (NHANES) and the

Continuing Survey of Food Intakes by Individuals (1994–96 CSFII) indicated that the majority of people don't get near adequate levels. The average American over fifty years old only takes in 130 mcg of folic acid per day. (The recommended daily allowance is 400 mcg a day.) Sure, they've "fortified" cereals with folic acid to try to correct the problem, but I'm not sure cereal grains are the best choice of food for everyone on the planet (in fact, I'm pretty darn sure they're not). Most are high-sugar nightmares that have their own set of problems.

Foods that contain folate include beans, leafy green vegetables, citrus fruits, beets, wheat germ, and meat. Up to 90 percent of folic acid can be destroyed by many kinds of processing, including cooking, so a raw salad made from dark greens is a good way to go. In addition, most multivitamins have at least 400 mcg of folic acid, though I'd like to see more in everyone's diet.

Don't forget that B vitamins work best when they work together. Folic acid is, after all, a B vitamin and it needs its partners—B12 and B6— to effectively carry out its functions. You can easily take extra folic acid (as in an additional supplement), but be sure to get a foundation of the other Bs, either in a B complex or multiple vitamin.

The Navy's Secret Weapon

If you were trying to pick a population of folks who are really in danger of losing their hearing, you couldn't come up with a better group than members of the military. Think about it. They shoot weapons. They're in battle. The noise level is phenomenal. As Dr. Wang on *Grey's Anatomy* might say, "That can't be good." It's no accident that in every movie you've seen where someone is practicing shooting at a firing range he's wearing headphones!

"About 10 percent of military personnel will suffer noise-induced hearing loss, even though they use hearing protection," says Brenda Lonsbury-Martin, director of science and research for the American Speech-Language-Hearing Association. So on what better group of folks to test a "hearing pill"?

You heard me (no pun intended). In 2004, the country's first clinical trial began at a California military base to test a compound that just might prevent noise-induced hearing loss. They're calling it the Hearing Pill. Its active ingredient is a powerful compound called N-acetyl-cysteine (NAC), which is known to have a number of positive effects on the body, not the least of which is to protect the liver. In a study at the University of Michigan, researchers blasted unfortunate guinea pigs with rock concert-level noise for five hours, resulting in a hearing loss of up to 50 db. But the piggies that had been given NAC prior to the experiment had only minimal hearing loss. NAC is also one powerful antioxidant.

Which makes sense because loud noises produce damaging molecules called *free radicals* in the ear, and antioxidants help fight the damage from free radicals, NAC (as well as other antioxidants) could conceivably be useful in preventing, minimizing, or slowing hearing loss. One free radical in particular—an especially nasty fellow named superoxide anion radical—appears in the inner ear of experimental animals after damage caused by noise-induced trauma. (The antioxidant *superoxide dismutase* goes after this one. You can help your body make it by taking some key nutrients like zinc and manganese.)

Recently, researchers from the Technion-Israel Institute of Technology in Haifa, Israel, attempted to find out whether antioxidants have a restorative or protective role in the inner ear. Their findings? They do. Adding a mere 800 mg of just vitamin E (a powerful antioxidant) to a group of patients who had suffered sudden hearing loss resulted in an improvement of 75 percent or more at the time of discharge. That recovery rate compares to only 45 percent in the group not given the vitamin E.

There appear to be many causes of hearing loss, and probably this natural prescription won't "cure" all of them. But it might make a significant difference in some cases, and if you happen to be one of them, you'll be happy you tried it.

Black Cohosh and Dong Quai

for Hot Flashes

OF ALL THE SYMPTOMS that accompany menopause, hot flashes would probably be at the top of the list of most bothersome. Between 50 percent and 85 percent of U.S. women going through menopause experience hot flashes, and 40 percent of those women suffer from them severely enough to seek medical attention. Hot flashes, including night sweats, occur because of an imbalance in the ratios of two primary female hormones, estrogen and progesterone.

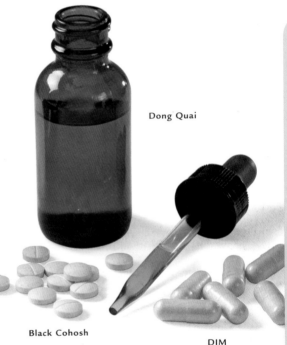

Dong Quai

Black Cohosh

DIM

Off-Balance Hormones and Their Effects

Winding your way through the maze of information related to hormones and their physical effects is simply mind-numbing: Too much estrogen can cause weight gain, headaches, insomnia, bloating, and heavy periods, while too little progesterone can cause anxiety, depression, insomnia, pain, inflammation, osteoporosis, decreased HDL (or "good") cholesterol, and breakthrough bleeding. (A full discussion of the female hormonal environment is way beyond the scope of this book, and certainly beyond the scope of this chapter, but please check the resources and recommended readings for some of the outstanding books that can help you learn more.)

During menopause, both estrogen and progesterone decline, but progesterone can sometimes decline more dramatically than estrogen, throwing off the balance and harmony of the two hormones. The result is a condition called *estrogen dominance*, which can set women up for all the uncomfortable menopausal symptoms that they know and hate.

When a woman has an excess of estrogen compared to progesterone it's usually because of a number of reasons, such as lack of exercise, a diet low in fiber, or environmental factors. Many things in the environment that we're exposed to daily—such as substances in our food or breakdown products from plastics—can act as "hormone mimics," behaving like estrogens in the body and aggravating the imbalance further. (For an excellent discussion of this phenome-

non, see the book *Hormone Deception: How Everyday Foods and Products Are Disturbing Your Health* by D. Lindsey Berkson.)

Then there's the little matter of the fat cells, tiny hormone factories that can make matters even worse when you've got too many of them. An overweight, postmenopausal woman has more estrogen circulating through her body than a skinny premenopausal woman does, according to the World Health Organization.

The Risk of Hormone Replacement Therapy

Traditionally, moderate to severe menopausal complaints have been managed with hormone replacement therapy (HRT) using synthetic hormones. This is absolutely not the place to get into the enormous controversy generated by preliminary findings from the Women's Health Initiative that reported a slightly increased risk of heart attacks and breast cancer for women on HRT.

I just want to point out two things and then urge you to speak to a knowledgeable health-care practitioner about them: One, the findings are controversial, and may apply only to women who started taking the hormones later in life. Two, further analysis has shown that taking hormones for a short time (a few years) during the "worst" of the transition phase does not appear to be a problem. I'd also urge—repeat *urge*— you to talk to a health practitioner who is knowledgeable about bioidentical hormones (see below) and nutrition. You are not going to get the full story on this speaking to a doctor

Natural Prescription for Menopausal Hot Flashes (and Other Nasty Symptoms)

Black cohosh: The German product Remifemin uses an extract standardized to 1 mg of 27-deoxyactein per 20 mg tablet; *The British Herbal Compendium* recommends 40–200 mg dried rhizome daily in divided doses. Use each product as directed on package label.

Dong quai: Can be used together with black cohosh, as directed on product label

DIM (diindolylmethane): A balancer of estrogen metabolism. 100–200 mg per day

★ FOR ADDED EFFECTIVENESS:

Cruciferous vegetables: Cabbages, cauliflower, mustard greens, bok choy, broccoli, Brussels sprouts, radishes, and turnips

Flax/high fiber: Ground flaxseeds, any other fiber, 35 g

Fermented soy: Miso, tempeh, and natto

Vitamin E: 400 IU, twice daily. Up to 1,000 is tolerable, but do not increase if you are on anticoagulants.

Essential fatty acids: Evening primrose oil or gamma-linolenic acid (GLA) 250–500 mg

ALSO USEFUL:

Hormone therapy: Work with a health-care provider to determine appropriate levels. Choose natural hormones like Tri-Est, which contains all three forms of estrogens plus natural progesterone cream.

Acupuncture: Work with a qualified acupuncturist

Exercise: Studies show that hot flashes decrease immediately after aerobic exercise. Exercise also keeps you "happy" and increases bone density. Walking briskly every day for 30 minutes cuts hot flashes by 50 percent while improving your heart and bone health at the same time.

Note: The above dosages are daily and in pill or capsule form unless otherwise noted.

who is firmly planted in the mainstream. (For help on finding a doctor, see Recommended Reading and Resources.)

Bioidentical hormones are compounds that have exactly the same chemical and molecular structure as those produced in your body. They're usually made by compounding pharmacies and prescribed by doctors knowledgeable in nutrition who take a holistic approach to hormone replacement and human health. Don't believe for a minute that bioidentical hormones are the same thing as the synthetic hormones used by conventional practitioners, and don't buy hook, line, and sinker into the conventional orthodoxy that they haven't been "tested" enough. The synthetic ones have been tested to death and we're still not sure how safe they are. The body knows what to do with the ones it makes—it's been using them just fine for as long as you've been alive.

The idea that synthetic and bioidentical hormones are the same thing doesn't pass the smell test. Synthetic hormones, made from the urine of pregnant mares, may be similar to the ones your body makes, but they're not identical, else they couldn't be patented. In biochemistry, if two substances vary by even a few molecules, they can be vastly different compounds.

But I digress.

Regardless of the issues involved in HRT—and they are many and they are thorny—it's pretty safe to say that a large number of people would prefer to use natural substances to manage whatever symptoms they have, especially when some of those natural substances have a good track record of safety and efficacy.

The Benefits of Black Cohosh

Black cohosh is a plant native to the United States and Canada and cultivated widely in Europe. That it has a medicinal effect is not in question; Native Americans used it for a wide variety of conditions, including menopausal symptoms. It's been used for pain and inflammation in Korean folk medicine. And the German Commission E has approved it for premenstrual discomfort. It's one of the best-selling herbs in the United States and a popular and accepted therapy in Europe.

A 2006 study in *Obstetrics and Gynecology* reported that a combination of St. John's wort and black cohosh appears to be especially useful for women who suffer from menopause-related depression, especially interesting since recent research suggests that compounds in black

cohosh bind to serotonin receptors in the brain. Another recent study in the journal *Gynecological Endocrinology* reported that black cohosh is as effective as the low-dose estrogen patch for relieving most symptoms and can also have a positive effect on cardiac risks.

"Since 2003 there have been about ten clinical studies on black cohosh, and all were positive," according to Gail Mahady, Ph.D., an associate professor of pharmacognosy at the University of Illinois and one of the principal authors of the black cohosh monograph for the World Health Organization.

One of the best-known commercial products containing a standardized extract of black cohosh is Remifemin, which seems to have an excellent track record in helping with hot flashes. The company's website (www.remifemin.com) explains what you can expect using a standardized black cohosh product and provides abstracts of research for those who want more information.

Other Plants Give Relief, Too

Dong quai has been used in Asian medicine for thousands of years and remains one of the most popular herbs in Chinese medicine where it is used primarily for "female" issues. It's even acquired a reputation as the "female ginseng." Despite its long tradition of use, the hard-core research on using dong quai for hot flashes—and other issues around menstruation and menopause—is weak.

It's worth noting, however, that in Chinese medicine, dong quai is almost always used in combination with other medicines and herbs. Dong quai may be one of those herbs or compounds that's used best as part of an overall treatment plan or formula, where it might have a synergistic effect. It doesn't seem to have too much of an effect on its own, though.

Soy has long had a reputation as good for hot flashes. I wrote about soy in my previous book, *The 150 Healthiest Foods on Earth*, and if you read it, you probably know I'm not a big cheerleader for the "all soy all the time" brigade. (For one reason, the form we tend to eat it here—as soy junk food—bears little resemblance to the soy in the traditional Asian diet.)

Fermented soy foods like miso and tempeh are fine. Asian women, who, by the way, have very few menopausal symptoms, eat *fermented* soy as accompaniments to a nutrient-rich diet built around seafood and vegetables. If you walk around Tokyo, you won't find them consuming soy milk, soy yogurt, soy cheese, soy burgers, soy chicken, soy chips, and soy lasagna. Get my drift?

Female versus Male Hormones

Jeffrey Bland, Ph.D., is known to virtually every health-care practitioner in America who practices integrative medicine. A nutritional biochemist, he's the cofounder of The Institute for Functional Medicine and has been in the forefront of educating doctors, chiropractors, nutritionists, and other health-care professionals about nutrition, biochemistry, hormones, and health for more than twenty-five years. There's very little about hormones and endocrinology that Jeffrey Bland doesn't know.

A few years ago, I attended his seminar on nutritional neuroendocrinology, a daylong affair devoted to the discussion of female hormones, health, and behavior. I remember Bland starting the day by saying, "We have a lot to cover today. We're going to talk about female hormones and we only have eight hours—we won't even be able to scratch the surface."

He then paused for a second and added, "If we only had to cover male hormones, we could be out of here in forty-five minutes."

Isoflavones are plant-based, estrogen-like compounds that are found in soy; they're also known as *phytoestrogens* (*phyto* means "plant"). Phytoestrogens in soy resemble real estrogen but have weaker properties. The reason they're thought to be good is that they can fit into the parking spaces meant for estrogen without doing any of estrogen's potential damage.

When estrogen levels are low, as in peri- and postmenopause states, phytoestrogens act as estrogen supplements. When they're high, phytoes-trogens can help bring them down gently (they're generally thought to be about $\frac{1}{16}$ as strong as the real deal). Phytoestrogens can therefore help balance either excess estrogen or insufficient estrogen. But unfermented soy products have more powerful estrogenic properties and can lead to further imbalances and unwanted effects

Bottom line: If you're going to eat soy, do as the Asians do. Don't overdo it and make sure it's fermented.

Enzymes and Bugs
for Heartburn

IN 1983, ONE OF MY favorite writers, Nora Ephron (you may know her films *Sleepless in Seattle* and *When Harry Met Sally*), published a novel that was in fact a thinly disguised autobiography. She called it *Heartburn*. It seemed an appropriate metaphor for a story about a crumbling marriage, heartache, and lots of what we Jews call *tsuris* (unhappiness). Not coincidentally, throughout the book was a there was a running theme: food.

Yogurt

Probiotics HCl

No one thought the title inappropriate. More than fifty million Americans have heartburn at least twice a week (even if it isn't caused by a cheating husband), and about twenty-five million have it daily. For almost a hundred years, many of us have relied on antacids to quench the flames of fire in the belly, and products such as Tums, Tagamet, Maalox, and Mylanta produce annual sales of more than a billion dollars.

When those aren't enough, we turn to prescription drugs that block the production of stomach acid even longer than their over-the-counter cousins. Prevacid and Nexium are among the five top-selling prescription drugs in the country, and heartburn drugs are now among the most widely prescribed medications in the United States, producing more than $13 billion in sales in 2004.

But consistently taking acid suppressors like heartburn drugs over time as a way of managing symptoms is a really, really horrendous idea. (Don't kill the messenger here.) Fortunately, there are other, much better (and much healthier) options. Keep reading.

Heartburn, Indigestion, and Reflux Explained

Heartburn is actually not associated with the heart at all but was labeled and named "heartburn" because it can feel like a heart attack. For some, that burning sensation can become unbearable.

The terms *heartburn* and *indigestion* are often used interchangeably, but there is a clear distinction between the two. Though they both have similar triggers, and treatment may be the same in many instances, indigestion isn't the same thing as heartburn. Indigestion is, in fact, a condition. It is a feeling of discomfort and pain in the upper abdomen and chest and may also be accompanied by a feeling of fullness, bloating, and belching.

Heartburn, which is described as a burning sensation in the chest and stomach, is a *symptom* of indigestion. The burning sensation may even travel up toward the neck. It's also a symptom of another common condition called *gastrointestinal reflux disease*, also called GERD, or acid reflux. In addition to heartburn, symptoms of acid reflux may include persistent sore throat, hoarseness, chronic cough, asthma, heartlike chest pain, and a feeling of a lump in the throat.

Natural Prescription for Heartburn

Digestive enzymes or digestive enzymes with hydrochloric acid: (take with every meal, dose dependent on improvement)

Note: if you have an ulcer, work with a health professional. Don't self-treat.

Probiotics: 10 billion. Keep refrigerated. (Note: Probiotics are available in either pill form or as a powdered supplement that can be mixed in water.)

Optional: Deglycyrrhizinated licorice: 380 mg or 1 to 2 tablets chewed and swallowed on an empty stomach, three to four times a day as needed

Diet: Avoid refined sugar, caffeine, alcohol, and citrus fruits (see above). Eat slowly and chew well. Eat yogurt and drink water.

Smoking: Stop.

Note: The above dosages are daily and in pill or capsule form unless otherwise specified.

The Role of Acid

So it might seem like an open and shut case. Hydrochloric acid "causes" heartburn—knock out the hydrochloric acid production with a pill, symptom gone, case closed. Right?

No.

"The myth that underlies the conventional treatment of 'acid indigestion,' and the implied message in all these commercials,

Acid for Acid?

An excerpt from an interview with Jonathan Wright, M.D.

Q: What can alleviate indigestion?

Wright: The large majority of indigestions (and I want to underline that I did not say *all* but *a large majority* of indigestions) are caused by a *lack* of acid in the tummy, not *too much*.

When folks past forty come into the clinic and tell me they have heartburn and indigestion, I tell them that I want to do these stomach tests. Upwards of 95 percent of those people come back with test results showing that they don't have enough acid in there.

So we tell them to take these replacement HCl acid with pepsin capsules with every meal. Of course, I get a lot of stares. They say, "Are you some kind of crazy doctor? Here I've got this acid coming up in my stomach, and you want me to take HCl? I'll burn myself to death!"

We tell them, "No, no, no, please look at your test. Even if you are a hard-to-please Boeing engineer, this is hard data. Now look at a *normal* test, and look at the difference. *Please,* even if you have to keep a glass of bicarbonate of soda handy in case I made a mistake, you do that, but *please* take these HCl capsules with meals."

People come back and say, "I never would have believed that taking HCl with pepsin with every meal would take care of my acid indigestion. How'd that happen?" I have to tell them that I don't *know* the molecular mechanism, I just know that it *works,* especially when we have an abnormal test in front of us."

Reprinted from Franklin Sanders's *The Money Changer* (www.the-moneychanger.com) with permission.

---

is that heartburn happens because we've got too much acid in our stomachs," writes integrative medicine icon Jonathan Wright, M.D. Wright has been in the forefront of the movement to educate people about the overwhelming importance of hydrochloric acid in human health—he even wrote a book about it called *Why Stomach Acid is Good for You*, which I highly recommend.

Here's how it works, and why suppressing acid is such a bad idea: Hydrochloric acid (HCl) is responsible for activating enzymes in the stomach that then allow us to break down the proteins that we've eaten. With limited HCl, those enzymes are not activated and the proteins are not broken down. Result? Badly impaired digestion. Stomach acid stays in the stomach and builds up, so we end up with more acid in our stomach that can potentially reflux back up into the esophagus.

Low hydrochloric acid is a major factor in many digestive disorders. Wright believes that diseases as disparate as rheumatoid arthritis, childhood asthma, osteoporosis, chronic fatigue, and depression all have in common low stomach acid. Childhood asthma is a good case in point: More than 80 percent of children diagnosed with asthma have exhibited low HCl levels. In fact, according to Wright, hydrochloric acid can be a significant part of the cure for children with asthma.

"In hundreds of cases," he says, "I have found that more than 50 percent of children who come to me with asthma can have their wheezing cured by simply normalizing their stomach acid and properly administering vitamin B12, with no bronchodilators and no corticosteroids."

Most bacteria can't survive an acidic environment, so killing off acid production creates nirvana for bacteria. Without acid to kill them off, they have a party and reproduce like rabbits. Bacterial overgrowth in the stomach and small intestine can lead to a host of symptoms, including gas, constipation, diarrhea, and even infections. Overgrowth of bacteria can also interfere with the absorption of vitamin B12 and can interfere with the proper digestion and absorption of fats and sugars. And low acid can contribute to food allergies. Why? Because if we don't have enough acid in our stomachs to digest food, we can't adequately break down foods, and we develop what's called a leaky gut. With a leaky gut, incompletely digested food particles escape back into our system. Our immune cells go "Hey, what's this? We don't recognize these dudes," and then proceed to attack what they perceive as "foreign invaders." This can easily be the birth of a food allergy.

Maybe you figure, okay, acid does all these good things for me, but it's still giving me serious heartburn. Don't I need to get rid of it for that reason alone? If you think this way, you're hardly alone. Most people think the way to get rid of acid reflux is to simply get rid of the acid. (Pharmaceutical companies and those making $13 billion a year from the sale of antacids are counting on you thinking this way.) If you're one of the many, many people who think an antacid is the answer to your acid problem, I hope you'll reconsider after reading this section.

What's Wrong with Acid Suppression? A Lot

The problem isn't that there's too much acid—in fact, it's sometimes the opposite (read on). The problem is that the acid sometimes goes to the wrong place, flowing back—or "refluxing"—into our esophagus where it can really burn the delicate tissues. This reflex reaction may in part be due to a muscle in the lower part of the esophagus (called the LES, or lower esophageal sphincter) that is weakened or stops working correctly. As long as the LES stays closed like it's supposed to, you're good to go. No heartburn symptoms, no burning.

"Given the right environment and enough time to heal itself, an irritated or injured LES often returns to its normal, healthy state, eliminating heartburn. Even the more severe condition of GERD can often [but not always] be brought under control by this approach to treatment," Wright says.

And here's the kicker: Heartburn can also occur—in fact, it frequently does occur—when hydrochloric acid levels in the stomach are too low! According to Wright, the overwhelming majority of people with indigestion have stomach acid deficiency. Keep in mind that a healthy gut and optimal digestion depend on adequate acid in the stomach. After all, acid promotes the digestion and utilization of critical nutrients and amino acids, not to mention vitamin B12, folic acid, and calcium. If there isn't enough acid to trigger the activation of the important digestive enzyme pepsin, you're out of luck. Your digestion is impaired and with it, your body's ability to extract healing nutrients from your food.

If you're still not convinced that the problem isn't too much acid, consider this: The incidence of heartburn and GERD increases as you get older. But as we age, we produce less hydrochloric acid, not more. (The elderly have the least HCl of all.)

"If too much acid were causing these problems, teenagers should have frequent heartburn while grandma and grandpa should have much less," notes Wright. Of course we know that just the opposite is true.

So while it may bring temporary symptom relief, acid suppression isn't the answer. A far better way to permanently cure heartburn and indigestion is to improve the digestive process and heal the lower esophageal sphincter so it works properly. With a few changes in your diet and with the use of safe, effective supplements like those in the natural prescription I'm

WORTH KNOWING

The next time you experience heartburn, take one tablespoon of apple cider vinegar or lemon juice. If the heartburn goes away, you are probably deficient in HCl. You can continue to use apple cider vinegar and water with meals (slow sipping). If the heartburn gets worse after sipping the vinegar, you may have an excess of HCl.

Cayenne pepper can also stimulate HCl, but if you're really deficient—many people are—you'll need supplements.

Another way to go is this: To test whether you're low in HCl, try taking one betaine-HCl capsule with a meal. If you don't notice any effect, you needed that HCl. Up the dosage on the next meal and continue to do so with each meal until you notice a slight burning. At that point cut back, and you're good to go. Jonathan Wright, M.D., recommends betaine hydrochloride with pepsin, which usually comes in capsules labeled "10 grains" or 650 mg. The full adult replacement dose can be as high as six or seven capsules per meal. "Some of us need that full replacement and some of us don't," Wright says.

If you are pregnant or have chronic digestive complaints or high blood pressure, use gentian and HCl only at the advice of a licensed health-care professional. Avoid HCl, pepsin, or gentian if you have a peptic ulcer or if you are in the midst of an acute episode. Work with your health-care professional instead.

going to tell you about, you can restore healthy digestion, heal the gut, and produce improvement in a wide variety of symptoms and health conditions.

By creating a healthy gut environment, which includes a healthy amount of stomach acid, and not triggering inappropriate behavior on the part of the LES (usually by simply eliminating foods that do just that), you are well on the way to banning heartburn symptoms from your life.

Step One: It Starts with Food

The first thing you want to do is eliminate known triggers that cause the LES to pop open inappropriately (allowing any amount of acid, even a little, to bounce back into the esophagus).

Off the food list comes caffeine, including caffeinated soft drinks, tea, and chocolate—all of which are known for relaxing the LES, allowing stomach contents to reflux back up into the esophagus. Chocolate contains concentrations of *theobromine*, a compound that occurs naturally in many plants such as cocoa, tea, and coffee plants, and which is known for relaxing the LES. Other foods that also relax or weaken the LES are tomatoes, spicy foods, onions, citrus fruits and juices, alcohol, and tobacco.

And then there are foods that slow down digestion, keeping the food in your stomach longer. This can result in increased pressure in the stomach, which in turn puts more pressure on a weakened LES, allowing reflux of stomach contents. These include fried or fatty foods and large meals.

Many people try drinking milk to ease heartburn before sleep, but milk may end up causing more heartburn distress. Drinking milk and eating a big meal at dinner can be a recipe for disaster. It's a myth that milk can "coat" the stomach or help heartburn. On the contrary, it can aggravate the heck out of it. And the higher the fat content in the milk, the worse it can be.

Here's one thing you *can* have: water, pure and clean (I know it's not the most exciting thing in the world, but it works). Some researchers theorize that heartburn is a sign of an internal water shortage, especially dehydration in the upper part of the GI tract. So try drinking up first before you overload your system with antacids and medications, but do this *in between* meals, not *during* meals: You'll want to drink only about 4 ounces of water with a meal so that you don't further dilute HCl, which will be needed to digest incoming proteins.

Step Two: On to Enzymes and Probiotics

The natural cure for heartburn is a two-step process. First, get the food triggers under control (see above). Then add the "big guns" of the natural prescription: digestive enzymes and probiotics.

Digestive enzymes are made in your body naturally (and turned on in the presence of stomach acid), but many of us make less of them as we get older. Fortunately, they can be taken as a supplement, and there are many terrific formulas on the market (check my website, www.jonnybowden.com, for ones I like and recommend). Digestive enzymes have been shown to be extremely beneficial in the treatment of heartburn. Also called bitters, they've been around for centuries in the form of plants and herbs.

Gentian root is one well-known bitter. Gentian improves digestion by increasing appetite and stimulating digestive juices and pancreatic activity. It also stimulates the secretion of hydrochloric acid and bile and is known for relieving gallbladder problems and indigestion. Most supplements these days contain a mix of enzymes like bromelain, found in pineapple, papain from papaya, and proteolytic enzymes, which are animal-derived enzymes that break down proteins.

I recommend a digestive enzyme supplement that also contains HCl; many good supplements do. Alternately you can take an HCl supplement on its own. The most common form of HCl supplement is called betaine-HCl. Betaine-HCl is a combination of betaine—a product derived from sugar beets—and hydrochloric acid. (Note: Plain betaine is also known as trimethylglycine, or TMG, the chemical name for betaine. Don't confuse the two. Betaine, or TMG, is a valuable supplement used to bring down the body's levels of an inflammatory compound found in the blood called homocysteine. But it has nothing to do with digestion. For that you need betaine bound to hydrochloric acid, i.e., Betaine-HCl.)

Probiotics, also known as "good bacteria," are wonderful for promoting healthy digestion. In fact, they're essential for it. Remember, your gut is a garden balanced between the "good" bacteria (the flowers) and the "bad" (the weeds). Everyone has some of both—the trick is to keep them in balance. The "good" bacteria—probiotics—are beneficial bacteria, such as *Lactobacillus acidophilus* and *Bifidobacterium bifidum*. Probiotic bacteria favorably alter the intestinal microflora balance, inhibit the growth of harmful bacteria (like *Candida albicans*, or "yeast"), promote good digestion, boost immune function, and increase resistance to infection. Probiotics also contain enzymes to help break down and digest dairy products like lactose in milk. The best place to find probiotics is in yogurts that contain "active cultures." But you can also increase the content by purchasing a high-quality probiotic formula. (I have several excellent ones listed on my website, www.jonnybowden.com). Take the probiotics as a pill or buy in powder form and stir it into water or yogurt.

Smaller meals can also help, as can looser-fitting clothes—you don't want pressure around the abdomen. In fact, see whether you can eat smaller meals in general, even if you have to eat more frequently. (Remember that large meals can put pressure on a weakened LES and cause the dreaded reflux.) Smaller meals rule.

And don't lie down after eating, particularly after a big meal. Keep the meal small and then wait a couple of hours before retiring with the remote.

This Just In

Just as this manuscript was being completed and sent in to my editor, I received an email that my good friend, the great integrative medicine guru Leo Galland, M.D., was appearing on the *Today* show. Galland went on national television to speak about virtually everything we've discussed in this section—why you need stomach acid to be at the top of the list, and why acid-lowering drugs are a really bad idea. You can see his *Today* show appearance online at www.fatresistancediet.com.

The Awesome Foursome

for Heart Disease

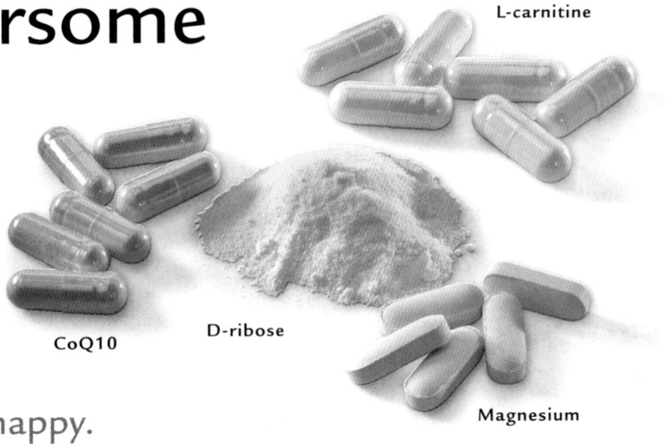

HERE'S A STORY I'll never forget. My mother was admitted to the hospital in the last week of her eighty-seven-year life, which up to then had been extremely healthy and pretty happy. The doctors diagnosed her with congestive heart failure. I immediately asked that, in addition to whatever treatment the doctors prescribed, she be put on a high dose of coenzyme Q10 (CoQ10). The first doctor told me he didn't know what that was. The second doctor said he had heard of it but it couldn't do any good and wasn't on their hospital pharmacy list. And the head nurse said, "Oh, that's some kind of enzyme that the heart makes when it's in trouble, right?" I knew right there we were in for trouble.

L-carnitine

CoQ10

D-ribose

Magnesium

It didn't matter that I faxed them fifty pages of peer-reviewed literature from the National Institute of Medicine. They wouldn't budge.

And my mother, bless her heart, was of the generation that believed that if the doctor told you something, that was it. You didn't question, you didn't go against their advice, Doctor Knows Best, and that was that.

Let me be blunt: The doctors who told me that they didn't know what CoQ10 was or that it couldn't possibly help were idiots.

"Although coenzyme Q10 represents one of the greatest breakthroughs for the treatment of cardiovascular disease as well as for other diseases, the resistance of the medical profession to using this essential nutrient represents one of the greatest potential tragedies in medicine," says my friend, board-certified cardiologist, nutritionist, and noted author Stephen Sinatra, M.D.

CoQ10 has been an approved drug in Japan for congestive heart failure since 1974. And several studies have demonstrated a relationship between depleted CoQ10 levels and heart disease.

So What Is CoQ10, Anyway?

CoQ10 isn't a vitamin; it actually belongs to a family called *ubiquinones*, and it's found in most tissues in the body. It's essential for the manufacture of the body's energy molecule, ATP (adenosine triphosphate). Virtually every one of the studies investigating the effect of CoQ10 on heart muscle function have reported significant and positive results. "If there is just one thing you do to help maintain your heart's health," says Sinatra, "make sure you're taking CoQ10 daily."

Every cell has a little structure in its nucleus called the mitochondria, which can be thought of as Ground Zero for energy production. This is where all the action takes place—where

cellular energy in the form of molecules like ATP is created.

Think of L-carnitine, a vitamin-like compound that can be obtained from the diet and also made in the body, as a shuttle bus. Its job is to escort fatty acids into the mitochondria of the cells where they can be "burned" for energy. Because the heart gets 60 percent of its energy from fat, it's critically important that the body have enough L-carnitine to "shuttle" the fatty acids into the muscle cells of the heart.

Nutritionists have long used the combination of L-carnitine and CoQ10 as an "energy" cocktail for just this reason. Though it doesn't necessarily make you feel more "get up and go" (although for many people it does just that!), it definitely helps give your heart muscle the tools it needs to function optimally.

If you think of your body as an automobile, then L-carnitine and CoQ10 can be thought of as agents (like spark plugs) that help turn the gas in the tank into energy to make the car go.

D-ribose, the third component of this quartet (which Sinatra calls the Awesome Foursome), can be thought of as the actual gas. D-ribose is a five-carbon sugar that seems to accelerate the recovery of energy during and following cardiac ischemia, a condition in which blood flow to the heart muscle is obstructed. One of Sinatra's coauthors, James Roberts, M.D., is a marathoner who began using D-ribose on himself and found that taking it before and after a run eliminated many of the problems, like pain, soreness, stiffness, and fatigue, associated with long-distance runs. He began putting his patients on D-ribose and found that his sickest patients improved within days.

"Giving D-ribose to patients both before (as a cardioprotective) and following (to restore lost energy) cardiac intervention has proven to be an effective way to improve clinical outcome," says Sinatra.

D-Ribose: A Mighty Molecule

D-ribose is made in the cells, and the body uses it in a variety of ways that are all critical to cellular function. When blood flow and oxygen are compromised as in, for example, ischemia, hearts can lose a lot of their stores of ATP (the energy molecule), and it can take up to ten days to normalize cardiac function. When you give D-ribose to patients with ischemia, energy recovery and function can return to normal in an average of one to two days, according to Sinatra.

Ribose can be of great benefit to people without heart disease, including athletes. Athletes place a lot of strain on their muscles' energy metabolism, according to Sinatra. While it might take a lot for trained athletes to subject

their muscles to this kind of stress and strain on energy reserves, a less-conditioned person might experience it gardening or participating in a "weekend warrior" tennis match.

Any time the energy reserves of the muscle are depleted, whether through exercise or a heart condition, ribose supplementation can help. "An adequate dose of ribose will usually result in symptom improvement very quickly," says Sinatra. "Remember that ribose therapy directly supports the heart's ability to preserve and rebuild its energy pool," he says.

Natural Prescription for Heart Health

Coenzyme Q10: 100 mg–300 mg

L-carnitine: 500 mg–4,000 mg

D-ribose: 5 g

Magnesium: 400 mg–800 mg

★ **FOR ADDED EFFECTIVENESS:**

Multivitamin

1 g fish oil

Vitamin E from mixed tocopherols or gamma-tocopherol: 400 IU

Taurine: 1–3 g

Note: All dosages are daily dosages and in pill or capsule form unless otherwise noted.

L-Carnitine: Energy for a Weak Heart

The strongest research evidence for the benefit of L-carnitine supplementation comes from studies of patients being treated for various forms of cardiovascular disease. People who take L-carnitine supplements soon after suffering a heart attack may be less likely to suffer a subsequent heart attack, die of heart disease, experience chest pain and abnormal heart rhythms, or develop congestive heart failure (a condition in which the heart loses its ability to pump blood effectively). A well-designed study of seventy heart-failure patients found that three-year survival was significantly higher in the group receiving 2 g a day of L-carnitine compared to the group receiving a placebo.

Carnitine also appears to really improve exercise capacity in people with coronary artery disease. In one study, the walking capacity of patients with intermittent claudication—a painful cramping sensation in the muscles of the legs due to decreased oxygen supply—improved significantly when they were given oral L-carnitine. In another study, patients with peripheral arterial disease of the legs were able to increase their walking distance by ninety-eight meters when supplemented with carnitine, almost twice what those given a placebo were able to do. Congestive heart failure patients have experienced an increase in exercise endurance on only 900 mg of carnitine per day. It also appears to help alleviate the symptoms of angina.

The Perfect Quartet

Vegetarians often lack L-carnitine in their diets (and most certainly lack D-ribose, which is

primarily found in red meat and veal). Carnitine (*carnis* means "meat" or "flesh") is found in mutton, lamb, beef, red meat, and pork and in only tiny amounts in plant foods.

Though certain vegetables, meats, and fish contain CoQ10, we only consume a tiny amount in our diet, not nearly enough to have a clinically important benefit. Many people feel a lot better on an "energy" cocktail of L-carnitine and CoQ10.

Rounding out the quartet with D-ribose and magnesium, as suggested by Sinatra, is a great idea, especially for heart patients. (Magnesium helps because it is critical for the making of ATP, has an important effect on cellular metabolism, has been found helpful in a wide range of cardiac

---

WORTH KNOWING

Ribose and Fibromyalgia

Just as we went to press, my friend and go-to guy for all things related to Fibromyalgia and Chronic Fatigue Syndrome, Jacob Teitelbaum, M.D., wrote to tell me of a just-published study showing that in Chronic Fatigue and Fibromyalgia patients, ribose increased energy an average of 45%. "It is even more incredible in heart disease," he wrote. Teitelbaum told me that he suspects Ribose "will be the most important nutritional discovery of the decade."

According to Teitelbaum, dosing is critical. He recommends 5 gms 3 x day for 3-6 weeks, then 2 x day. "This is too important of a nutrient discovery to be missed," says Teitelbaum.

conditions, and because approximately three-fourths of the population are deficient in it!)

Let me be perfectly clear: The combination of CoQ10, L-carnitine, D-ribose, and magnesium doesn't "cure" heart disease. But to not use it as part of a treatment protocol to strengthen and protect the heart would be a huge mistake.

A Powerful Combo
for Hepatitis C

HEPATITIS C IS close to my heart and interests because I have it. The only way I *know* I have it is because of a routine blood test taken about twenty years ago. I've never had a symptom. I've never missed a day of work. I've never had any of the classic problems like fatigue, jaundice, and lack of energy. I only know it's in there somewhere because a blood test—and subsequent liver biopsy taken back in the mid-90s—tells me so. The universe willing, I expect to live a long, healthy life and die of old age. My hepatitis C can come along with me for the ride if it likes.

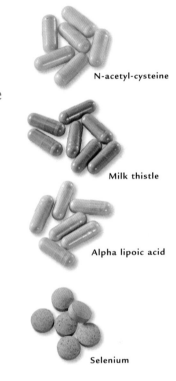

N-acetyl-cysteine

Milk thistle

Alpha lipoic acid

Selenium

Okay, maybe this sounds flippant. But my experience has given me great optimism when it comes to dealing with hepatitis C in a "natural" way. I'm not saying my way is perfect for everyone, but it has worked for me and it cannot possibly hurt anyone to try what I and others have tried. It might even keep you symptom-free. At the very least, it will help your liver.

This is a disease in which many outcomes are possible, and I believe fervently that what you do and the choices you make can have a profound influence on the course the disease takes.

Let's get this out of the way right off the bat: The single best thing you can do is to stop drinking. Completely. No kidding. I consider myself very lucky that I did this in 1982, because I believe that if I hadn't, there would have been considerably more damage to my liver by the time I found out I had hepatitis C, and it would have been that much more difficult to keep under control.

A Medical Hero Takes on the Establishment

I first learned about the "natural cure" I'm going to tell you about from Burt Berkson. I'll introduce him so you'll understand why I paid as much attention as I did to his recommendation, and why I'm going to pass it on to you with a ringing, unqualified endorsement. I consider Burt Berkson a medical hero. After reading this, you may agree with me. It's worth pointing out that his story is also a microcosm of everything that's wrong with the business of conventional medicine and why we need mavericks like Berkson more than ever before.

Years ago, Berkson was doing his internship at a hospital in Cleveland when two people were brought in by ambulance in pretty dire condition. They had been hiking, had eaten some highly poisonous mushrooms, and were pretty close to death. Berkson remembered reading some research on a substance called alpha lipoic acid, which was being used with great results on insulin resistance syndrome. But Berkson also remembered that alpha lipoic acid, in addition to being great for blood sugar, was an amazing

> ## Natural Prescription for Hepatitis C
>
> **Alpha lipoic acid:** 900–1,200 mg
>
> **Selenium:** 200–400 mcg
>
> **Milk thistle (silymarin):** 900 mg
>
> **ALSO HIGHLY RECOMMENDED:**
>
> **N-acetyl-cysteine:** 1,000–2,000 mg
>
> **Whey protein powder:** 1–2 servings
>
> **Dandelion tea:** Frequently
>
> **Phosphatidylcholine:** 3 g
>
> **Optional:** Olive leaf extract has some antiviral properties and may be useful as well; 500–1,000 mg, three times a day. Use a capsule containing at least 10 percent extract of the active ingredient, oleuropein.
>
> **Note:** All dosages are daily dosages and in pill or capsule form unless otherwise noted.

free-radical scavenger. He appealed to the hospital to let him try alpha lipoic acid on the couple, but was turned down since no one had ever heard of it and it wasn't in the hospital's pharmacy. He was basically told there was nothing that could be done for the couple and if there was, the powers that be at the hospital would certainly have known about it. What did a mere intern think he could do with some nutritional supplement no one had ever heard of? And besides, what could an intern know that a resident or attending physician didn't?

Well, quite a lot actually.

Berkson, who is not only an M.D. but just happens to have a Ph.D. in microbiology with an advanced specialty in mushroom toxology, knew a bit about liver disease. Risking censure and loss of his internship, he called an old colleague, Fred Bartter at the National Institutes of Health, who arranged to fly in some alpha lipoic acid. He administered it to the dying couple.

And they're alive and well today.

That, by the way, is medical courage.

When Burt Berkson talks about the liver, I listen.

Back in 1999, Berkson published a paper called *A conservative triple antioxidant approach to the treatment of hepatitis C. Combination of alpha lipoic acid (thioctic acid), silymarin, and selenium: Three case histories.* In it, he suggested a basic protocol that would protect the liver from free-radical damage, increase the levels of other fundamental antioxidants, and interfere with viral proliferation. That protocol is the core of the "natural cure" for hepatitis C.

That has been the basis of my supplement regimen for the liver every day since I heard that lecture, and I believe every single person with hepatitis C should be on it.

You can support the liver in four major ways:

1. **Don't add to its burden.** Number one on the list of the liver's biggest burdens is alcohol, so stop drinking. Immediately. No kidding. And stop taking acetaminophen (found in Tylenol and other medications). Acetaminophen poisoning is the number-one cause of hospital admissions for liver failure in the United States. Think what people who drink and then take Tylenol for a hangover are doing to their poor liver. Though many establishment medical types will tell you acetaminophen is "safe" in reasonable doses, I'm a hardliner on acetaminophen: If you have—or suspect you have—liver problems, the only safe dose of acetaminophen is zero. I rank it right up there with trans fats.

2. **Do a periodic detoxification.** There are dozens of ways to do this, using just raw foods, lightly steamed vegetables, broths, fresh vegetable juice, medical foods like Metagenics Ultra-Clear, or any combination thereof. Many excellent books give details. One of my favorites is *The New Detox Diet* by my friend, Elson Haas, M.D.

3. **Eat a liver-friendly diet.** Obviously, the fewer chemicals, preservatives, and artificial ingredients the liver has to get rid of, the better. Some foods are particularly liver friendly. Turmeric, the spice that makes so much of Indian food yellow, contains natural anti-inflammatory curcuminoids, has anticancer activity, and is one of the best liver-friendly spices. Put it on everything. Wheatgrass juice and all the other "green drinks" that are high in chlorophyll are excellent. Coconut oil contains lauric acid, a well known antimicrobial and antiviral fatty acid. Beets and

beet juice have long had a reputation for being excellent for the liver, and in any case buying a juicer and making fresh vegetable juice on a daily basis (with some fruits thrown in if you like) is probably the best gift you can give your liver.

4. **Take liver-friendly supplements.** See below.

Antioxidants and Others Also Assist

Alpha lipoic acid is a powerful antioxidant that not only scavenges free radicals and helps protect cells but also helps regenerate vitamins C and E. It has multiple uses (see also diabetes and metabolic syndrome, page 47), but it is one of the most powerful liver nutrients available. Berkson wrote a book about it called *The Alpha Lipoic Breakthrough*. Read it.

Alpha lipoic acid also helps regenerate glutathione, arguably the body's most important antioxidant. Lester Packer, Ph.D., professor and senior researcher at the University of California for more than 40 years and author of *The Antioxidant Miracle*, has called alpha lipoic acid "probably the most potent naturally occurring antioxidant known to man."

By the time you read this, selenium's reputation will probably be even greater than it is today, and it's already held in pretty high esteem. This vitally important mineral is a premier cancer fighter (it decreases the rate of prostate cancer) and in January 2007, one of the most conservative publications in medicine, *The Archives of Internal Medicine*, published an article showing that daily selenium supplements appear

to suppress the progression of the viral load in patients with HIV infection. It's essential for those with hepatitis C. "Selenium acts as a birth control pill to the virus," Berkson told me.

The herb milk thistle (silymarin) is a premier liver nutrient. The active ingredient in milk thistle is silymarin, which is believed to be responsible for its medicinal qualities. Milk thistle has been used in Europe as a treatment for liver disease since the sixteenth century.

The Supporting Cast of Liver-Friendly Nutrients

There are a number of other really important nutrients you should consider as part of a liver health/hep-C-fighting program.

N-A-C (N-acetyl-cysteine). This derivative of the amino acid L-cysteine is a precursor to the formation of the powerful antioxidant glutathione. It's one of the best ways to increase glutathione in the body (since glutathione isn't well absorbed orally, you have to make it). Recommended: 1,000 mg daily

Whey protein powder. Though not technically a supplement, whey protein is another powerful way to increase the body's stores of glutathione and boost the immune system. Be sure to get a pure, high-quality powder made by a reputable company that markets to health professionals. You don't want one of the God-awful "fancy" protein shakes sweetened with sugar or some artificial chemical hazard that lines the shelves at the mall. (One brand I like is PaleoMeal by Designs for Health, which has whey from grass-fed animals, is carefully prepared, and is fortified with omegas and other heart-healthy nutrients. I have links to it, as well as several other first-rate brands, on my website, www.jonnybowden.com.)

Vitamin C. This vitamin has antiviral activity, and intravenous vitamin C has long been used by practitioners of nutritional and integrative medicine for a variety of conditions. It has been championed for hepatitis by Robert Cathcart, M.D., a California physician who was recognized by the Society for Orthomolecular Health-Medicine as recipient of the Linus Pauling Award.

"Since acute hepatitis A, B, C, etc. is easily cured with massive doses of ascorbate (vitamin C) intravenously and with follow-up with oral ascorbic acid (vitamin C), it is tragic that it is not properly utilized. Hepatitis C is a special problem because only about a quarter of cases present as acute (when it would be easily cured). Chronic hepatitis C is more of a problem; however with massive doses of ascorbic acid orally, a no-sugar diet, vitamin E, selenium, silymarin (an antioxidant from milk thistle), and alpha lipoic acid, among other nutrients, I have never seen a case to go onto acute hepatic necrosis or cancer of the liver," Cathcart says.

Olive leaf extract. This supplement may have some antiviral properties.

SAMe (S-adenosyl-methionine). SAMe is a naturally occurring molecule present in all living cells, and is made in the body by a reaction between methionine and another compound called adenosyntriphosphate (ATP). It has many incredible benefits, including a positive effect on depression and arthritis pain. For our purposes, it helps the liver to replenish important substances, notably the all-important glutathione. In one double-blind trial, people with cirrhosis of the liver due to alcoholism who took SAMe for two years had a 47 percent lower rate of death or need for liver transplantation compared with those who took a placebo.

Neominophagen. A component of licorice known as glycyrrhizin seems to have significant antiviral action. Neominophagen (also known as stronger neominophagen C or SNMC) is a kind of "superglycyrrhizin." Research published in Asia (available online at www.pubmedcentral.nih.gov) shows that it can inhibit HIV. It is widely used in Japan to treat hepatitis. Some cutting-edge practitioners in the United States have used it as well. It's injectable, so it has to be administered by a doctor.

Vitamin E. This vitamin has a place at the table in a liver-health protocol because of its antioxidant effects.

Artichokes. This vegetable has a long folk history in treating many liver diseases. Their active ingredient is cynarin, which has demonstrated liver-protecting effects. Artichoke extract is in a lot of liver-protection supplement formulas.

Dandelion root. Many people living healthily with hepatitis C swear by this herb and use it to make a tea.

Reishi and shiitake mushrooms. Chinese herbalists prize Reishi mushrooms for their protective effect on the liver. The bitterer the mushroom, the higher the level of triterpenoids, which give it its potency. It's usually made into a tea or taken as an extract.

Phosphatidylcholine. The active ingredient in the popular supplement lecithin is actually a substance called phosphatidylcholine. In animal research, it protects against cirrhosis and fibrosis. We know that choline—the prime constituent of phosphatidylcholine—is essential for normal liver function, and phos choline is an excellent "delivery system" for choline. In one double-blind study in England, chronic active hepatitis C patients were treated with 3 g of phos choline each day; they had significantly reduced symptoms compared to the control subjects. Many researchers have postulated that phosphatidylcholine has an ability to repair the membranes of liver cells.

You can die of old age *with* your hepatitis C (or even better, without it, if you're one of the lucky people who can clear it on your own). You don't have to die *from* it.

That's what I plan to do. I hope you do, too.

CoQ10, Whey Protein, and the DASH Diet

for Hypertension

WHEN IT COMES to hypertension, it's hard to come up with a more authoritative source than Mark Houston, M.D.

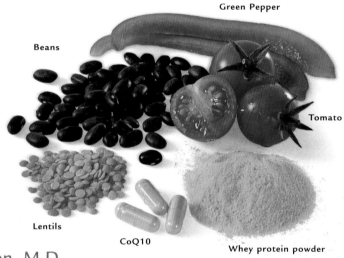

Beans
Green Pepper
Tomato
Lentils
CoQ10
Whey protein powder

Pretty much everything I know of value about hypertension I learned from Mark Houston, as did most of the nutritionists and doctors with whom I've trained. He's an associate clinical professor of medicine at Vanderbilt University School of Medicine and director of the Hypertension Institute in Nashville. In addition, he is a staff physician at Saint Thomas Medical Group and the Vascular Institute of Saint Thomas Hospital in Nashville. With both an M.D. and a master's degree in nutrition, he's uniquely qualified to speak about natural cures and the integration of conventional and nutritional medicine. And if you have hypertension, are at risk for it, or just want to know more, there's no better place to begin than with his book *What Your Doctor May Not Tell You about Hypertension.*

When I asked Houston to single out a few basics for a combo cure for hypertension, he replied that it would be tough to single out the superstar performers. After all, the basics of the Hypertension Institute Program involve a sophisticated vitamin regimen, exercise, weight maintenance, stress reduction, and the DASH diet (more on that in a moment). But several elements of the program stood out, and it's those three elements that form the core of our combo cure for hypertension: the DASH diet, coenzyme Q10, and hydrolyzed whey protein.

The DASH Diet

In 1997, the National Heart, Lung and Blood Institute funded research on the effects on blood pressure of groups of nutrients as they're found together in foods. The name of this study was Dietary Approaches to Stop Hypertension, or DASH, for short. The first study, known as DASH-1, investigated three dietary regimens: the standard American diet (with the apt acronym SAD), SAD plus some extra fruits and vegetables, and finally, the DASH-1 diet, which is high in fruits, vegetables, and low-fat dairy products, but low in cholesterol, saturated fat, and total fat. The results? Adding fruits and vegetables to the crummy SAD reduced blood pressure, demonstrating that simply eating more fruits and vegetables is helpful. But those on the DASH-1 diet enjoyed the greatest reduction in their blood pressure.

The thing of it was that the DASH-1 diet didn't control for sodium, and each of the three tested diets (including the DASH-1) contained about 3,000 mg of the stuff. So the researchers decided to do a second study, called the DASH-2 Sodium (or DASH-2 for short) diet. In this study, which involved both prehypertensives and hypertensives, half the subjects ate the DASH-2 diet; half ate the SAD. But every single subject consumed a specific level of sodium for one month at a time: 4,300 mg per day for the first month, 2,400 mg per day for the second month, and 1,500 mg per day for the third. The results showed that simply cutting back on sodium intake reduced blood pressure, no matter which diet someone followed. But those on the DASH-2 diet showed greater reductions in blood pressure at each level. And the biggest reductions were in those who were hypertensive before starting the diet.

Making Modifications

So we know that the DASH diet works for lowering blood pressure and works even better when you lower sodium in the diet as well. But at the Hypertension Institute, they've gone the DASH diet one better.

"I give my patients a specially modified version of the DASH that I believe is the best diet possible for people with hypertension," Houston told me. "The main change is to increase the amount of protein, vegetables, and 'good' fats consumed every day, while decreasing the grains, fruits, and dairy products. It's much lower in refined carbohydrates and has a lower glycemic index and glycemic load. Otherwise it's the same great, pressure-reducing program that's helped so many."

So here's what the best *dietary* "natural cure" for hypertension looks like:

- **Cereals, grains, pasta:** 3 to 4 servings a day, all from whole grains with no sugar or salt added
- **Vegetables:** 6 to 8 servings a day
- **Fruits:** 4 servings per day
- **Meat, poultry, and cold-water fish:** 2 to 4 servings per day
- **Dried beans, seeds, and nuts:** 1 to 2 servings per day
- **Low-fat dairy products:** 1 to 2 servings per day
- **Fats and oils:** 4 to 5 servings per day of polyunsaturated and monounsaturated fats; no trans fats; low saturated fat
- **Sweets:** none
- **Fiber:** mixed (soluble and insoluble) 50 g a day

(You can read more about the specifics of this diet in Houston's book, mentioned above.)

Note: With all this talk about salt and the dangers of sodium for people with high blood pressure, it's important to note that this is not true for everyone. Houston estimates that up to 60 percent of those with elevated blood pressure are salt sensitive—that is, their blood pressure rises when they consume more salt and falls when they take in less. African Americans, the elderly, and the obese are more likely to be salt sensitive. But many people are not.

Couple the DASH diet, especially in its Houston-modified form (above), with a couple of superstar nutrients, add exercise and some

Natural Prescription for Hypertension

DASH diet: Houston modification

Coenzyme Q10: 50–300 mg

Hydrolyzed whey protein powder: 1 serving of 30 g

★ FOR ADDED EFFECTIVENESS:

Magnesium chelate: 500 mg, twice a day

Calcium citrate: 1,000 mg

Taurine: 1,500 mg, twice a day

Omega-3 fatty acids: 2–3 g

Vitamin D: 2,000 IU

L-arginine: 2 g twice a day

L-carnitine: 1,500–4,000 mg per day in divided doses

High-quality multiple vitamin with vitamin E and vitamin C

ALSO RECOMMENDED:

Exercise

Stress reduction

Celery, garlic, and extra virgin olive oil

Hawthorne berries: 80–300 mg per day

Note: All dosages are daily dosages and in pill or capsule form unless otherwise noted.

form of stress reduction (try the Relaxation Response on page 291, any form of meditation or yoga, or even warm relaxing baths), and you're well on your way to making a big difference in your health. Here are the superstar nutrients that form the basis of the combo cure for hypertension.

Coenzyme Q10 is widely given in Europe and Japan to millions of people suffering from cardiovascular disease. People with essential hypertension are more likely to have a CoQ10 deficiency than those without hypertension. It's been an approved treatment for congestive heart failure in Japan since 1974, and Houston considers it one of the best natural treatments for high blood pressure.

In addition to being a superb source of high-quality, absorbable protein, hydrolyzed whey protein is a natural ACE inhibitor. ACE inhibitors, short for *angiotensin-converting enzyme inhibitors*, help reduce blood pressure by interfering with an enzyme that causes muscles surrounding the arteries to constrict, thus raising blood pressure.

"Hydrolyzed whey protein lowers blood pressure," says Houston.

The Supporting Cast

Though CoQ10, whey protein, and the DASH diet form the core of a natural cure for high blood pressure, they're far from the only elements of a hypertension reduction program. Calcium, magnesium, and potassium (and a reduced amount of sodium) work in concert to optimize blood pressure. Interestingly, much research has shown that the overwhelming majority of Americans are deficient in magnesium (see Desert Island Cures, page 303). And

as far back as 1928, studies have suggested that a high potassium intake could reduce elevated blood pressure. Since then, numerous population, observational, and clinical studies have demonstrated that blood pressure falls when dietary potassium is increased. Omega-3 fatty acids are the kind of fats that can help lower blood pressure the most and improve overall heart health to boot. And especially in people with high blood pressure, vitamin C improves endothelial dysfunction (a dysfunction of the cells that line the inner surface of all blood vessels) in people with hypertension.

A diet high in fruits and vegetables can do wonders for high blood pressure. So can certain foods. Celery, for example (see page 186) can lower blood pressure when you consume four sticks a day, as can garlic. (For more on how garlic works its magic, see my book *The 150 Healthiest Foods on Earth*.)

Finally, resveratrol has made news for the last decade or so as one of the key "antiaging" compounds in red wine and grapes. "It lowers blood pressure, blood fats, and glucose," Houston says, "and it relaxes the vascular smooth muscles."

And just in case you were living on another planet for the last few decades—stop smoking. Immediately. Do it now. No excuses.

(For more information about the full hypertension reduction program of supplements and lifestyle changes, visit www.hypertensioninstitute.com.)

Hold the Soda, Pass the Water: Prevention of

Recurring Kidney Stones

I'VE NEVER HAD kidney stones, but I've heard people describe the pain of passing them as akin to pulling your upper lip over the back of your head. (Or maybe that was a description of childbirth.) In any case, no one I know who's ever had them—kidney stones, that is, not kids—is eager to repeat the experience.

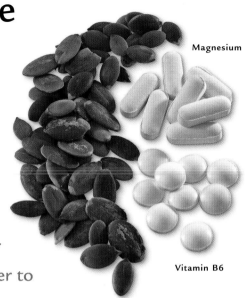

Magnesium

Vitamin B6

Pumpkin Seeds

Kidney stones are hardly a modern ailment. Scientists have found evidence of kidney stones in 7,000-year-old Egyptian mummies. Today, they're one of the most common disorders of the urinary tract, causing 2.7 million visits to health-care providers and more than 600,000 emergency room visits yearly.

Kidney stones are hard masses that can grow from crystals forming within the kidneys. Women get them, but men are more likely to get them. About three-quarters of the stones are made out of calcium oxalate (more on that in a moment), but stones can also contain uric acid, cysteine, calcium phosphate, or struvite (magnesium ammonium phosphate). The uric acid stones are most commonly found in gout.

How to Treat Kidney Stones

So what do you do when you have a kidney stone, or what can you do to prevent another excruciatingly painful stone from ever forming again?

"Start by drinking a ton of water," advises my friend, naturopathic physician Andrew Rubman, N.D. Water will make calcium oxalate more soluble and a lot less likely to form crystals. Water and lemon juice—a standard, all-purpose healing drink used for a variety of purposes—may help as well, since a half cup of lemon juice a day will raise citrate levels, which can help fight stone formation. (Soda, on the other hand, does the opposite—see below.) And research shows that grapefruit juice raises the risk of stones by as much as 44 percent, so if you're prone to stone formation, avoid it. Ditto with salt. In one review paper in the journal *Nutrition Reviews*, researchers theorized that stone formers may be more sensitive to salt than non-stone formers and that for those folks, a reduced intake of salt may decrease the risk of kidney stones.

Conventional treatment advocates pain relief medications, such as nonsteroidal anti-inflammatory drugs (such as ibuprofen or aspirin) or narcotics like Percocet. Diuretics are also sometimes prescribed for prevention of calcium oxalate stone formation. Besides medication, lithotripsy is an ultrasound treatment that breaks the stones into pieces that are small enough to pass in the urine. This procedure has largely replaced surgery as the preferred method for stone removal. (Note: If you're going to get surgery, it might be worth it to try acupuncture. It may not make the stone come out any more easily, but it's been shown to decrease the anxiety and anticipation of the ultrasound procedure.)

Because 75 percent of kidney stones are formed from oxalates, you'll want to avoid foods that are high in oxalates: nuts, tea, chocolate, beets, rhubarb, and wheat bran are all on the list. Phosphate-based soft drinks are also a big problem for stone formers. A study in the *Journal of Clinical Epidemiology* examined 1,009 male patients who formed kidney stones and were also consumers of a significant amount of soda to see what effect soda might have on stone recurrence. The guys who consumed the largest quantities of phosphate-based sodas had the highest rate of stone recurrence.

We know that most stones are made from calcium oxalate, and we know limiting high-oxalate foods is a really good idea. But what about limiting the other half of this duo—calcium? On the face of it, it sounds like a good idea. But it isn't, even though it's still given as advice by people who don't know what they're talking about.

"There's actually an inverse relationship between calcium intake and stone formation," Rubman says. In one study, calcium restriction led to an increase in the absorption and excretion of oxalate in the urine, and this happened both in people with and without kidney stones. You can ensure this doesn't happen by making sure you get enough calcium in the first place. (Note that calcium supplements should be taken with meals rather than on an empty stomach; that way, they have the best chance of binding to oxalates found in food.)

Natural Prescription for Kidney Stones

To reduce recurrences and prevent new calcium oxalate stone formation

Magnesium citrate: 500 mg

Vitamin B6: 40 mg

Pumpkin seeds: 510 g

Diet: Reduce intake of oxalate-containing foods, increase water and fiber, reduce salt and caffeine. Avoid grapefruit juice.

Note: The above dosages are daily and in pill or capsule form unless otherwise noted.

If you need more data to put the urban legend about restricting calcium to rest, consider this: The largest prospective epidemiological study ever published on calcium and kidney stones (*New England Journal of Medicine*) concluded that high calcium intake is associated with a decreased risk of symptomatic kidney stones. The 1993 study, which followed more than 45,000 men, found that those who consumed less than 850 mg of calcium per day were at an increased risk for kidney stones. The authors concluded that calcium may actually have a protective effect by binding to oxalate in the gut and preventing its absorption in a form that leads to kidney stones.

Animal protein and coffee have gotten a bad rap because both extra protein and coffee can cause calcium to be excreted in the urine, and some early studies showed that a lot of stone formers (about 24 percent) also have high amounts of calcium in their urine. But later research has shown that as far as kidney stones go, urinary oxalate is way more important than urinary calcium. In fact, in the Nurses' Health Study, the risk of stones was decreased by 8 to 10 percent for each 8 ounce serving of coffee (caffeinated and decaffeinated) per day.

Putting increase of urinary calcium aside for the moment, a *British Medical Journal* study in 2002 suggested that animal protein may increase the urinary excretion of oxalate, and that's something we definitely don't want. Animal protein will also likely increase the risk of uric acid stones. Moderate amounts of protein are probably fine, though all my usual precautions about

WORTH KNOWING

There's a persistent urban legend about the connection between vitamin C and kidney stones, and many people are still afraid to take vitamin C because of it. Don't be. There's not a shred of evidence that vitamin C increases actual stone formation. In fact, vitamin C will bind up calcium, which may decrease the formation of calcium oxalate. And because vitamin C is a powerful infection fighter it may help break up bacteria that usually forms around a "nucleus of infection," which eventually leads to a stone.

One large-scale, prospective study followed 85,557 women for fourteen years and found no evidence to support that vitamin C causes kidney stones. Some women took 250 mg of vitamin C; others took 1.5 g or more. There was absolutely no difference in their incidence of kidney stones. And a large, similar study on men found that vitamin C could actually reduce the incidence of kidney stones. It's time to put this urban legend to bed.

factory-farmed meat still apply for other reasons. and if I were a stone former, I'd probably keep protein to a reasonable amount—say 20 percent or so—of my diet for a while.

The Magic of Magnesium

What about supplements? Glad you asked.

My friend, integrative medicine icon Alan Gaby, M.D., has written that research results "strongly suggest that supplementing with modest doses of magnesium and vitamin B6 can greatly reduce the recurrence rate of calcium oxalate kidney stones."

In one study, 149 patients with long-standing stones received 100 mg of a cheap form of magnesium (magnesium oxide) three times a day, equal to 180 mg per day of elemental magnesium. They also received 10 mg of B6 once a day at the same time. Would you like to know what happened?

The mean rate of stone formation dropped by 92.3 percent.

Yes, you did read that right. Without a single significant side effect, the average rate of stone formation went from 1.3 stones per patient per year, to $^1/_{10}$ of a stone per year. (Remember, this is a mathematical average, like 2.5 children!) Point is, this is pretty dramatic. And it's not the only time it happened.

Another study published in the *Journal of the American College of Nutrition* showed that supplementing with 500 mg of magnesium a day (even without the B6) dropped stone formation by 90 percent.

"Unfortunately, many doctors remain unaware of this simple, safe, effective, and inexpensive treatment for recurrent kidney stones," Gaby says.

Herbs and Nutrients Work Together in This Cure
for Migraines

WHETHER YOU'VE BEEN hit with a classic low-grade migraine or a full-blown migraine complete with aura and flashing lights, these are the worst type of headaches and can be debilitating for many people.

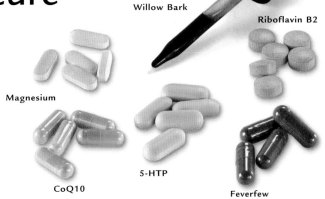

Willow Bark

Riboflavin B2

Magnesium

5-HTP

CoQ10

Feverfew

Not to be confused with tension headaches, migraines are much more severe and incapacitating, lasting anywhere from four to seventy-two hours. More women experience migraines than men, most likely because of the role that hormones play (consider the fact that most women get them either right before or during menstruation and that most migraines actually disappear after menopause).

But there's hope. Research has shown that a number of nutrients—and a couple of powerful herbs—may significantly help sufferers of migraines (and perhaps headaches in general). And it's those nutrients—CoQ10, riboflavin, and magnesium—and herbs—butterbur and fever-few—that form the backbone of the natural prescription for migraines. With maybe some 5-HTP thrown in for good measure. Read on.

How a Migraine Begins

No one really knows for sure what causes a migraine; the triggers can be different and varied for each person. When that switch is flipped on, a series of events takes place within the nerve cells of the brain. Substances called excitotoxins overstimulate these nerve cells. They also cause the warning signs that commonly precede a migraine: depression, irritability, restlessness, loss of appetite, and an aura that most describe as brightly colored lights. As this is happening, the nerve cells send out impulses to the brain's blood vessels and release substances that cause inflammation and swelling.

So what causes the nerve cells to get excited in the first place? Truth is, the list is long and

---

Natural Prescription for Migraines

CoQ10

Children/Adolescents: 1–3 mg per kg of body weight per day in a single dose. Liquid gels are best.

Adults: 100 mg per day, three times daily

Magnesium: 200–600 mg

Vitamin B2 (riboflavin): 400 mg per day for three months. Take with a B-complex supplement.

5-HTP: 200–600 mg

Combo herbs: Butterbur, 50 to 150 mg; feverfew, 300 mg, twice daily for 12 weeks; white willow bark (300 mg, twice daily for 12 weeks)

Diet: Avoid refined sugar, alcohol, caffeine, aspartame, smoking, salt, and tyramine-containing foods

Reduce stress and get enough sleep

Check for food allergies

Note: The dosages are daily and in pill or capsule form unless otherwise noted.

---

varied, and differs from person to person. Some of the usual suspects include anxiety, stress, lack of food, lack of sleep, exposure to light, and hormonal changes in women. And then there are food triggers (more on that in a moment) and the possibility of missing nutrients in the diet. There is even some information that suggests a link to the bacterial infection *H. pylori*.

One promising line of research suggests that people who are prone to headaches may benefit by supplemental 5-hydroxytryptophan or 5-HTP. (You can read about 5-HTP as a natural cure for depression on page 42.) 5-HTP is made in the body from the amino acid tryptophan and then converted into serotonin, the "feel good" brain chemical. Low levels of serotonin are associated with everything from depression to aggressive behavior to obsessive-compulsive disorder to carbohydrate cravings—and also, it seems, with headaches. In one study there was a significant decrease in the consumption of painkillers with a group treated with 300 mg of 5-HTP a day, as well as a significant decrease in the number of days with headaches in the two weeks following the study. The patients in this study suffered with chronic tension-type headaches, but there's reason to think 5-HTP might be a useful adjunct for those with migraines as well.

The excellent evidence-based monograph on 5-HTP—written as a collaboration between Natural Standard (www.naturalstandard.com) and the faculty of Harvard Medical School—states that "there is evidence from several studies in both children and adults that 5-HTP may be effective in reducing the severity and frequency of headaches, including tension headaches and migraines. 5-HTP may be most effective for treating headaches in people with a history of depression or those who experienced severe headaches before the age of 20 years."

Diet: Avoiding the Trigger Foods

Then there are food triggers, some of which you might not want to hear about but I'll tell you anyway: chocolate and alcohol come to mind. (Hey, isn't it worth a trial period without them just to see if it helps? It really might.) Maybe it's not chocolate or alcohol—maybe it's salt. It could be sugar. It could be milk. It could be wine. In fact, it could be anything that flips that brain switch and releases those excitotoxins.

And by the way, I didn't pick on chocolate and alcohol just to annoy you—truth is, they're among the most common culprits largely because they contain tyramines. Tyramines are chemicals derived from the amino acid tyrosine. For many people, tyramines are a huge trigger for migraines. In addition to chocolate and alcoholic beverages, high-tyramine foods include anything fermented (like aged cheeses, fermented soy sauce, and sauerkraut) and processed meats like pepperoni and sausage.

Individuals who have *reactive hypoglycemia*—low blood sugar that occurs one to three hours after a meal—may find that being on the blood-sugar roller coaster triggers severe headaches. Reducing refined sugar and eating smaller, more frequent meals (with more protein, fat, and fiber) will help balance blood sugar and keep it on a more even keel. But for goodness' sake, don't reach for aspartame instead of sugar: It contains an amino acid called phenylalanine, which also has the potential to be a migraine trigger. (I won't even get into the whole aspartame story—let's not go there. Suffice it to say, I don't recommend it even if you don't suffer from headaches.)

I wish there were an easy formula for determining what your individual triggers are, but there isn't. But make like Columbo and do some good detective work. If you systematically note what triggers, e.g., environmental, food, interpersonal, etc. seem to precipitate an attack, you'll eventually hit pay dirt.

And it's not just the things you're eating (but maybe shouldn't be) that can trigger an attack—it could also be the absence of things in your diet that should be there. (Since we can't know for sure just what those missing elements might be, the best advice is to make your diet as rich in whole foods, antioxidants, minerals, omega-3 fats, and plant phytochemicals as possible. It's the ultimate "can't hurt, might help!" strategy.)

Now Add in the Combos: Three Nutrients, Two Herbs

Riboflavin (vitamin B2), magnesium, and coenzyme Q10 (CoQ10) have been researched, reviewed, and studied for their effectiveness in managing migraines. They are all good, effective alternative treatments and can help to prevent migraines. CQ10 is a nutrient that is normally associated with energy: It helps the cells utilize oxygen. Andrew Hershey, M.D., Ph.D., associate director of neurology research at Cincinnati Children's Hospital Medical Center, looked at its relation to migraine in a recent study done at the University of Cincinnati.

He examined 1,552 children and adolescents between the ages of three and twenty-two and found that most had insufficient CoQ10 levels. After supplementing with CoQ10, the frequency of headaches fell significantly. Those affected went from having migraines an average of 19.2 days per month to 12.5 days per month. That's a big difference when you are experiencing a migraine, and when you're a teen whose state of mind and feeling of well-being play a big role in determining how successful your social life is.

Another study done in 2005 examined CoQ10's effect on adult migraine sufferers. Those who took 300 mg of CoQ10 for four months experienced a 50 percent or greater reduction in frequency of migraine attacks, significantly different from those just using a placebo. As for side effects in the groups in both these studies: none.

Riboflavin, or vitamin B2, is another nutrient that has been shown to be effective in the treatment of migraines. It can potentially decrease the number of migraine days by about 25 percent and lower the frequency by 30 percent. Similar to CoQ10, riboflavin is needed to convert food into energy. Dairy products, eggs, and meat contain significant amounts of B2 but wouldn't come close to providing the high doses you would need to treat a migraine. Remember that all the B vitamins work synergistically; when taking any single B vitamin therapeutically, it's best to also take a B-complex vitamin as a base and then, at a different time of day, add that extra therapeutic dose of B2.

Magnesium plays an important role in migraine prevention and reduction. Like 5-HTP, it has an effect on serotonin, so when magnesium levels are low, the risk for a migraine may increase. Magnesium also improves energy production in the heart, plus it dilates the arteries, helping blood deliver oxygen more effectively. Up to 50 percent of patients who experience acute migraines have been shown to have a magnesium deficiency. This is actually not surprising because most adults in the United States—75 percent by some estimates—are deficient in this important mineral. The National Academy of Sciences recommends that all women over the age of thirty take 320 mg of magnesium daily, but half of them consume only 230 mg or even less. The academy suggests more for men: 420 mg, yet only half of men over thirty get more than 330 mg.

Beneficial Herbs

Two herbs stand out when it comes to treating migraines: butterbur (*Petasites hybridus*) and feverfew (*Tanacetum parthenium*). Compelling evidence from human trials suggests that butterbur may have real benefits in preventing migraines. One hundred and eight children and adolescents between the ages of six and seventeen tried butterbur root extract for four months and experienced a decrease in the frequency of migraine attacks. In addition, they all reported feeling better.

The same results were found in adults. In one study, Pedadolex—a patented, high-quality butterbur preparation that you can buy in stores—was used at the dosage of 25 mg twice daily for twelve weeks. The frequency of migraine attacks decreased by a whopping 60 percent—and no side effects were reported to boot.

The most frequently used herb for the long-term prevention of migraines is feverfew. A number of well-done studies have suggested that feverfew may prevent migraine headaches. In studies, feverfew users seem to have milder headaches, fewer headaches, and less vomiting and nausea (though the herb doesn't necessarily shorten the length of time each headache lasts). Using feverfew together with another herb, white willow bark, also reduces the frequency, intensity, and duration of migraine attacks, by up to 60 percent.

Vitamin B6, Magnesium, and Evening Primrose Oil

A Natural Cure for PMS

LET ME BE perfectly honest. As a man who has been on this planet for more than a few decades, I've lived with my share of women prior to meeting the love of my life, with whom I'm now happily living.

Magnesium

Vitamin B6

Evening Primrose Oil

Melatonin

I've experienced PMS—on the receiving end of the spectrum—in many of its forms and intensities with a variety of women. And I can honestly say that my discovery of the "PMS cocktail" I'm about to tell you about probably saved my neighbors from having to be interviewed on the evening news and hearing themselves say things like, "Gee, that Jonny Bowden was such a nice fellow, who would have ever thought he'd do something like *this*?"

As anyone who has experienced it knows well, PMS is no picnic. It's also—let me be very clear—not "all in your head." It's the product of a real hormonal turbulence that accompanies the menstrual cycle, more in some people than in others, and it can cause significant mood swings, crying jags, depression, anger, and irritability, not to mention a compendium of physical symptoms like bloat and constipation. That hormonal storm, which can be a light tropical rain for some folks and Hurricane Katrina for others,

also affects neurotransmitters like serotonin, influencing mood and cravings and behavior.

For various reasons the combination of nutrients I'm about to tell you about works wonders.

The Dynamic Duo: Magnesium and Vitamin B6

Let's start with magnesium. Taking magnesium seems to relieve symptoms of PMS for many people. Supplementation with magnesium can improve mood and also help with fluid retention. Women with PMS have reduced magnesium levels.

In one of many studies, supplementation with 360 mg of magnesium three times a day (just a little more than the amount in my recommended PMS cocktail) produced significantly improved scores on the Moos Menstrual Distress Questionnaire, leading the researchers to conclude that magnesium supplementation could represent an effective treatment of premenstrual symptoms related to mood changes.

Vitamin B6 has long been observed to be part of a comprehensive nutritional support package for PMS. I suspect that one reason for this is that the body needs B6 to make serotonin out of the amino acid tryptophan, and many people may be low in B6 (as well as other B vitamins) because of the high level of B-eating stress. And who couldn't use more relaxing, calming, crave-busting serotonin? But whether it's the serotonin connection or something else, research shows that supplementing with B6 up to 100 mg a day is very likely to be of benefit in treating premenstrual symptoms and premenstrual depression.

One study in the *Journal of Women's Health and Gender-Based Medicine* tested various combinations of B6 and magnesium and found that both B6 and the B6-magnesium combo were helpful in reducing mild PMS-related anxiety symptoms. This study was all the more interesting because even though it used a really crappy kind of magnesium—magnesium oxide—and a low dose to boot, it still reported improvements. A high-quality magnesium at the 800 mg dose I recommend, together with B6, would be likely to produce even better results.

Evening primrose oil (like borage oil and black currant oil) is a natural source of a fatty acid called GLA—gamma-linolenic acid. Most of the health benefits of these oils can be attributed to the GLA content. However, the research on evening primrose and PMS has been mixed. Though some studies have shown it to be beneficial for PMS, many have not, though that may be because a great deal of the research used a preparation that contained only 40 mg of GLA. The average 1,000 mg dose of evening primrose oil contains about 100 mg of GLA. My "cocktail" would provide at least 200 mg (if not more) of GLA a day. It may also be true that GLA works best in combination with B6 and magnesium and is not quite as effective on its own. Because GLA is a natural anti-inflammatory, and because many people find it helpful for PMS, I think you should include it in the cocktail.

What about Calcium?

You can take plenty of other things as part of a natural prescription for PMS. First and foremost is calcium and vitamin D. A lot of research suggests that calcium and vitamin D supplements may reduce the severity of PMS, and there appears to be a link between PMS and low dietary calcium intake. Taking 1 to 1.2 g of calcium daily seems to really reduce depressed mood, water retention, and pain.

In one study, women consuming an average of 1,283 mg of calcium a day from foods had about a 30 percent lower risk of developing PMS compared to women consuming much less (529 mg). A more recent study, in the *Archives of Internal Medicine*, saw a 40 percent lower risk of PMS developing in women with high intakes of vitamin D and calcium. Considering all the other great things vitamin D does—such as its role in cancer prevention and bone health—and considering that most of us get far too little of it, vitamin D supplements are a good idea.

Remember, if you want to increase your calcium intake, dairy is hardly the only way to do it, though the dairy industry would have you believe it is the best way. It's not. Adding more dairy to your diet opens up a whole other can of worms that you may not want to open (see the section on dairy in my book *The 150 Healthiest Foods on Earth*), and it may even aggravate PMS symptoms. Green leafy vegetables, sardines, and seeds (such as sesame or pumpkin) are full of calcium, and there are always supplements (be sure to take magnesium at the same time).

Neptune Krill Oil is a very high-quality source of omega-3 fats and has been found in research to significantly reduce PMS symptoms when you take 3 g a day. Considering all the other benefits of omega-3s, there's no way this isn't worth a try. The single downside: Neptune Krill Oil is expensive.

Other Helpful Nutrients

The herb chasteberry (vitex) has been used for more than 2,500 years in Egypt, Greece, and Rome for a variety of conditions, not the least of which was decreasing libido (making it popular among celibate clergy but kind of a drag for the rest of those folks). It's widely prescribed in Germany, where the esteemed German Commission E approves it for irregularities of the menstrual cycle and PMS.

Taurine, an amino acid, is a natural diuretic and the best way I know to reduce bloat. One product I use (available through my website) is called Water Ease, and it's almost pure taurine

---

Natural Prescription for PMS

Vitamin B6: 50 mg, twice a day

Magnesium: 400 mg, twice a day

Evening primrose oil: 1,000 mg, twice a day (or GLA, 320 mg, twice a day)

ALSO HIGHLY RECOMMENDED:

Melatonin (at night): 1–3 mg

Neptune Krill Oil: 3 g

Vitex (herb), also known as chasteberry: Use as directed on label or as instructed by a health practitioner. Studies have used anywhere from about 4 mg per day of the dried extract all the way up to 1,800 mg per day of the dried fruit (in three divided 600 mg doses).

Taurine (if bloating is an issue): 1,000 mg

Consider: Natural progesterone

Note: All dosages are daily dosages and in pill or capsule form unless otherwise noted.

(with a little B6 thrown in for good measure). For water retention I recommend 900 to 1,000 mg of taurine when needed.

And don't forget diet: A great deal of research supports the idea that diet can profoundly affect PMS symptoms. Coffee and alcohol may make things worse. Sugar almost certainly does. Tory Hudson, N.D., a highly respected expert in the field of women's health, wisely recommends a diet of fruits, vegetables, whole grains, legumes, nuts, seeds, and fish, and the avoidance of refined sugar, dairy, salt, tobacco, and caffeine. It might be hard to follow, but it's sure to work.

Dr. Starbuck's Fruit Peel Candy, etc.

for Seasonal Allergies

"THERE'S POLLEN in the air." That's hardly music to the ears of anyone suffering from seasonal allergies. The symptoms are all too familiar: itchy and watery eyes, runny noses, sneezing, headache, and swollen sinuses. And while none of those are exactly life threatening, they can certainly ruin your day.

Candied Citrus Peel

Quercetin

Vitamin C

Stinging Nettles

Seasonal allergies are characterized by inflammation of the mucous membranes in the nasal passages. Airborne pollens from grasses, flowers, weeds, trees, or ragweed are the culprits, so allergy season officially begins whenever trees and grasses start to pollinate in your area of the country. (In the South, trees can start as early as late February while grass may start around the end of April. Meanwhile, in the Midwest, things may not kick in until May. In the West, you have longer pollination time for grass and some weeds that will hang on all the way into the fall.

And ragweed—another major cause of seasonal allergies—doesn't even get started in the Northeast till late summer or early fall.)

So why do these innocuous little molecules cause so much suffering in the first place? Well, these airborne little buggers, which can be pollens or even chemicals, get absorbed through the lungs or skin into the blood and cause the white blood cells of allergy-prone folks to produce a ton of an antibody known as IgE (immunoglobulin E). These molecules then travel through the bloodstream and hit cells called mast cells, which are major storage sites for histamine. Once the mast cell takes a hit from the IgE antibody, it begins "leaking" histamine all over the place, producing the familiar and annoying symptoms everyone who suffers from seasonal allergies knows all too well.

Conventional medicine doesn't have a lot to offer. Antihistamines like Benadryl and Tavist D can help, but they can cause drowsiness (no wonder the labels tell you not to use them while operating cars or machinery!). Nasal decongestants can help, but they're also not without possible side effects (restlessness, irritability, and insomnia are among the most common). And while most of these are probably safe, I can't help remembering that one "safe" nasal decongestant—phenylpropanolamine—was pulled off the market a few years ago after it was found to be linked to an increased risk of hemorrhagic stroke in women aged 18 to 49. Wouldn't it be great if there were some powerful natural treatments for seasonal allergies?

Well, there is. And it's a bioflavonoid called quercetin. Combined with a few other things, it just might be your most powerful natural weapon against the annoying symptoms of seasonal allergies.

Quercetin to the Rescue

I've talked about the reasons quercetin is effective for asthma (see page 101)—it's effective against seasonal allergies for similar reasons. For one thing, it's a powerful anti-inflammatory. For another, it has an "affinity" for mast cells, tending to stabilize their membranes and helping to

---

Natural Prescription for Seasonal Allergies

Quercetin: 300 mg, three times a day (When symptoms are under control, you can go down to 500 to 1,000 mg once a day.)

Stinging nettles (optional): 600 mg, freeze-dried extract

Vitamin C: 1,000–2,000 mg

Dr. Starbuck's candied fruit peels: Several times a day

OPTIONAL:

Eyebright (tincture taken orally): 2–6 ml (1:5 in 45 percent alcohol), three times a day

Chamomile tea: Several times a day

Zinc: 15–30 mg

Note: The dosages above are for daily dosages and in pill or capsule form unless otherwise noted.

---

prevent them from pouring out histamine in response to the IgE antibody.

Jaimison Starbuck, N.D., a naturopathic physician and past president of the American Association of Naturopathic Physicians, is a huge fan of quercetin. "It strengthens the capillaries in the upper respiratory tract to make them less reactive to the kind of inhalants that trigger allergic symptoms," she says.

Sometimes people with hay fever simply have very reactive mucous membranes, meaning they have a low threshold for irritation. These membranes may be slightly inflamed to begin with, or tend toward inflammation at the slightest irritation.

"Quercetin tends to decrease inflammation, and it helps support the immune system at the same time," Starbuck told me. "I've had clients who just used quercetin alone and it makes a huge difference in their symptoms and suffering." And according to my friend Cathy Wong, N.D.—www.about.com's alternative medicine expert—adding the supplemental enzyme bromelain increases the amount of quercetin absorbed in the digestive tract.

Accompanying Allergy Aids

Nettles—also known as stinging nettles—are a type of flowering plant native to Europe, North America, and Asia. Freeze-dried extract of nettles is gaining in popularity as an adjunct treatment for allergies, even though research on it is scant. Nonetheless, a study at the National College of Naturopathic Medicine in Portland back in the 1990s indicated that it may be helpful, though the effect is mild. But nettles have a long traditional use of being used for allergies (as well as other conditions), and many health practitioners recommend nettles as part of a total natural prescription for allergies; nettles do have a mild anti-inflammatory effect. The standard dose is 600 mg of freeze-dried nettles a day, though some people use more. It's also most effective if you start using it at the first onset of symptoms. "I use about two caps every two to three hours to calm things down," Starbuck told me. Note that nettles may react with blood-thinning medications like Coumadin. Patients with diabetes should check with their health-care practitioner before taking them.

Eyebright is an herb that's been used for hundreds of years as a compress against eye infections and other irritations, but according to Starbuck, it's effective orally to treat inflammation of nasal mucous membranes and sinuses.

"I often have clients take the tincture by mouth," she says. "Topically it's great as a compress against the eyes for irritation and watery eyes." She also suggests drinking chamomile tea, as it has an anti-mucus action that allergy sufferers will find soothing. (Eyebright can be used according to the label directions, and chamomile tea can be brewed to taste.)

And don't rule out homeopathy. A recent four-week double-blind study published in the *Annals of Pharmacotherapy* tested homeopathic preparations against a placebo during allergy season in the Phoenix area. The study subjects were forty men and women ranging in age from twenty-six to sixty-three with seasonal allergic symptoms of varying degrees of severity. Test results from three different questionnaires used to measure quality of life, well-being, functionality, and activity, showed significant positive changes on all three. No one reported any adverse effects from the homeopathic medicine.

Food Allergies

Most people think that seasonal allergies and food allergies (or sensitivities) are two distinctly different things. Guess again. Seasonal allergies are definitely aggravated by food allergies.

Starbuck told me about an eight-year-old kid who was brought into her office by his mother, who said, "He's got really bad allergies this year!" Starbuck took a history and found out that the kid had had dairy allergies when he was younger, but according to the mother, "not anymore."

"Just for fun, why don't you take him off dairy for a while?" Starbuck suggested.

Can you guess what happened?

Wheat, dairy, corn, soy, or any of the other common foods that produce sensitivities can aggravate a seasonal allergy and send it into overdrive. Remember, too, that dairy, wheat, and soy are all potentially mucus-producing foods. A nice, low-tech "elimination" diet might be just the ticket, at least during the allergy season. Take the offending foods out of the diet for a while and see whether your hay fever symptoms get better. Better yet, combine an elimination diet with the natural prescription for allergies and you might find you can throw your over-the-counter medications away, or at least reduce your use of them significantly.

I've saved the best for last: Starbuck generously offered to allow me to reproduce the recipe for her homemade decongestant "brew," which not only tastes amazing but is incredibly effective in fighting seasonal allergy symptoms (particularly when used in conjunction with the rest of the natural prescription for seasonal allergies). If you're wondering why it would work so well, the answer is simple: The peels of these fruits are among the richest natural sources of quercetin and other active bioflavonoids. Here's a delicious way to get them into your body:

- Wash and peel an orange, a grapefruit, and a lemon (use organic fruits, because you're going to be eating them!).

- Cut the peels into bite-size pieces (you're welcome to eat the fruit, but it's not part of this concoction).

- Mix water and organic honey together (in a 50-50 mix based on the amount you want to make).

- Bring the mix to a simmer, but don't boil it since boiling will kill the bioactive bioflavonoids in the peels.

- Add the peels and simmer until they are soft and coated with the honey mix.

- Cool in the fridge and eat like candy. They're beyond delicious.

Antioxidants
for Vision

THERE ARE A LOT of things I don't want to be when I grow older, but one of them is blind. Especially when it's preventable—which, in a huge number of cases, it is.

Omega-3

Multi-Vitamin

Zinc

Lutein

The leading cause of blindness in adults under the age of sixty is diabetic retinopathy, caused by complications of long-term diabetes. But the leading cause of adult blindness and vision loss in adults over sixty is something called macular degeneration. And a few simple supplements can significantly reduce the risk of your ever getting it.

You may recall from high school biology that the retina contains two types of photoreceptors—cones and rods. Cones are the ones that provide color sensitivity, and most of them are located in the central area of the retina in a structure called the *macula*. So when the macula "degenerates," you're in trouble—color vision and vision sharpness both deteriorate significantly, and in the worst case scenario, you can be looking at blindness (excuse the pun!).

The cause of macular degeneration is not really known, but it's believed that there is an insufficient disposal of waste materials from the cells. Cell waste is normally carried off, but in this case some is left behind and it blocks the light. Essential vision decreases; you always have peripheral vision, but you lose your central vision. In other words, you can't recognize faces or watch TV.

Risk Factors and Solutions

Macular degeneration is estimated to affect 1.75 million Americans as of 2006, a figure that is expected to grow considerably. Smoking, poor diet, and obesity all increase the risk, as do high blood pressure and a number of factors that you can't control (like family history, aging, and the newly discovered *complement factor H (CFH) gene*, which is strongly associated with macular degeneration). But what you eat—and the supplements you take—affect the macula, and research shows that diet and supplements can be used to treat or prevent the condition.

In 2001, the National Eye Institute conducted the Age-Related Eye Disease Study (AREDS), which involved more than 3,600

Natural Prescription for Preventing Macular Degeneration and Preserving Vision

Multivitamin: Containing at least 500 mg vitamin C, 400 IU vitamin E, and 15 mg beta-carotene

Zinc: 30–80 mg

Omega-3 fatty acids: 1,000 mg (1 g)

Lutein (and zeaxanthin): 10 mg for general prevention, 20–40 mg for someone who already has macular degeneration

Note: All dosages are daily dosages and in pill or capsule form unless otherwise noted.

people. Researchers found that supplementation with certain nutrients reduced the risk of progressing to advanced macular degeneration by 25 percent, especially in groups at highest risk. They reported a significant 27 percent reduction in risk for vision loss in these higher-risk groups.

What were those nutrients? A simple antioxidant combo consisting of 500 mg vitamin C, 400 IU vitamin E, 15 mg beta-carotene, and 80 mg zinc.

But there are two important nutrients for the eye that were not included in the study. Why? Because not much was known about them at the time of the research. Not anymore. We now know that lutein and zeaxanthin—two members of the carotenoid family that are emerging as the superstars of eye nutrition—

are vitally important for vision. Lutein and its related compound, zeaxanthin, are highly concentrated in the macula, providing a yellow color known as the macular pigment, which protects the macula. You want that pigment to be dense, the better to protect your eyes.

A 1997 study found that subjects fed a diet high in spinach and corn experienced nearly a 20 percent increase in macular pigment density. What's the connection with those foods? That diet effectively boosted the subjects' consumption of lutein about 400 percent and zeaxanthin about 300 percent. That same year it was found that the use of a lutein supplement can also increase the density of the protective macular pigment. You can, of course, get some lutein from foods such as spinach, kale, broccoli, and Brussels sprouts, though probably not enough to get the full therapeutic effect of supplements.

In 2004, the Lutein Antioxidant Supplementation Trial (LAST) found that subjects receiving lutein or lutein plus antioxidants showed a significant increase in macular density and in some measures, visual function. Virtually every expert now includes lutein and zeaxanthin (they are usually found together) in any formula for eye health and for the prevention of macular degeneration and adult vision loss.

The Power of Antioxidants

Both antioxidants and omega-3 fatty acids can help protect your eyes and preserve your vision in a variety of ways.

Oily fish—and the omega-3 fatty acids found in them—can help protect against macular degeneration. A review of omega-3 functions in the retina from the National Eye Institute's Division of Epidemiology and Clinical Research suggests that omega-3 fatty acids play a pivotal role in protecting the retina. They should be included in any program for eye health and vision preservation. And while you're at it, take a multivitamin. An analysis of data from the Physicians Health Study shows that taking a multivitamin supplement can decrease the risk of cataracts.

Antioxidants protect cells throughout the body, not just in the eyes. And some have multiple effects. Zinc, for example again, is critical for the functioning of the immune system. An interesting and little noted "side effect" of AREDS was that participants who received zinc, either alone or with the other antioxidants, had lower rates of death than those not taking zinc. Hey, an extra few years of healthy life is a nice "side benefit" of taking a few antioxidants that can preserve your vision!

In addition to being an antioxidant, zinc improves the transport and use of cysteine, an amino acid needed to manufacture glutathione, arguably the most important antioxidant in the body.

WORTH KNOWING

Michael Geiger, O.D., a nutritionally minded optometrist and author of *Eye Care Naturally,* also recommends garlic. "Garlic helps with circulation," he told me. "One of the problems with macular degeneration is the buildup of waste products, so you want to get the blood flowing."

Interestingly, eye problems can be a predictor of other health issues and even mortality. According to Harvard researcher Johanna Seddon, M.D., sick eyes are especially likely to show up in people who are sick with other illnesses. There's a well-established link between macular degeneration and cardiovascular disease, for example, and the two share a number of risk factors, including obesity, smoking, and inflammation.

HCA, CLA, EGCG, and Chromium

for Weight Loss

BACK IN 2004, when I wrote *Living the Low Carb Life: Choosing the Diet That's Right for You from Atkins to Zone,* I wrote the following sentence in the chapter on supplements: "Memorize this: There are no supplements you can take for weight loss that will cause the pounds to just melt off without you having to do anything at all."

L-carnitine

CLA

Green Tea

Cromium Picolinate

Hydroxycitric Acid

Now, I've been "America's Weight Loss Coach" for more than a decade, and I've written a ton of stuff about how to lose weight in a healthy way; in the past fifteen years or so I've probably addressed more questions about weight loss supplements (on www.AskJonnyBowden.com and other sites) than I have about any other topic I've ever been asked about. Hundreds. Probably a thousand. (But who's counting?) And for the most part, to tell you the truth, I haven't been exactly sanguine about weight loss supplements in general. Most people have unrealistic expectations of what weight loss supplements can do, fueled in part by outrageous hyperbole in late-night infomercials. Those expectations are almost never met when people continue to do all the wrong things and simply pop the latest

"miracle" weight loss pill expecting flab to "melt off" by itself.

Guess what? It doesn't.

So let's be clear: If a person is going to eat 7,000 calories of fast food a day, then these four supplements aren't going to do a thing. But if you're serious about losing weight and are willing to make some basic lifestyle changes, then the supplements I'm going to tell you about can really make a difference.

Start with Hydroxycitric Acid

Garcinia cambogia, also known as the Malabar tamarind, is a small, sweet tropical tree fruit shaped like a pumpkin. (It's also the source of the spice tamarind, which is used in all sorts of curry dishes.) In the late 60s, scientists discovered an acid in the fruit that's somewhat similar to the citric acid found in fruits like oranges and lemons. That acid is called hydroxycitric acid, or HCA, and it may well turn out to be a terrific adjunct to a weight loss program. (Note: Hydroxycitric acid is also commonly referred to as *hydroxycitrate*. They are interchangeable.)

Folks were very excited about hydroxycitrate for a while back in the 90s because of a number of studies that showed that it causes weight loss in animals. One thing we know is that HCA blocks a portion of an enzyme called citrate lyase, which—long story short—helps turn sugars and starches into fat. It also seems to somewhat suppress the appetite. My friend Shari Lieberman, Ph.D., C.N.S., suggests that the metabolic change brought on by HCA may send a signal to the brain that reduces appetite and food intake.

But the buzz on HCA faded out pretty quickly after a large study published in the prestigious but conservative *Journal of the American Medical Association* showed that it didn't work so well in humans. This 1998 study found HCA had basically "no effect." But more recent research, notably by Georgetown University Medical Center professor Harry Preuss, M.D., and his colleagues, is pointing in a very different direction. And because of this new information, I now think HCA has real potential as a weight loss supplement.

I asked Preuss—who wrote glowingly about hydroxycitrate in his excellent book *The Fat-Loss Pharmacy*—why he thought the previous studies were discouraging.

"You have to take the right dose of the right product, and you have to take it properly," he told me. "In the *JAMA* study, they used whatever the dose was at the time, and they never even mentioned the type of citrate that they used. You have to give enough so that it reaches the sites in the body that it needs to reach." Preuss points out that there are different forms of hydroxycitrates. "If you have almost a pure calcium hydroxycitrate, it's just not going to work," he told me. He prefers hydroxycitrate bound to both calcium and potassium, which dramatically increases the absorption and effectiveness of HCA. (One brand that meets that requirement is Super CitriMax. Note that plain old CitriMax does not.)

In one study, Preuss and his colleagues looked at thirty healthy but overweight people ages twenty-one to fifty over an eight-week period. All participants ate a diet of 2,000 calories a day and walked for a half an hour five days per week. One group was given Super CitriMax, and the other group was given a placebo. At the end of the study, the placebo group had lost an average of three pounds, but the hydroxycitrate group had lost an average of twelve pounds—a whopping 400 percent more weight. Their average BMI fell by 6.3 percent (in the placebo group it fell only 1.7 percent). To top it off they had an 18 percent drop in triglycerides and—interestingly—an almost double boost in serotonin levels compared to the placebo group. (Higher serotonin levels are associated with fewer cravings and a greater sense of calm.) In a second similar study using sixty people and published in the journal *Diabetes, Obesity and Metabolism*, the HCA group lost an average of 10¹/₂ pounds compared to the placebo group, which lost only 3¹/₂ pounds.

"Perhaps the most remarkable result was in appetite control," Preuss says. "The placebo group had no change, but the HCA group had a 16 percent reduction in the amount of food they ate per meal!"

Remember, besides using the right form of HCA, you have to use the right dosage. Preuss and his research team have determined that the ideal dose for weight loss is likely to be about 2,800 mg a day of HCA. Super CitriMax (also known as HCA-SX) for example, is 60 percent HCA. If you do the math you'd find that to deliver that amount, you'd need about 4,667 mg of Super CitriMax in divided doses of 1,555 mg each. (No need to be obsessive—1,500 mg, three times a day, is just fine.) Studies show it's best absorbed on an empty stomach, so Preuss suggests taking it thirty minutes before each of the three big meals of the day.

Add Conjugated Linoleic Acid

Then there's CLA (which stands for conjugated linoleic acid). Whenever I'm asked to comment about trans fats and I go into the whole speech about "the right amount of trans fats in the human diet is zero," I always have to remind myself to add this caveat: I'm talking about *man-made* trans fats (e.g., partially hydrogenated oils). There's actually one trans fat, believe it or not, that's found naturally and is one of the most beneficial fats you can consume. It not only has

an impressive research history showing it has anticancer properties, it also has an emerging body of research behind it showing it's quite effective for fat loss. The name of the trans fat in question? CLA.

I'll never forget seeing a series of photos years ago that came out of an early study on overweight rodents given CLA in their diets. After euthanizing the rats, the researchers did the equivalent of a rodent autopsy and took photos of their inner abdominal areas. The rats that ate only regular rat chow had huge amounts of white abdominal fat around their middle, while the CLA rats had almost none. It was dramatic, and I still remember the pictures. The question, of course, was does CLA do the same for people?

There's been a lot of research on CLA since then, and the results show it has a lot of potential. In one study, published in the *Journal of Nutrition* in 2000, researchers wrote, "The beneficial effects of CLA with regard to body fat mass and lean body mass … are promising." It appears they were right. In a number of studies since then, CLA has been shown to whittle away abdominal fat.

Just as this manuscript was being submitted, a new randomized, double-blind intervention trial was published in the *British Journal of Nutrition*. The researchers divided 118 overweight subjects into two groups and gave one of them about 3¹/₂ g per day of CLA and the other group a placebo. Those assigned to the CLA group lost a little more than 3 percent of body fat mass (compared to about a tenth of 1 percent in the placebo group).

Natural Prescription for Weight Loss

Hydroxycitric acid (from a product like Super CitriMax or Citrin K): 2,800 mg a day of HCA, taken in divided doses, three times a day, 30 minutes before a meal. (Remember to calculate the percentage of HCA in the supplement you're taking to arrive at the right supplement dosage. If it's 60 percent HCA, as in Super CitriMax, you'll need about 1,500 mg, three times a day, of the supplement.)

Conjugated linoleic acid (CLA): 3.4 g (again, check the percentage: if the pill is 80 percent CLA, you'll need about four pills a day)

EGCG (green tea extract): 270 mg per day and/or green tea, three cups a day (let it steep 3–5 minutes or more)

Chromium picolinate or chromium nicotinate (ChromeMate): 1,000 mcg (Jonathan Wright, M.D., uses much higher doses—3,000 to 4,000 mcg a day—with patients and then tapers down to 1,000 mcg for maintenance)

High-fiber diet: 35 mg or more daily from food or supplements

Adequate protein: A good guideline to start with is 30 percent of daily calories or one-third of each plate of food

Low-carb diet of moderate calories: 1,400 for women (105 g protein), 1,800 for men (135 g protein)

L-carnitine: 1,500 to 4,000 mg

Daily exercise: The more the better

Note: All dosages are daily dosages and in pill or capsule form unless otherwise noted.

But here's the thing: Compliance is always an issue in weight loss studies, and not everyone in this study complied with the CLA regimen. When the researchers adjusted for that fact and only included the folks who actually *took* the CLA as prescribed, the results were even more impressive: a loss of 5.6 percent body fat mass over six months. (Note to self: You have to take it for it to work!) Most fat loss was from the legs, primarily in women who were obese at the beginning of the study, and waist size decreased by more than one inch in the CLA group. Remarkably, these changes were independent of alterations in calorie intake or exercise level. The researchers stated, "This trial confirms several previous reports showing that CLA reduces body weight without reducing lean body mass."

Now without going into a lot of boring and technical stuff on biochemistry, it's important to note that CLA comes in a number of different forms, called *isomers*. (Isomers are chemical compounds that have exactly the same number and type of atoms, but in different arrangements—like, for example, the chemical equivalent of the words dog and god). The two most common isomers of CLA are called trans,9-cis,11 and trans,10-cis,12. Of course that's completely useless information for the majority of people in the world, certainly those who are not doing biochemical research. But what you *should* know is that studies can show different results depending on the form of CLA used. In some of the latest and most promising studies, researchers have used Tonalin CLA, which is a fifty-fifty mix of the two isomers.

Tonalin CLA is found in many brands of CLA (including the CLA product on my website, www.jonny bowden.com).

The dose of CLA that seems to be most effective is around 3.4 g a day. "But pay close attention to the label on the supplement," advises Preuss. "For example, a pill may be 1 g (1,000 mg), but contain only 80 percent CLA, thereby delivering 800 mg of CLA. Four of those pills a day would equal an intake of 3.2 g." (That should be fine for most purposes.)

CLA is a perfect example of why you can't always get what you want from food. It's only really found in serious amounts in milk and meat from ruminant animals, especially in products that come from grass-fed cows. Even then the average intake from those sources is tiny (less than 200 mg a day on average). To get the weight loss benefits (3 to 4 g a day), take a supplement with Tonalin CLA.

By the way, the benefits of CLA go way beyond the loss of fat. "In 2005, nearly 300 studies were published on CLA, including studies in which CLA slowed the spread of cancer cells, helped stop bone loss in postmenopausal women, calmed the inflammation of asthma, was linked to lower rates of colon cancer, and boosted immune function," Preuss says.

Two more supplements figure into our little combo cure for weight loss: green tea and chromium. Let's look at them one by one.

The Many Benefits of Green Tea

When I recorded my audio program, *Twenty-Three Ways to Improve Your Life*, I came up with close to two dozen relatively easy things you could do on a regular basis that would make a measurable and significant difference in your health and well-being. Since there are so many great things you can do to improve your health (and your life), it was hard to select which ones to include—but one that was a really easy choice, near the top of the list in fact, was this one: Drink green tea. Frequently. Every day if possible.

Green tea has more benefits than we can possibly cover in this one section, so let's just concentrate on its effect on weight and metabolism. We've known for a while that regular tea drinking seems to be associated with less body fat. In *Obesity Research* back in 2003, researchers investigated the relationship between tea drinking, body fat percentage, and body fat distribution and found that folks who drank tea on a regular basis for more than ten years had a 19.6 percent reduction in body fat and a 2.1 percent reduction in waist-hip ratio compared to non-tea drinkers. Now that could be due to any number of factors other than the tea drinking, but other research since then has pointed to the likelihood that there is indeed something in tea that helps you lose fat.

Green tea contains a plant compound called epigallocatechin gallate, mercifully abbreviated EGCG. This compound—a member of the catechin family—has multiple health benefits, but one of them is that it appears to increase metabolism. Some researchers have theorized that EGCG blocks the action of an enzyme that breaks down noradrenaline; noradrenaline stimulates many metabolic functions including heart rate and the release of energy from fat, so by allowing more of it to stick around, EGCG may actually "boost" your metabolism. And green tea contains a bit of caffeine, which may work synergistically to help get the job done. In one study, done by Abdul Dulloo, Ph.D., and his colleagues, subjects were given caffeine alone (50 mg), green tea extract plus caffeine (90 mg EGCG plus 50 mg caffeine), or a placebo. Dulloo then measured the subjects' energy expenditure (a measure of metabolic rate). Those who got the EGCG-caffeine combo had a significant increase in their energy expenditure, leading Dulloo to conclude that "green tea has thermogenic properties and promotes fat oxidation beyond that explained by its caffeine content per se."

More recently, Canadian researchers tested out different doses and mixes of EGCG and caffeine. They gave subjects 200 mg of caffeine together with either 90, 200, 300, or 400 mg of EGCG to be taken three times a day; the control group got a placebo. They found that there was a significant increase in energy expenditure for all the EGCG-caffeine mixtures, and interestingly, the results were pretty much same for all four doses. This led the researchers to conclude that 90 mg * 3 (or 270 mg) was the "optimal concentration" to produce calorie burning. It's worth pointing out that a lot of the antiobesity drugs on the market boost heart rate and blood pressure (in addition to helping you burn more calories). Green tea doesn't, at least not in any significant way.

"I highly and wholeheartedly recommend green tea as a supplement for the metabolically challenged, especially since it appears to have no adverse effects and so many health benefits," says my dear friend and author of *The Real Vitamin and Mineral Book*, nutritionist extraordinaire Shari Lieberman, Ph.D., C.N.S.

Last but Not Least: Chromium

Finally there's chromium. I talked about chromium's effect on blood sugar elsewhere in the book (page 46), but it's worth mentioning here as well. Though studies correlating chromium supplements with actual body fat loss are rare, it's still an important part of an overall fat-loss regimen, and here's why: Chromium absolutely helps insulin, the fat storage hormone, do its job more efficiently. That's a big deal.

Since high levels of insulin keep you from "burning" fat—essentially locking the doors to the fat cells and preventing fatty acids from being released into the bloodstream so they can be transported into the muscle cells and "burned" for energy—anything that helps keep insulin levels down is an important adjunct to a fat-loss program. Jonathan Wright, M.D., an icon in the field of integrative medicine for thirty years, regularly uses high doses of chromium to help curb carbohydrate cravings. And Harry Preuss, M.D., is a fan as well.

"Chromium plays a key role in the regulation of your insulin system," he says. For that reason alone, I think it makes sense to include chromium as part of the "natural cure" for being overweight. By itself, it's not going to melt off pounds. But it's a valuable adjunct to an overall strategy for fat loss.

Oh, one more thing. When I wrote the chapter on supplements for *Living the Low Carb Life: Choosing the Diet That's Right for You from Atkins to Zone*, I stated that the number-one supplement for weight control was … (drum roll, please) … fiber. Plain, old-fashioned, grandmother-endorsed fiber (which in grandma's day was called *roughage*). I've changed my opinion about a few things since writing that book—notably on CLA and HCA—but I haven't changed my mind about fiber. It's not expensive, it's not exotic, it's not sexy, but it works like a charm. More than a dozen clinical studies have used dietary fiber supplements for weight loss, most with positive outcomes.

When you take fiber supplements with water before meals, the water-soluble fiber binds to water in the stomach, making you feel full and less likely to overeat. Fiber supplements have also been shown to enhance blood sugar control and insulin effects and even to reduce the number of calories the body absorbs. A study in the prestigious *New England Journal of Medicine* found that a diet with 50 g of fiber a day lowered insulin levels in the blood. And another study, by David Ludwig, M.D., Ph.D., published in the *Journal of the American Medical Association*, found that people who consumed the most fiber gained the least weight over a period of ten years.

My friend, naturopath physician Andrew Rubman, N.D., is bullish on konjac fiber. The main ingredient in konjac root is a water-soluble dietary fiber called glucomannan, which is made from mannose and glucose sugars. However you get it—from food or supplements—a diet with at least 35 of mixed fiber a day is likely to produce a number of health benefits and will most likely help you in the battle of the bulge.

The Yeast Killers

for Candida albicans

THERE'S A FUNGUS among us. And its name is *Candida albicans*. Also known as candida vaginitis, candidiasis, thrush, and "that-annoying-itch-that-is-making-me crazy," yeast infections are just not fun.

Garlic

Caprylic Acid

Oil of Oregano

Probiotics

They are an overgrowth of the *Candida albicans* bacteria and are one of the most common reasons women consult health-care professionals. But if you're thinking we're just talking "female problems," think again. A yeast infection may sound like girl talk, but the mischief done by *Candida albicans* goes way beyond that most obvious of syndromes. That mischief affects both men and women, and it's hardly limited to private parts.

And it's serious.

A Gut Course in Ecology

Your gut, which is one of the most important and complex systems in the body and which Michael Gershon, M.D., aptly nicknamed "the second brain," is really akin to a complex ecological system. Think of it as a garden, populated by all sorts of beautiful flowers but plagued by annoying little weeds. If you keep those weeds in check, you've got a gorgeous garden. If you ignore them, they'll take over the garden,

squeeze out the roots of the flowers, and leave you with something that looks like the lawn in *Nightmare on Elm Street*.

The flowers in that garden are analogous to the "good" bacteria in your gut. Collectively known as probiotics, these include such beneficial species as *Bifidobacterium bifidum* and *Lactobacillus acidophilus*. But that gut garden of yours also has its weeds—chief among them, *Candida albicans*. When the ecology gets out of balance, candida grows and multiplies like weeds (or rabbits). While a vaginal yeast infection is one common symptom of that, it's far from the only damage yeast can do. Yeast can actually travel throughout the body and become a systemic infection, producing symptoms both mental and physical. And candida, being a living organism, produces waste products that can be allergenic for some people. Simply put, an overgrowth of candida is not your friend.

So how does this imbalance happen in the first place? Let's start with candida's favorite

COMBO CURES

food: sugar. Yeast thrives on sugar. Loves the stuff. Processed carbohydrates like breads and cereal are like "Miracle-Gro" for yeasty bugs.

Next, there are antibiotics, also known as candida's best friend. Why? Because, like a powerful weed killer that also kills your roses, antibiotics kill everything, making it even easier for candida to pop back up and overtake the farm. (Just like in your garden, it's easier for the weeds to come back than the roses.) Anyone on antibiotics for more than two weeks is at increased risk for an overgrowth of candida. Oral contraceptives, alcohol, caffeine, and immune suppressant medications (including corticosteroids) add to the problem. Put a high-sugar diet together with a course of antibiotics and you can pretty much guarantee you've got a serious candida problem.

It's a particularly insidious problem to have. Only in some cases are the symptoms localized and obvious—a vaginal yeast infection, for example, or a case of thrush, which is an overgrowth in the mouth. Most of the time the symptoms are general and somewhat ambiguous. You could experience anything from brain fog to fatigue to GI distress, rashes, hives, skin problems, or sinus infections—the connection to candida can be elusive. With such a wide range of diffuse symptoms, most people have no idea that they're infected with the little bugs. (One tip-off: Check under your toenails. If there's a fungus there, there's a good likelihood you've got yeast in your system.)

How Does Your Garden Grow?

What to do, what to do?

First thing is, you want to send some reinforcements for the good bacteria in your gut. Start with supplements of probiotics. These guys live in the small and large intestine and happily make vitamins for us, while keeping the overgrowth of the bad bugs in check. They boost the immune system and increase resistance to infection. Lactobacillus in particular is

Natural Prescription for Yeast Infections

Probiotics: 10-30 billion bacteria, in capsule or powder form. Take with food.

Diet: Eliminate sugar, alcohol, bread, moldy foods like cheeses, melons, and pistachios.

Caprylic acid: 500–2,000 mg, three times a day, with meals.

Oil of oregano: 250–500 mg, three times a day. Or drink oregano tea three times a day.

Garlic: 600–900 mg per day, in divided doses

★ **FOR ADDED EFFECTIVENESS:**

Boric acid suppositories: Insert into vagina. Never drink boric acid.

ALSO RECOMMENDED:

Pau d'arco tea: Steep for five minutes and drink three times a day. A natural antifungal agent.

Note: All the dosages above are daily and in pill or capsule form unless otherwise noted.

a species of friendly bacteria that is an integral part of normal vaginal flora; consider it a guard dog for candida overgrowth.

Probiotics offer a baker's dozen of health benefits. Remember that without a healthy, optimally functioning gut you can't properly absorb and utilize nutrients, so in a real sense a gut well tended to is the foundation of good health. Probiotics also have been shown to help prevent diarrhea and eczema, support the immune system, and reduce the frequency of the common cold.

Yogurt is the traditional source of beneficial bacteria; however, different brands of yogurt can vary greatly in their bacterial strain and potency. Look for something on the label that says "contains active cultures." Don't confuse that with "made from active cultures" because there may have been some living bacteria in the mix at one time, but heat and processing often kills them, so you want a product that actually contains active cultures, not just one that had them long ago. (And by the way, the only thing "frozen yogurt" has in common with real yogurt that contains probiotics is that they're both white.) I'm also a big fan of kefir (fermented milk), goat's milk yogurt, and Greek-style yogurt. And I'm not a big fan of the no-fat kind, which contains more sugar than the regular varieties.

Probiotics are also available in supplement form, in both capsule and powder. They're alive, so refrigerate them for best results.

Starve the Critters: The Anti-Yeast Diet

If you want to get rid of yeast, you have to starve them. And that means not giving them their favorite food: sugar. Remember, yeast thrives in a sweet, carbo-loaded environment. The best "anti-yeast" diets look like some version of the Atkins diet, at least for the first few weeks: no sugar, no processed carbs (grains, pastas, breads, and cereal products), no alcohol, vinegar, fruits, aged cheeses, peanuts, melons, and soy products, at least not in the beginning. Sorry to say, but beer is quite simply an infusion of yeast, so stay away. (Actually, except for the "no-fruit" rule, an anti-yeast diet is a pretty healthy way to eat. After you've gotten rid of them, you can always add back stuff, especially the fruit.)

Here are some suggestions for your anti-yeast arsenal.

Coconut Oil

If you read my previous book, *The 150 Healthiest Foods on Earth*, you know I am an unabashed fan of coconut oil, one of nature's leading antifungal foods. It contains medium-chain fatty acids that help the body eliminate yeast. As a cooking oil, it is unmatched in its ability to tolerate a wide range of heat without burning or scorching. For those with systemic yeast overgrowth, ingesting 2 to 4 tablespoons of coconut oil daily is very beneficial.

If you're mainly concerned with the more localized and specific form of a yeast problem, the common vaginal yeast infection, you can consider adding a douche to the natural prescription (above). Remember that the vaginal yeast infection is just one manifestation of candida, so it's a good idea not to skip the dietary and supplement recommendations. That said, a douche of one of the following may be a nice addition to the program. According to my associates, nutritionists Suzanne Copp, M.S., and Susan Mudd, M.S., C.N.S., these are all effective, so choose one that appeals to you and give it a try:

Boric acid: Studies show the effectiveness of boric acid as a douche is very high, especially in women with chronic resistant yeast infections. One study with 100 women showed a 98 percent success rate with this condition.

Boric acid suppositories, containing 600 mg of boric acid, have been used successfully as a treatment for vaginal yeast infections. The suppositories were inserted vaginally twice a day for two weeks, then continued for an additional two weeks if necessary. Boric acid should never be swallowed.

Garlic: Insert a garlic clove into the vagina in the morning and an acidophilus capsule in the evening for three to seven days.

Combo douche: Prepare a retention douche (in which the preparation of substances stays in the vagina and is not flushed out) with equal parts bentonite clay, pau d'arco tea, yogurt, tea tree oil, and goldenseal, and douche two times a day for seven to ten days.

Tea tree oil: Soak a tampon with diluted tea tree oil and keep it in the vagina overnight.

Caprylic Acid

Caprylic acid is one of the fatty acids found in coconut oil and is also available as a separate supplement. Nutritionists and natural health practitioners have relied on it for years as a dependable yeast slayer. Its antifungal effect has been demonstrated in clinical trials. Though the exact mechanism of its action against yeast isn't completely understood, we think it penetrates and destabilizes the yeast cell walls. Caprylic acid is absorbed very rapidly, so capsules should be enteric coated or timed release for best results

Garlic

Known as Russian penicillin, garlic is considered nature's premier antibiotic and antifungal, which makes it a perfect adversary for candida. It's like a stealth smart-bomb—it's effective against bad bacteria and yeast but leaves the body's normal, friendly bugs unharmed. Several studies demonstrate the power of garlic to combat candida, with some showing garlic to be more powerful than nystatin, gentian violet, and other standard antifungal agents.

Oil of Oregano

Oil of oregano has been used for years in the treatment of candida, and studies have demonstrated the effectiveness of oils in the destruction of candida. In fact, oil of oregano is such a powerful antimicrobial that it prompted one physician, Cass Ingram, D.O., to write a book on it, aptly titled *The Cure Is in the Cupboard*. Wild oregano as well as extracts of olive leaf are recognized for their potent antifungal, antibacterial, antiviral, and antiparasitic properties. Oregano can be made into a tea by steeping 1 to 2 teaspoons of the dried herb in hot water for ten minutes. You can drink the tea three times a day. You can also take both oil of oregano and olive oil extract as supplements. Note: If you're pregnant, don't use oil of oregano, as it may induce miscarriage.

FOOD CURES

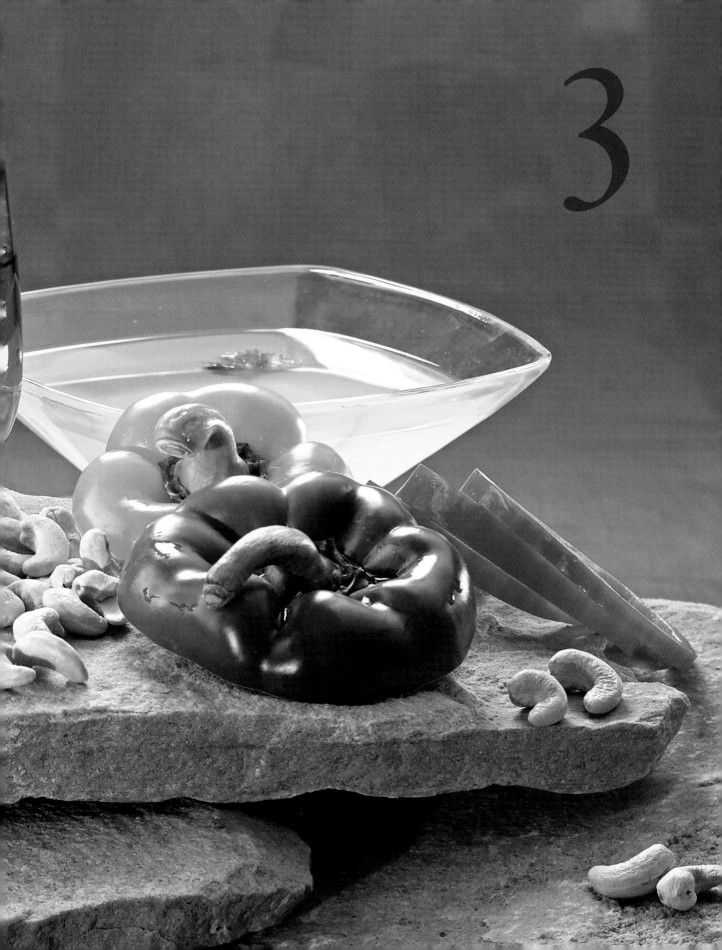

3

Celery
for High Blood Pressure

HERE ARE TEN WORDS you probably haven't heard your doctor say in a while: "Take four celery sticks and call me in the morning." But if you have high blood pressure, that's exactly what you should do.

Now let's be clear: Celery alone isn't going to "cure" hypertension. But peer-reviewed research has found that eating four sticks of celery a day lowers blood pressure. A Chinese study found that blood pressure fell significantly in fourteen out of sixteen people with hypertension when they were given celery. Mark Houston, my go-to guy for all things hypertension and the medical director of the Hypertension Institute in Nashville, recommends celery or celery extract as part of the institute's protocol for lowering blood pressure naturally.

The substances in celery that produce the benefits are phytochemicals called phthalides. When animals are given a dose of a phthalide (*3-n-butyl phthalide*) that is equal to four stalks of celery in humans, their blood pressure drops by a respectable 13 percent on average. Clinical studies show that phthalides work by relaxing the muscle tissue in the artery walls. Relaxed muscle tissue in the artery walls translates to increased blood flow and a reduction in blood pressure. As an added benefit, phthalides also lower stress hormones, which can contribute to and aggravate nearly every known disease and cause a few of their own.

For centuries, traditional Chinese medicine doctors have recommended celery for high blood pressure. It makes sense for anyone with this serious condition to include celery in their diet on a daily basis.

Celery also contains silicon, an important nutrient for bone health. Because of its silicon content, celery can help renew joints, bones, arteries, and all connective tissue. It also contains acetylenics, which have been shown to stop the growth of cancer cells, as well as *phenolic acids*, which block the action of compounds in the body known to encourage the growth of cancerous tumors.

And celery is also a dieter's best friend. Smear some peanut or almond butter on it for a stick-to-your-ribs snack and energy pick-me-up. It combines wonderfully with other vegetables, or with fruit, in a juicer. One of my favorite juice recipes: one pear, several stalks of celery, and a few inches of gingerroot, thrown together in a juice maker.

Cherries

for Gout

ONE ITEM I CAN guarantee you'll see on the recommended list of just about any integrative medicine approach to gout is this: Eat more cherries. More on that in a moment.

Gout, also known as metabolic arthritis, is a painful, largely inherited disorder in which the body can't properly metabolize uric acid. Usually the bloodstream contains a small amount of the stuff, but in gout there's a lot of it. The body doesn't know what to do with the excess so it bunches it up into nasty little crystals that get deposited in areas like the big toe and the joints, causing a lot of pain and discomfort.

Nutritionally minded health-care professionals and other healers have known for eons that cherries help relieve the pain of gout, but now we have a scientific explanation for why. Compounds in cherries lower levels of uric acid in the blood. Less uric acid, fewer disposal problems, fewer crystals, less pain. A study at the University of California–Davis showed that consuming two servings' worth of cherries daily (280 g total) after an overnight fast significantly lowered the blood uric acid of women by as much as 15 percent. And in another study, volunteers' blood levels of uric acid decreased significantly up to five hours after a breakfast meal of forty-five fresh, pitted Bing cherries.

The Power of Red: The Miracle of Anthocyanins

As with most natural cures in the plant kingdom, the secret is in the color. Nature gives fruits and vegetables protection against their natural predators and other destructive forces (like the sun), and many of these protective compounds are what give the fruits their color. The red in raspberries and cherries, the blue in blueberries, and the orange in peppers all contain powerful plant chemicals that have antioxidant, anti-inflammatory, and frequently anti-cancer activity.

The secret to the benefits of cherries and cherry juice are compounds called anthocyanins. These are the particular pigments in cherries that give them their bright red color and are considered to be the key to helping the body relieve inflammation. It's believed that the anthocyanins in the cherries cause the decrease in uric acid and the relief from the pain of gout.

Anthocyanins act like natural COX-2 inhibitors. COX stands for cyclooxygenase, which is produced in the body in two major flavors, COX-1 and COX-2. It's the latter that is responsible for signaling pain and inflammation. Aspirin tends to block both, but COX-1 has some valuable uses. Some years ago, a popular class of arthritis drugs was developed that were known as COX-2 inhibitors; they inhibited the pain-signaling COX-2 molecules without touching the non-inflammatory COX-1s. The problem was, there were some really serious side effects with some of these drugs—such as the increased risk of blood clotting and heart attack—and at least one, Vioxx, was taken off the market. But anthocyanins produce a similar effect with none of the side effects.

Cherries (and raspberries) have the highest yields of pure anthocyanins. In one study, the COX inhibitory activity of anthocyanins from cherries was comparable to those of ibuprofen and naproxen. And researchers feel that in addition to helping with pain and inflammation, anthocyanins may help lower heart attack and stroke risk if consumed on a regular basis. As a bonus, these same anthocyanins may significantly reduce your risk for colon cancer, the third leading cancer in the United States.

But That's Not All, Folks!

Besides anthocyanins, cherries have three other compounds in them that are of great interest to the field of natural healing: quercetin, ellagic acid, and perillyl alcohol.

Quercetin has been found to be a potent anticancer, as well as a powerful anti-inflammatory, agent (see page 101, allergies and asthma). And in animal research, ellagic acid inhibits the growth of certain tumors. The American Cancer Society's *Guide to Complementary and Alternative Cancer Methods* calls ellagic acid a promising natural supplement, largely because in lab studies it caused the death of cancer cells while leaving normal, healthy cells alone.

Perillyl alcohol inhibits tumor growth in animal models of pancreatic, stomach, colon, skin, and liver cancer. It's so promising that the Cleveland Clinic Taussig Cancer Center is currently running a multiple-dose trial of perillyl alcohol on healthy women who have a history of breast cancer.

Cherry juice is another way to get the gout-relieving benefits of cherries. In my book *The 150 Healthiest Foods on Earth*, I shared one of my favorite desserts: frozen cherries. (You can get them in almost any grocery.) I take them directly from the freezer, put them in a bowl, and mix them with raw milk or yogurt, which promptly freezes on the cold cherries, forming a kind of cherry-flavored sherbet. Top with slivered almonds and enjoy!

Chicken Soup
for Colds and Souls

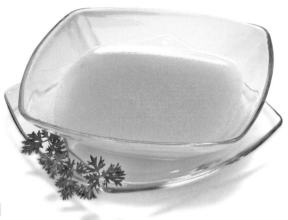

STEPHEN RENNARD, M.D., is the Larson Professor of Medicine at the University of Nebraska Medical Center. Bachelor's degree from Harvard, medical degree with honors from Baylor University, board certified in internal medicine and pulmonary disease, author of more than 300 scientific articles. Get the picture?

So one day this esteemed doctor and researcher was making chicken soup for the Jewish holidays with his wife, Barbara. And they started chatting about how good it is for colds.

Pause for a moment for editorial comment.

Years ago, when I was a "blond," I was having my hair bleached one day, and let me tell you, it burned. The hairdresser said, "Hey, let me put some sugar or Sweet'N Low on it; it takes away the burn." My reaction: Huh? Until she put it on. It was like magic. No burn, soothing as aloe vera gel. I've since shared this discovery with other folks, and every one of them reports the same thing.

Being a good academic, I did a literature search, and guess what: There's not a single piece of research anywhere in the world showing that sugar or Sweet'N Low, applied to the scalp while bleaching your hair, completely kills the burn.

But it works.

Consider how many things in life your grandmother knew about that "worked," even though no one had ever done a double-blind, randomized control study on them. My friend, the great nutritionist (and humorist) Robert Crayhon, used to say, "There's never been a double-blind study showing that water puts out fires. Yet the entire New York fire department considers that to be a pretty good working hypothesis!"

Back to the Rennard kitchen and chicken soup.

So there are the Rennards, preparing the soup in the kitchen and speculating on why it is a miracle remedy for colds. They theorized that maybe it has anti-inflammatory properties, which alone would make it good medicine if for no other reason than it would soothe sore throats and other inflammatory cold or flu symptoms. Being the researcher that he is,

Rennard got the bright idea that perhaps they could test the theory out in his lab.

Which they did.

And voilá—they found that the ingredients in chicken soup stop the movement of white blood cells called neutrophils that get released when you have an infection or cold. (Just for the record—and to bring a smile to your face—the title of the actual published study was *Chicken Soup Inhibits Neutrophil Chemotaxis in Vitro.* And no, I'm not making that up.) Neutrophils are the most abundant kind of white blood cell in the body and an important part of the immune system. (They're the predominant cells in pus, and the reason it's white. Thought you'd like to know.)

Now don't get me wrong—neutrophils are important to the immune system. Their job is to eat up microorganisms. You *want* them working for you when you get sick. But the movement of neutrophils toward the site of an infection is an inflammatory response. Neutrophils can also stimulate the release of

WORTH KNOWING

There's a reason chicken soup has a reputation as being good for the soul as well as for the body, and it's called TLC (tender loving care). As Stephen Rennard, M.D., Larson Professor of Medicine at the University of Nebraska Medical Center, told CNN, "You can't rule out the TLC factor.... If you know someone prepared soup for you by hand, that might have an effect."

mucus, which contributes to the annoying symptoms of upper respiratory infections like colds. The researchers suspected that slowing the movement of neutrophils might reduce activity in the upper respiratory tract that is responsible for many cold symptoms.

Not for nothing is chicken soup known as Jewish penicillin.

Grandma's Chicken Soup Recipe

Here's a recipe for chicken soup, adapted from the one Stephen Rennard and his wife made in their kitchen. Other versions of chicken soup also are effective, including many that are store bought.*

3 large onions
1 large sweet potato
3 parsnips
2 turnips
11 to 12 large carrots
1 (5- to 6-pound [2.3 to 2.7 kg]) stewing hen or baking chicken
1 (1-pound [455 g]) package of chicken wings
5 or 6 celery stems
1 bunch of parsley
Salt and pepper to taste

Chop the onions. Leaving the skin on, chop the sweet potato, parsnips, turnips, and carrots. Set aside.

Clean the hen or chicken, put it in a large stovetop pot, and cover it with cold water. Bring the water to a boil. Add the chicken wings, onions, sweet potato, parsnips, turnips, and carrots.

Reduce heat and simmer for $1^1/_2$ hours. Remove fat from the surface of the water as it accumulates.

Add the celery and parsley. Simmer the mixture about 45 minutes longer. Remove the chicken. The chicken is not used further for the soup. (The meat makes excellent chicken parmesan.)

With a measuring cup or ladle, scoop the broth and vegetable mixture into a food processor or blender. Purée the mixture in batches, setting the puréed mixture aside while puréeing the next batch. When all vegetables have been puréed, return the puréed soup to the pot and add salt and pepper to taste. Note: The soup freezes well.

Matzoh balls were prepared according to the recipe on the back of the box of Manischewitz matzoh meal. Add to soup as desired.

*Researchers tested thirteen different brands of commercial soup as well as the recipe above. Interestingly, five inhibited neutrophils and inflammation even more than Grandma's Chicken Soup Recipe, but two did nothing whatsoever and one actually worked in the opposite direction of the good stuff.

Cinnamon

for High Blood Sugar

"YOU HAVE HIGH blood sugar." Those are five words you'd really rather *not* hear from your doctor at your next checkup. High blood sugar is the first step down a road that can easily lead to metabolic syndrome (a kind of prediabetes that puts you at considerable risk for heart disease) or even diabetes itself. When your blood sugar is high, all kinds of metabolic events occur, none of them good.

Foremost among them is an overproduction of the "sugar-clearing" hormone insulin. One of the jobs of insulin is to clear the bloodstream of excess sugar. The more sugar in your bloodstream, the more insulin the pancreas has to send out to get the job done. While insulin is necessary for life, too much of it can set you up for high blood pressure. Insulin sends a message to the kidneys that says "Hold on to the sodium, dude!" This in turn means you have to hold on to more water to balance the excess sodium. Excess sodium plus excess water translates into high blood pressure—an enormous risk factor for heart disease. Insulin is also known as "the fat storage hormone." High levels of circulating insulin make it fiendishly difficult to lose weight.

Even more frightening, high blood sugar is being linked to a significant increase in the risk of cancer. A major European study, part of the Vasterbotten Intervention Project in Northern Sweden and published in the March 2007 issue of *Diabetes Care*, found that hyperglycemia (high blood sugar) was associated with an increase in total cancer risk in women. The researchers found that women whose blood sugar readings were in the top 25 percent of women tested had a 26 percent higher chance of developing cancer than those whose readings were in the bottom quarter. Another study, involving more than a million people and published in the *Journal of the American Medical Association* in 2004, found that men with the highest fasting blood sugar levels (greater than 140 mg/dl) were 29 percent more likely to die of cancer than those with blood sugar levels of 90 mg/dl or less. The association was strongest for pancreatic cancer. High blood sugar (greater than 125 mg/dl) almost doubled the risk for men and more than doubled the risk for women.

"It puzzles me why the simple concept *'sugar feeds cancer'* can be so dramatically overlooked in a comprehensive cancer treatment plan," says my friend, Joe Mercola, D.O., author of *Dr. Mercola's Total Health Plan*.

Have I convinced you yet that controlling your blood sugar should be one of your top health priorities?

The Proof is in the Phytochemicals

Enter cinnamon. Though cinnamon has a formidable reputation as a health-giving compound, the newest, hottest buzz about it has to do with its uncanny ability to moderate blood sugar. C. Leigh Broadhurst, Ph.D., a researcher at the U.S. Department of Agriculture (USDA), says many plants and individual phytochemicals can lower blood sugar, but many of them accomplish this at a price of imposing some nasty toxic costs on the body. Not cinnamon. Broadhurst and her team at the USDA have identified new phytochemicals in cinnamon called chalcone polymers that increase glucose metabolism in the cells twenty-fold or more. And with nary a side effect in sight.

USDA researchers tested the effects of forty-nine different herbs, spices, and medicinal plants on blood sugar metabolism and published their results in the prestigious *Journal of the American College of Nutrition* in 2001. Cinnamon was the star of the show. The active ingredient—*methylhydroxychalcone polymer*, or MHCP— seems to mimic insulin function, increasing the uptake of sugar by the cells and signaling certain kinds of cells to turn glucose (plain blood sugar) into glycogen (the storage form of sugar).

In 2003 researchers from the Department of Human Nutrition at NWFP Agricultural University in Pakistan, working with Richard Anderson, Ph.D., from the Beltsville Human Nutrition Research Center in Maryland, tested the effects of cinnamon on blood glucose as well as other important blood measures like triglycerides and cholesterol in people with type 2 diabetes: They found that even 1 g of

---

Natural Prescription for High Blood Sugar

Cinnamon tea: 8 oz, 2 or 3 times a day

Cinnamon: used as a spice as often as possible

Chromium: 800–1,000 mcg

★ **FOR ADDED EFFECTIVENESS:**

Low-carbohydrate diet

Gymnema sylvestre: 200 mg of extract twice daily (optional)

Magnesium: 400–800 mg

Biotin: 8–16 mg

For the management of diabetes, a fuller program is necessary, which should include omega-3 fatty acids, alpha lipoic acid, and a B-complex vitamin at the very least.

Note: All dosages are daily dosages and in pill or capsule form unless otherwise noted.

cinnamon a day reduced blood sugar (18 percent to 29 percent), triglycerides (23 percent to 30 percent), LDL cholesterol (7 percent to 27 percent), and total cholesterol (12 percent to 26 percent). Not bad for a little brown spice you can get in any grocery store for a couple of bucks.

More recently, in a series of ingenious experiments, Harry Preuss, M.D., C.N.S., and his colleagues at Georgetown University Medical Center found that cinnamon reduced the systolic blood pressure of rats with high blood pressure. Interestingly, in these particular experiments the cinnamon didn't reduce the rodents' blood sugar, but it *did* reduce their insulin levels.

Sip Your Medicine

Broadhurst says the best way to use cinnamon to help lower blood sugar and improve type 2 diabetes is to put three rounded tablespoons of ground cinnamon in ¹/₂ to 1 teaspoon of baking soda (less if sodium is a problem for you) in a 32-ounce (quart) canning jar. Fill the jar with boiling water and let it steep at room temperature until it's cool. Strain or decant the liquid, discard the grounds, put a lid on the jar, and stick it in the fridge. Drink one 8-ounce cup of the tea four times per day. After one to three weeks you can drop down to one or two cups a day, but you don't have to—it tastes good, it's a great way to increase your water intake, and it's healthy as can be.

People with type l diabetes can use it, too, but should start with only one or two cups per

<aside>

WORTH KNOWING

Because cinnamon can affect insulin and blood sugar, work with your health-care practitioner on adding this natural prescription to your routine if you currently take insulin or medications for high blood sugar.

</aside>

day and increase by one cup per week, all the while monitoring blood sugar closely. Licensed naturopathic physician Cathy Wong, author of *The Inside Out Diet*, recommends placing ¹/₄ teaspoon of ground cinnamon in a cup, adding 1 cup of boiling water, and steeping for ten minutes. (For variety, she suggests throwing in a bag of black tea with the cinnamon and sweetening with stevia.)

"If you don't like the look or texture of tea made with ground cinnamon, try bringing water to a boil with a piece of cinnamon bark added to it," she advises.

One of the coolest parts of the whole cinnamon story is that the best results are gotten with the cheapest stuff, according to Broadhurst. You definitely don't need the esoteric (and expensive) oil extracts. "Buying cinnamon in bulk is cost effective and highly recommended," she told me.

Meanwhile, I sprinkle the stuff on everything. (It's particularly good on oatmeal.) I even use it on my morning Starbucks, as it's thoughtfully provided by the company—right at the counter next to the half and half.

Cranberry Juice
for Urinary Tract Infection

IF YOU'VE EVER HAD a urinary tract infection (UTI)—and you'd know if you had—you know it's not particularly pleasant. Urinary tract infections are a serious health problem, and they affect millions of people. (They're actually the second most common type of infection in the body.) Though women are more prone to get them than men, men are hardly immune. An enlarged prostate gland, for example, can slow the flow of urine and raise the risk of infection. What to do, what to do?

For ages, people believed that cranberry juice was the answer, at least in the short run. When I was in college and not even thinking about a career in nutrition, I remember women advising each other to "drink some cranberry juice" whenever they had the familiar burning that signaled a UTI. Decades later, it appears the folk wisdom on cranberries, like so much of folk medicine, has a real basis in scientific fact. A great deal of research has supported the ability of compounds in cranberries and cranberry juice to help maintain the health of the urinary tract.

Here's how it works: Urine is normally sterile and free of bacteria, but sometimes tiny organisms like bacteria from the digestive tract make their way to the opening of the urethra. Then they do what bacteria like to do—they

multiply. When that happens, infection is right around the corner. (An infection that stays in the urethra is called *urethritis*, and if it moves up to the bladder it causes an infection called cystitis. It can even move further up the ureters and infect the kidney in which case it's called *pyelonephritis*, but that's a whole other story.)

Nature designed the urinary system in such a way as to help prevent infection; the flow of urine itself helps wash away bacteria. But like all defense systems, it doesn't always work properly, and urinary tract infections still occur. Frequently.

In 1999, UTIs accounted for more than 8 million visits to the doctor, and according to the 1988–1994 National Health and Nutrition Survey, 34 percent of adults over 20 in the

United States reported having at least one occurrence of a urinary tract infection.

Cranberry juice can—and does—help.

Cranberry Compounds to the Rescue

Cranberries contain important plant compounds called *proanthocyanidins* that are probably responsible for cranberry's remarkably positive effects on urinary tract infections. The bacteria responsible for the majority of UTIs are the ever popular *E. coli*. An 8 ounce serving of cranberry juice cocktail prevented *E. coli* from adhering to bladder cells in the urine of six volunteers, according to a study by Amy Howell, Ph.D., research scientist at the Marucci Center for Blueberry and Cranberry Research at Rutgers University, and Jess Reed, Ph.D., professor of nutrition at the University of Wisconsin–Madison. Interestingly, the equivalent amount of grape juice, apple juice, green tea, or chocolate—all rich sources of proanthocyanidins or related compounds—did not produce the same result.

"The cranberry's proanthocyanidins are structurally different than the proanthocyanidins found in the other plant foods tested, which may explain why cranberry has unique bacterial anti-adhesion activity and helps to maintain urinary tract health," Howell says.

Best of all, new research seems to point to the use of cranberries for preventing urinary tract infections in the first place. One study published in the *British Medical Journal* in 2001 found that women who regularly drank a cranberry juice beverage over the course of a year had a statistically significant 20 percent reduc-

Natural Prescription for Urinary Tract Infections

Unsweetened cranberry juice: 1–2 eight-ounce glasses per day

tion in the risk of getting an infection. Another study found that taking cranberry extract tablets or drinking unsweetened cranberry juice significantly reduced the number of patients having at least one symptomatic UTI per year.

"Cranberry appears to be a safe, herbal choice for UTI prophylaxis and has relatively good tolerability. The most recent studies have found that the use of cranberry for up to 12 months is safe and moderately effective," says Darren M. Lynch, M.D., of Beth Israel Medical Center in New York, writing in the peer-reviewed journal *American Family Physician*.

Healing Nutrients from the Plant Kingdom

My good friend Ann Louise Gittleman, Ph.D., C.N.S., the "First Lady of Nutrition" and author of the excellent *Fat Flush Plan*, has touted unsweetened cranberry juice diluted with water for as long as I've known her (going on ten years!). She points out that cranberry juice is a rich source of phytonutrients such as *anthocyanins*, *catechins*, *lutein* (the new superstar of eye nutrition), and *quercetin* (one of the most powerful natural anti-inflammatories in the plant kingdom). These phytonutrients act as antioxidants and, according to Gittleman, provide nutritional support for the detoxification pathways in the body.

The rich phytonutrient content of both cranberries and cranberry juice has been borne out by research and may have an awful lot of benefits that go beyond relief from urinary tract infection. In one study, biochemist Yuegang Zuo, Ph.D., from the University of Massachusetts Dartmouth, showed that cranberry juice cocktail had the highest total phenol content of twenty fruit juices tested. (Phenolic compounds are natural antioxidants. They help neutralize harmful free radicals in the body that are linked to most chronic diseases, including cancer, heart disease, and diabetes.)

Zuo and his team stated that "cranberry has the highest radical-scavenging capacity among the different fruits studied." Even more wonderful, Catherine Neto, Ph.D., assistant professor at the University of Massachusetts Dartmouth, found compounds in the berries that were toxic to a variety of cancer tumor cells. "The tumor cell lines that these compounds inhibited most in our assays included lung, cervical, prostate, breast, and leukemia," she says.

Debating the Dose

Different doses and formulations of cranberries have been used in studies on UTIs, and some researchers have argued that we don't really know the optimal dose, which is probably true. Gittleman, for example, has her "fat flushers" sip a "cran-cocktail" made of one part

---

WORTH KNOWING

One small study found that cranberry juice could raise urinary oxalate levels, prompting a caution that regular use of cranberry may increase the risk of kidney stone formation in patients with a history of oxalate stones.

I mention this only in the interests of being fair and balanced. Truth be told, cranberry juice has been a folk medicine treatment for kidney stones for a long time. The highly regarded naturopathic physician Michael Murray, N.D., says that for those prone to kidney stones, cranberry is the juice of choice.

The discrepancy probably comes from the fact that there are several types of kidney stones; the two most common are formed from either calcium or oxalate. Cranberry juice does contain oxalates, so theoretically it may increase the risk for those kinds of stones if you're prone to them. (Other foods contain way more—coffee, for example.)

On the other hand, Murray points out that cranberry juice reduces the amount of calcium in your urine. He even recommends two 8-ounce glasses daily as a preventive measure. In any case, three of the best things you can do to prevent kidney stones in the first place are to eat a diet high in potassium (fruits and vegetables), take magnesium and B6 supplements, and drink a ton of water. (For more on kidney stones, see page 154.)

---

unsweetened cranberry juice to three to four parts water all day long.

In one particularly respected study, the dose given was 8 ounces of unsweetened cranberry juice three times a day or one tablet of concentrated cranberry extract (300 to 400 mg) twice a day. That's an awful lot of cranberry juice. I can't prove it, but I suspect that you'd get some benefit drinking less than the three 8 ounce glasses a day used in that study, which in any case would be hard to do since the unsweetened kind—which is clearly the best—is pretty bitter.

Bitter or not, the unsweetened kind is the way to go. Most of the "cranberry juice drinks" in the supermarket are full of sugar and have no more than about 10 percent cranberry juice. Go for the real deal. Dilute it, drink it, sweeten if you must with xylitol or stevia, but get the powerful health benefits of this terrific berry.

Low-Carb Diet
for Polycystic Ovary Syndrome

WHEN I HEAR the three words polycystic ovary syndrome (PCOS), the first thing I think of is insulin resistance. And the next thing I think of is *low-carb* diet. Let me explain.

PCOS is both a metabolic and a hormonal disorder. No one knows exactly what causes it, but there are a number of risk factors (see below). As the name suggests, it's a *syndrome*, which means it's more like a collection of multiple symptoms than an actual *disease*. Many doctors who see women with these symptoms don't necessarily

connect the dots, and many women seek treatment for the individual symptoms from specialists who may miss the larger picture.

It can go completely undiagnosed because its symptoms overlap with so many other health concerns. Many women—and their doctors—wind up treating the symptoms of PCOS, such as acne or infertility, as separate and discrete problems. They'll go to a dermatologist about their acne, for example, and call it a day, never suspecting that the acne is just a symptom of a whole underlying process. The result? Many women who have PCOS don't actually know it.

The Insulin Connection

One thing that almost always goes with PCOS is weight gain, and women with PCOS find it fiendishly difficult to lose weight, even with dieting and exercise. One thing we know for sure is that women with PCOS are much more likely to have a condition called *insulin resistance*, which is also associated with metabolic syndrome and type 2 diabetes. (More on insulin resistance in a moment.) Our diet can significantly aggravate the condition of insulin resistance, which is why dietary intervention can be so effective in all conditions where insulin resistance is a problem.

In my opinion, a low carb diet is the absolute best strategy for dealing with PCOS naturally. It doesn't mean that other things won't help, but rather that the first place to begin is with diet. In fact, according to many experts, one of the biggest contributors to PCOS is poor diet, especially a high intake of refined carbohydrates. Because insulin resistance is such a huge contributor to the PCOS, a diet that helps control blood sugar and insulin is the first order of business. Too much sugar, or foods that convert quickly into sugar, like potatoes and starches, causes a rise in insulin, a hormone that not only aggravates PCOS but also contributes to weight gain.

The weight gain–PCOS connection is a classic chicken-and-egg dilemma. We're not sure whether women get PCOS because they are overweight (or obese) or whether they become overweight (or obese) because they have PCOS in the first place. We do know, however, that the two are intimately connected. Fifty percent of women with PCOS are overweight.

Do You Have PCOS?

No single blood test can determine whether you have PCOS, so it takes a bit of detective work to identify what's really going on. It's estimated that 5 to 10 percent of women of childbearing age have PCOS. Some of the symptoms include:

- Menstrual irregularities: infrequent periods, no periods, or irregular bleeding
- Infertility or the inability to get pregnant due to not ovulating
- Facial hair (or hair on chest, stomach, back, thumbs, or toes)
- Acne
- Weight gain or obesity
- Thinning hair (or male pattern hair loss)

PCOS sufferers have an increased risk for some very serious diseases. Later in life, women with PCOS are at higher risk for developing type 2 diabetes, high blood pressure, heart disease, and cancer.

Ovarian Cysts

As the name of the disorder suggests, women with PCOS frequently have many ovarian cysts. The cysts don't necessarily rupture, but if they do it can be agonizing, even though it's not necessarily medically dangerous.

Each month the ovaries cause a number of follicles to ripen. These follicles are actually cysts, pockets of tissue filled with fluid and hormones (mostly estrogen). Normally, one (or two) of these follicles become dominant and actually produce an egg. The egg pops out of the follicle and goes into the fallopian tube, which in turn triggers a whole bunch of hormonal events such as the secretion of progesterone that in turn will help support a pregnancy if the egg is fertilized. In this "normal" scenario, the egg becomes a little factory (the corpus luteum) for making progesterone, and the concentration of progesterone in the body can become a couple of hundred times higher than estrogen. That's normal. If there's no fertilization, the "factory" stops its hormonal production of estrogen and progesterone and the uterine lining sheds, resulting in a menstrual period. The low levels of hormones then cause the cycle to begin all over again.

But with PCOS, a lot of follicles are created but no one follicle becomes predominant. Ovulation is disrupted, making it very difficult to get pregnant. (Women with PCOS have a 10 to 15 percent greater risk of miscarriage than women without it.) Estrogen becomes dominant and isn't balanced by sufficient progesterone, and other hormones, called androgens, remain high. The result is a host of symptoms, triggered by or aggravated by a hormonal imbalance characterized by elevated levels of male hormones and low levels of progesterone.

These hormonal imbalances prevent ovulation from taking place regularly and cause the ovaries to form multiple cysts. Adding to the difficulty in identifying the underlying problem is the fact that 30 percent of women with PCOS don't actually present with cysts.

Enter insulin.

A Low-Carb Diet Is the Answer

High-carbohydrate diets stimulate high blood sugar, which in turn stimulates high levels of insulin, especially in susceptible people. High levels of insulin then stimulate the androgen receptors on the outside of the ovary, which may lead to more cysts as well as other problems related to too much androgen production. And high insulin levels are thought to increase the production of male hormones. Thus high levels of insulin are intimately connected to the typical PCOS symptoms of excess facial hair, thin hair on the head, and acne. The high level of insulin

Natural Prescription for Polycystic Ovary Syndrome

Low-carb (low-glycemic) diet

Goes well with:

Chromium picolinate or polynicotinate: 1,000 mcg

Biotin: 8–16 mg

Note: All dosages are daily dosages and in pill or capsule form unless otherwise noted.

also further increases the risk of obesity. Bringing down insulin (and the blood sugar that drives it up) becomes a priority.

You know, when we talk about insulin resistance, we tend to forget that not all tissues and cells become resistant at the same time. In fact, some don't become resistant at all. For example, overweight people may—at least in the beginning—have very nonresistant fat cells. In fact, far from being resistant to its siren call, their fat cells may just love insulin and sugar. Their *muscle* cells may refuse to take any more sugar, but the fat cells say, "Hey, bring it on!" These fat cells are said to be insulin *sensitive*.

And guess what? The ovaries also tend to remain insulin sensitive. That means that if there's a genetic predisposition for the ovaries to overproduce androgen hormones—as there is with women who have PCOS—the excess insulin that's sent into the bloodstream to deal with the excess sugar winds up bathing these nonresistant tissues in an ocean of insulin that's way too much for their needs. And one of the responses to all that insulin hitting the ovaries is that they produce even more testosterone and androstenedione, which leads to hair loss, acne, obesity, infertility, and other symptoms of PCOS.

Enter the low-carb diet, the perfect "natural" solution to high levels of insulin and to the problem of insulin resistance.

Conventional Medicine: An Incomplete Answer

Conventional medicine usually treats PCOS with drugs that lower levels of male hormones (androgens) or with diabetes medications that help the body to utilize insulin better. For women who don't want to become pregnant, docs will sometimes use birth control pills to help regulate menstrual cycles, clear up acne, and reduce levels of male hormones, but the Pill does not cure PCOS.

Metformin, a drug known by its trade name of Glucophage, is often given to people with diabetes or metabolic syndrome because it helps the body utilize insulin more effectively. Research published in the *British Medical Journal* and elsewhere shows that metformin is effective in helping women with PCOS achieve ovulation, and it reduces insulin concentrations and blood pressure as well. It also helps patients lose

Without getting into the complex biochemistry of the sympathetic nervous system, understand that stress can elevate hormones that in turn contribute to excessive insulin and blood sugar. Biofeedback, stress reduction, and meditation have been shown to reduce a hormone that stimulates many of the physiological processes that can aggravate or contribute to PCOS. Depression frequently accompanies PCOS, perhaps because good mood is one of the serious casualties of hormone imbalances. Consider meditation or any other stress-reducing technique as well as exercise, which elevates mood, as important natural components of any treatment plan for PCOS.

weight. On the other hand, it's also associated with a higher incidence of nausea, vomiting, and other gastrointestinal disturbance. That said, it might be helpful.

Biotin and Fenugreek

Yet many experts consider it something of a Band-Aid on the problem, which doesn't get to the cause of PCOS. Remember that the main thing metformin does is help the body use insulin better. Chromium picolinate (see page 46) does the same thing and is a great supplement to use together with a low-carb diet to help manage both blood sugar and insulin.

In addition to chromium, which improves glucose tolerance, decreases fasting blood sugar, and has been shown to help insulin resistance in people with diabetes, two other supplements may be helpful. Though not normally thought of as the first nutrient you'd take for PCOS, biotin in high doses (8 to 16 mg) should be considered because it has the potential to be of great help in normalizing and lowering blood sugar.

And then there's fenugreek, an herb that also has a beneficial effect on blood sugar. It reduces fasting blood glucose (blood sugar) when used at the dosage of 1.5 to 2 mg per kg of body weight. (Note: Just to be on the safe side, I wouldn't use fenugreek while pregnant; be aware of this, since many people may first discover they have PCOS while trying to conceive.)

Weight Loss: Slow but Successful

The single most effective thing you can do to help the symptoms of PCOS is to lose weight. Some research shows that it really doesn't matter what kind of diet you use to accomplish this—high protein, low protein, etc.—but losing weight absolutely helps normalize the symptoms of PCOS.

Most holistic or complementary health practitioners favor a low-carb (or low-glycemic) diet for anyone who has blood sugar or insulin problems. That means high-quality protein, good fats, such as olive oil, coconut oil, some butter, avocado, flaxseed oil, fish oil, and nuts, and some low-sugar fruits, such as grapefruit and berries. Get the sugar out of your diet and reduce calories, something that will be a lot easier to do on a higher-protein, lower-carbohydrate diet.

It's just way easier to manage blood sugar and bring down insulin levels with a diet higher in protein, fiber from vegetables, and good fats than it is on a diet high in refined carbs, flour, and sugar, even if it's lower in calories.

Keep in mind, however, that weight loss for an individual with PCOS may be slower than weight loss for someone without the condition. It will take time for your metabolism to "heal itself" before the weight comes off. So be patient and stay committed to a healthy diet for the long haul.

Paleo Diet

for Acne

TELL JOHN MCDOUGALL that acne has nothing to do with diet and be prepared to see him fighting mad. "Next time you hear that, ask for the evidence," he says.

McDougall, a legendary physician, nutrition expert, and medical director of the renowned McDougall Wellness Center, traces this wrong-headed information to a seriously flawed study by James Fulton, M.D., in the *Journal of the American Medical Association* way back in 1969. Fulton, aided by the Chocolate Manufacturers Association of America, tested thirty adolescents and thirty-five young adult male prisoners. He gave the subjects one of two sugar- and fat-loaded candy bars—one with and one without chocolate. Then, at the end of the study, he counted their pimples. The complexions of forty-six of the sixty-five subjects stayed the same, ten actually improved, and nine showed more acne. Based on this highly suspect and flawed study, the claim that "diet has nothing to do with acne" was born and remains the "conventional wisdom" to this day.

But don't get me started.

Opposing Forces Create Confusion

I hate to be cynical, but one reason that doctors and dermatologists say that diet doesn't cause acne is because they can't sell a healthy diet. In addition, they were trained to believe that there's no connection between what you eat and what your face looks like. Plus, there's constant pressure from the pharmaceutical industry to prescribe creams, drugs, and other "remedies."

The problem is muddied further by the fact that there isn't a perfect correlation between diet and acne—some people can eat crap all day long and have perfect skin and others eat quite well and still have outbreaks.

"Acne sufferers are not a homogenous group," says my friend Richard Fried, M.D., Ph.D., author of *Healing Adult Acne*.

That said, there is overwhelming evidence—both clinical and theoretical—that diet is a huge contributor to acne.

The Causes of Acne

First, let's talk about what causes acne in the first place. Two events conspire to create or aggravate most forms of acne. One is blockage, two is infection. Here's how it works: Keratin is a fibrous protein that's the main component of the outermost layer of the skin. Sebum is part of the oil found on the surface of the skin and is produced by the sebaceous glands, most of which open into a hair follicle. When either too much keratin or too much sebum is produced, they can block the skin pores. Those overstuffed pores then can become infected by bacteria, which literally eat up the sebum and thrive.

But if diet has nothing to do with acne, why is the incidence of acne in underdeveloped countries eating natural, native diets almost zero while the incidence of acne in Western countries is in the double digits?

Read on.

Eating Locally and Healthfully

The idea that the Western diet has nothing to do with acne should have been given its walking papers years ago. Back in 1971, O. Schaeffer published a reporting that acne was completely absent in the Inuit (Eskimo) population when they were eating and living in their traditional manner, but as soon as they adopted the Western way of eating, acne showed up. Local physicians in Okinawa prior to World War ll reported that "These people had no acne vulgaris."

According to one published report, only 2.7 percent of almost 10,000 rural Brazilian school kids have acne. There's far less acne in Kenya, Zambia, Malaysia, and rural Japan than is common in Western societies.

But if there was any doubt left about the diet-acne connection it should have been erased by the seminal research paper published in the *Archives of Dermatology* in 2002 by respected

researcher Loren Cordain, Ph.D., of Colorado State University.

Cordain and his team studied two nonwesternized populations: the Kitavan Islanders of Papua New Guinea and the Ache hunter-gatherers of Paraguay. Are you ready for the number of cases of acne observed by these trained researchers?

Natural Prescription for Acne

Paleo Diet: No grains, dairy, beans, or soy; high in protein (fish, grass-fed meats), vegetables, fruits (especially berries), nuts, and omega fats

See also: Saw palmetto for acne, page 256

Clearogen as directed (www.clearogen.com) or saw palmetto (make sure to get a high-quality formula from a reputable company): 320 mg

★ **FOR ADDED EFFECTIVENESS:**

An antioxidant supplement

Zinc: 30 mg, two to three times daily, taper off to 30 mg as maintenance

Essential fatty acid supplement or fish oil: 1–2 g

GLA: 320 mg

Topically: Tea tree oil (an antiseptic)

Azelic acid (an anti-inflammatory): Use as directed.

Note: The above dosages are daily and in pill or capsule form unless otherwise noted.

None.

Of 1,200 Kitavan subjects and 115 Ache subjects examined, *not a single case* of active acne was observed.

Tubers, fruit, fish, and coconut represent the dietary mainstays in Kitava and, according to Cordain, dietary habits are virtually uninfluenced by Western foods in most households. Similarly, the diet of the Ache of eastern Paraguay contains wild, foraged foods, locally grown foods, and only about 8 percent Western foods.

Ancestral Advantages

In other words, they were eating the diet of our hunter-gatherer ancestors: food you could hunt, gather, pluck, or fish, what Cordain, author of a well-respected book by the same name, calls *The Paleo Diet*. In another of his books, *The Dietary Cure for Acne*, he lays out some tasty options for a diet based on whole foods—salmon, sirloin, strawberries, walnuts, carrots, and the like— which may well be the cornerstone of a natural prescription for getting rid of acne. (The Paleo Diet is absent of grains and dairy and high in grass-fed meats, vegetables, fruits, and omegas.)

Cordain hypothesizes that a diet that produces high levels of the hormone insulin is partly the culprit when it comes to acne. Here's how it works: High-sugar foods (processed carbs and the like) produce higher levels of a hormone called insulin, which in turn elicits a rise in another hormone called IGF-1 (Insulin-like growth factor). IGF-1 has a high potential for stimulating growth in *all* tissues, including the follicles. Both insulin and IGF-1 stimulate more hormones in both ovarian and testicular tissues, meaning they stimulate more testosterone (in both men and women). And more testosterone— with its especially nasty metabolite DHT—may well be acne's best friend. (More on the testosterone connection in a moment.)

Choose the Right Carbs

It's not just a "high-carb" diet that's responsible for the surge in insulin and its resulting effect on acne. The Kitavan Islanders ate a diet almost 70 percent carbohydrate—but they never saw a Twinkie or a processed breakfast cereal. Their carbs came from tubers, fruits, and vegetables, which is considered a low-glycemic, or low-sugar, diet.

While no one has investigated this directly, factory-farmed meat and chicken contain hormones and hormone-like compounds that can affect the body's hormonal balance and could certainly be part of the problem. Meat eaten in the native cultures where acne is virtually absent comes from wild game and pasture-fed (grass-fed) animals, *not* from factory farms where cows are routinely given large doses of hormones.

One study in the *Journal of the American Academy of Dermatology* investigated the relationship between diet and teenage acne and found a significant positive association between acne and milk (skim and whole). The researchers hypothesized that the association may be because of the "presence of hormones and bioactive molecules in milk."

While no one is claiming that diet is the *only* cause of acne, no responsible nutritionist or health practitioner should deny the overwhelming evidence that a bad diet makes matters much worse. There are probably some genetic factors that make one susceptible to excess keratin and sebum production, and to the inflammation and infection that can contribute to acne. But eating in a way that produces excessive amounts of hormones that do the same thing may "turn on" those genes; eating a natural, traditional diet lower in sugar and processed foods does not.

Selling Health to Your Teens

Acne is also promoted by a diet low in the antioxidants found in abundance in vegetables and fruits. "Acne may be the best angle you will ever use to sell a healthy diet to your teenage children," says McDougall. "After all, millions of people living in Papua New Guinea, Paraguay, and rural Africa and Asia who eat a plant-based diet are acne-free throughout their lives—so why can't you also be acne-free, if you behave like they do?"

A diet rich in plant foods provides huge amounts of antioxidants and natural anti-inflammatories. Whole foods are also high in fiber and low in sugar, and do not raise insulin to any levels that are likely to be problematic. Research going back to 1977 suggested that patients with acne may not metabolize sugar very well. Back in 1959, researchers writing in the *Journal of the Canadian Medical Association* went so far as to refer to acne as "skin diabetes." It appears they were on to something.

When eating meat, grass-fed, hormone-free choices are at the very least less likely to contribute to the problem of acne since they don't add hormones to the diet. According to Robert Ivker, D.O., a diet of 45 percent protein appears to restrict the conversion of testosterone to "son-of-testosterone," a metabolite known as DHT (which is hypothesized to play a big part in this whole scenario—see saw palmetto for acne, page 256). My guess is simply reducing sugar and processed carbs—even if they weren't replaced with protein—would accomplish the same thing. The take-away message is that the processed foods that are rampant in the Western diet create a hormonal situation that is likely to seriously aggravate acne or even, in some cases, actually cause it.

Pomegranate Juice

for the Heart ... and More

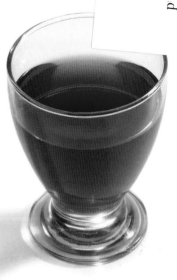

THE POMEGRANATE HAS always been associated with love and erotica. Just look at it—it's beautiful, purple, luscious, and sensual. In Turkey, brides throw the fruit to the ground and believe that the number of seeds that pop out predicts how many children they're going to have. The ancients connected the fruit with procreation and abundance. Aphrodite, the goddess of love, is said to have planted the pomegranate on the isle of Cyprus. And pomegranate's reputation as a love food wasn't exactly hurt by recent research in the *Journal of Urology* that suggested that pomegranate juice just might be a "natural Viagra."

So now that I've got your attention, let's talk about heart disease.

Pomegranate juice may just turn out to be one of the great natural weapons against heart disease. A daily dose of this delicious juice may go a long way toward keeping you from becoming a statistic. Studies in Israel have shown that, taken daily, pomegranate juice prevented the thickening of arteries. It also slowed down the oxidation of cholesterol by almost half—which to me is more impressive than just reducing cholesterol, since cholesterol is only a problem in the body when it's oxidized. And it makes sense that pomegranate juice would have that effect because of its stunning antioxidant content.

"Pomegranate juice contains the highest antioxidant capacity compared to other juices, red wine, and green tea," says Michael Aviram, D.Sc., a professor of biochemistry and medicine at the Rappaport Family Institute for Research in the Medical Sciences in Haifa, Israel, who led the team of Israeli researchers.

What the Research Reveals

He's not alone in his opinion. Research at the University of California confirms that the antioxidant capacity of pomegranate juice is two to three times that of red wine or green tea.

The research on pomegranate juice is mounting, and it's impressive. In one study, lished in the *American Journal of Cardiology*, forty-five participants—all of whom had some form of ischemic heart disease—were divided into two groups. For three months, one group received 8 ½ ounces of pomegranate juice daily while the other group got a placebo drink with the same number of calories, coloring, and flavor. The researchers found that blood flow to the heart improved by about 17 percent in the pomegranate group while *declining* about 18 percent in the placebo group. And this benefit was realized without any negative effects whatsoever.

Dean Ornish, M.D., senior author of the study and the author of the classic book *Dean Ornish's Program for Reversing Heart Disease*, said this of the results: "Although the sample in this study was relatively small, the strength of the design and the significant improvements in blood flow to the heart observed after only three months suggest that pomegranate juice may have important clinical benefits in those with coronary heart disease."

The Protection of Plant Pigments

Pomegranate juice is loaded with health-giving plant compounds like anthocyanins and tannins. Anthocyanins are pigments found in plants that act as a kind of "sunscreen," protecting the plants from sun damage and acting as powerful antioxidants.

They have a similar protective function in the human body. Tannins are bitter-tasting plant compounds found in tea, wine, and certain fruits, notably pomegranate. The most abundant tannins in pomegranate are called punicalagins,

> ### Natural Prescription for Heart Disease
>
> **Pomegranate juice:** Drink 6 oz unsweetened juice daily.

and they're believed to be one of the major reasons why pomegranate juice packs such a powerful antioxidant wallop.

At the Twentieth Annual Convention of the American Association of Naturopathic Physicians, Risa Schulman, Ph.D., visiting assistant professor at the University of California, Los Angeles, gave a presentation called "Breakthrough Findings in Pomegranate Juice Research." In it, she called attention to published research showing that pomegranate juice significantly increased levels of nitric oxide.

Nitric oxide is an important molecule that plays a critical role in vascular disease. A lot of medications—and the amino acid L-arginine—work by increasing nitric oxide in the system, a very good thing indeed. (If you guys need any more motivation for including pomegranate juice in your daily diet, consider this: Nitric oxide is also involved in erectile dysfunction, since not having enough of it doesn't allow enough blood flow into the penis.)

A Natural ACE Inhibitor

You may have heard of the class of medications known as ACE inhibitors, which are used in the treatment of both hypertension and congestive heart disease. ACE stands for angiotensin-converting enzyme, an enzyme that "converts" angiotensin l to the blood vessel–narrowing angiotensin ll, which in turn raises blood pressure. Schulman presented research that shows that pomegranate juice functions like a natural ACE inhibitor, reducing ACE by 36 percent and reducing systolic blood pressure as well. Since hypertension—high blood pressure—is a serious risk factor for heart disease, the ability to act as a natural ACE inhibitor is an important addition to pomegranate juice's heart-protective résumé.

Scientists have also tested the juice in mice and found that it combats atherogenesis (hardening of the arteries). According to study author Claudio Napoli, a professor of medicine and clinical pathology at the University of Naples, Italy, their research—published in the *Proceedings of the National Academy of Sciences*—

established that polyphenols and othe[r] compounds contained in the pomegr[anate] may retard atherogenesis. "The prote[ctive] effects of pomegranate juice were higher than previously assumed," Napoli says.

Best of all, you don't have to have existing heart disease to benefit from pomegranate juice's antioxidant wallop. Researchers at Hammersmith Hospital in London are currently trying to determine whether pomegranate juice could be an effective prevention measure against heart disease in people with healthy arteries. Ornish himself has commented that the juice may have the potential to help prevent cardiovascular disease in people who don't already suffer from it.

Because cardiovascular disease is the number-one killer in many Western countries, including the United States, this could be good news indeed.

Rotation Diet
for Food Allergies

FOOD ALLERGIES ARE one of the hottest topics in nutritional and integrative medicine, partly because no one can agree on exactly what they are. In the most general sense, an allergy is an exaggerated response by the immune system to a food, a drug, or an environmental trigger (like ragweed or pollen), which is usually harmless under most conditions. But conventional medicine has narrowed the definition to mean a very specific type of immune reaction—an inflammatory response that's triggered by a very specific type of soldier in the immune system known as an IgE immunoglobulin.

The word *allergy* originally comes from two Greek words—*allos* (meaning "other") and ergon (meaning "work" or "activity"). It was coined by a European pediatrician named Clemens von Pirquet back in the early part of the twentieth century. Von Pirquet noticed that some of his patients had a kind of "hypersensitivity" to substances that didn't seem to bother others. So the term *allergy* originally referred to any undesirable action of the immune system (from mild to severe) usually in response to a relatively innocuous stimulus (e.g., pollen, dust mites, peanuts, and so on). The definition soon became narrowed and the term *allergy* now means only immune responses triggered by IgE antibodies. The IgE response is the only kind of reaction that conventional medicine regards as a true "allergy," leaving people who experience a host of unwanted symptoms in response to foods and things in the environment frustrated with the inability of conventional medicine to treat them. Because conventional medicine sees only an IgE response as a true allergy, it's woefully inadequate when it comes to treating a host of other "bad responses" to foods and environmental substances that don't fall strictly into this category.

If you go to a conventional allergist's office to be tested for an allergy, you'll usually get one of two tests. The first is a skin prick test (where a small amount of the substance is introduced to the skin either with small scratching or with a series of pricks. Usually symptoms, like a rash, redness, or hive-like bumps, show up within a half hour, indicating an allergy. Alternately, you might get a RAST, or radioallergosorbent, test where they take a little of your blood and expose it to the suspected allergen and then measure the amount of IgE contained in the blood sample. A high amount of IgE means you've likely got an allergy. Using these definitions and standards, only about 2 percent of adults and about 5 percent of children have real allergies. And therein lies the rub.

A "true" (in the classic sense) food allergy will indeed produce a dramatic and usually quick reaction like hives. But here's the thing: There are many *other* ways your body can react to a food to let you know that it doesn't like it— fatigue, bloating, "brain fog," energy crashes, and even delayed aches and pains are all common examples. Folks in integrative or nutritional medicine have taken to calling these symptoms "delayed food sensitivities" or "food sensitivities" to avoid a turf war with the conventional allergists and distinguish these kinds of reactions

from classical, true allergies. Even so, many people still use the word *allergy* to describe this kind of reaction to food.

Here's a Better Way to Test for Food Allergies

There are a million tests for food allergies or "sensitivities," and everyone has their favorites— blood tests where they expose a little of your blood to ninety different foods and see what happens, saliva tests, you name it. All have their partisans and all have their detractors. Many are expensive (most, in fact). Many are confusing (you show up "allergic" to a food you've never eaten in your life). Many are inconsistent. Some are outright silly.

But there's a better way. It's low tech and— best of all—free. Plus it's likely to give you just as useful and meaningful a result as the most expensive of the "food sensitivity" tests.

It's called the rotation diet. And it's by far one of the best and most reliable methods for identifying foods that might cause you a variety of health problems.

Most people use rotation diets as a first plan of attack when they suspect a food allergy, but a rotation diet can also be a good all-around starting point for other symptoms that just can't be explained any other way: fatigue, achy joints, eczema, irritable bowel, or a depressed immune function. If you've already been diagnosed with certain food allergies or sensitivities, a rotation is the very best place to start.

Notice that I didn't say that the rotation diet was easy. It's not. It can actually be pretty overwhelming when you're trying to sort out what to have for breakfast, lunch, and dinner while coordinating the fact that similar foods can't overlap within a given time period. But if you can stick it out and stay with it for thirty days, the benefits can be enormous. For the first time, you may have answers to many questions about your own health that you've been unable to get anywhere else.

And what can be more empowering than that?

The Rotation Diet Explained

A rotation diet simply means that you are *rotating* the foods that you eat every four to five days, or longer, depending on how you react to each food item. In the classic version, you first eliminate the common offenders—sugar, wheat, and dairy—for thirty days. (That little trio of "usual suspects" is responsible for more unexplained symptoms than you can possibly imagine.)

Then, at the start of the second month, you would, for instance, eat wheat on Day 1. You would not be able to eat any kind of wheat again until Day 5 or 6. You may find that you can eat some of the foods that are on rotation every fourth day with no problems, but that others must be rotated at longer intervals for you to tolerate them. Eating the allergenic foods on a rotated basis reduces your exposure to them and also reduces your sensitivity to them so that you are better able to tolerate them. The general thinking is that after four or five days you have completely excreted the food from your body, so there is no risk of a buildup of allergenic toxins.

Allan D. Lieberman, M.D., director at the Center for Occupational and Environmental Medicine in South Carolina, is one of many practitioners who believe we should all think about rotating our foods. Rotation not only helps to reveal hidden food allergies and prevent new allergies from developing, but by allowing us to identify offending foods—and then putting a temporary "off limits" sign on them—we give our immune systems a needed break, Lieberman says. Hidden food allergies can cause digestive problems that will send the immune system on an all-out alert, creating inflammation and a host of other symptoms. By removing the problem foods the immune system is better able to heal and stay strong. Best of all, rotation diets allow us to eventually eat the foods we love—just less of them. And less frequently.

Lieberman has a kinder, gentler way of doing the rotation diet than starting right off with wheat, dairy, and sugar. He suggests easing into a rotation diet slowly, so that it doesn't seem so overwhelming. Starting with rotating proteins—like fish, lamb, meat, and the like—on a four- or five-day basis. So, for example, if you eat lamb on Monday, you don't eat it again till Friday or Saturday (depending on the severity of the allergy). On Tuesday, you can eat fish—and so on down the line. Your body gets a four- to five-day "rest" from each food in the category—in this case protein. Then add a fruit rotation; then vegetables. You might have to keep a chart to keep things straight for a while, but how hard can that be? Then try the big guns: wheat, then dairy. By the time you get to the wheat and dairy categories—the biggest offenders for most people—you're practically a pro at the whole rotation thing.

Anecdotes and Investigations

I've seen a host of problems disappear just by eliminating a food or food group. One of my very first "successes" when I first started seeing clients privately was quite by accident. A woman named Lucy came to see me at the Equinox Fitness Clubs in New York where I had an office. She was in great shape, very happy, toned, fit, and generally healthy. She actually came to me to try to lose a few pounds. (She also happened to mention—*incidentally*—that she had these terrible headaches that she'd had for almost all of her adult life. No doctor had been able to help her.) As a weight loss strategy, I suggested she cut out bread and cereal. Lo and behold, she came back a week or two later and the headaches were gone. A complete accident, but a fortuitous lesson—dump the wheat, lose the headache. It was the first time I saw it myself, but it was an experience to be repeated so many times over the years that I've long ago lost count.

But there's more than anecdotal evidence out there about food allergies. The European Congress of Allergology and Clinical Immunology (1999) conducted a study of 275 patients and found food connections to a wide variety of conditions including migraines, depression, hypertension, angina, irritable bowel syndrome (IBS), and eczema. For instance, people with IBS showed "remarkable" improvement with the elimination of pineapple,

WORTH KNOWING

Because this is detective work, it would be wise to keep a food journal while you begin your program. After all, Holmes and Watson always used one to crack their crimes. This is no different. You must find the culprits. Writing down how you feel after you eat and paying attention to any symptoms will give you clues and lead you to the cause.

Food allergy websites, books, and magazines can be helpful. For more information, see Recommended Reading and Resources, page 331.

I hope it goes without saying that I'm not suggesting you try the rotation diet with foods that have ever triggered serious, potentially life-threatening reactions. (If you've gone into anaphylactic shock when eating peanuts, don't eat peanuts. Period.) We're talking here about foods that produce annoying, vague, hard-to-pin-down symptoms that you may not even have suspected as being food related. For goodness' sake, do *not* try this with any foods that have triggered a life-threatening response in the past. I'm sure you know this, but it's worth mentioning anyway.

citrus, cantaloupe, bread, pork, and cheese (not necessarily all for the same patient!). In another study of fifty-seven patients with asthma, fruits were the most common triggers and—combined with milk, beef, lamb, pork, fish, and grain products—were by far the most common cause of food-related asthma symptoms.

Natural Prescription: Guidelines for a Four-Day Rotation Diet

Day One. Choose your menu from the following list:

- Lemon, orange, grapefruit, lime, or tangerine
- Banana, coconut, or date
- Carrots, parsnips, celery seed, dill, anise, fennel, cumin, parsley, coriander, or caraway
- Pepper, peppercorn, nutmeg, or mace
- Brazil nuts
- Chicken, turkey, duck, goose, or eggs
- Juices (preferably fresh) made from fruits and vegetables listed above

Day Two

- All varieties of grapes and raisins
- Pineapple, strawberries, raspberries, or blackberries
- Watermelon, cucumber, cantaloupe, pumpkin, squash, or zucchini
- Beets or spinach
- Peas, dry beans, green beans, carob, soybeans, lentils, licorice, peanuts, or alfalfa
- Cashews, pistachios, or mangoes
- Filberts or hazelnuts
- Flaxseed
- All pork products
- Snails, squid, clams, or scallops
- Crab, crayfish, lobster, prawns, or shrimp
- Juices made from the fruits and vegetables listed above

Day Three

- Apples, pears, quince, currants, or gooseberries
- Buckwheat or rhubarb

- Lettuce, chicory, endive, escarole, globe artichoke, dandelion, sunflower seeds, or tarragon
- Potatoes, tomatoes, eggplant, peppers (red and green), chile pepper, paprika, cayenne, or ground cherries
- Onion, garlic, asparagus, chives, or leeks
- Tapioca
- Basil, savory, sage, oregano, horehound, catnip, spearmint, peppermint, thyme, marjoram, or lemon balm
- Walnut, pecan, hickory nut, butternut, sesame, or chestnut
- Herring, anchovy, cod, sea bass, sea trout, mackerel, tuna, swordfish, flounder, sole, sturgeon, salmon, whitefish, bass, or perch
- Any juices from any combination, unsweetened

Day Four

- Plums, cherries, peaches, apricots, nectarines, almonds, wild cherries, blueberries, huckleberries, cranberries, wintergreen, pawpaw, papayas, or papain
- Mustard, turnips, radishes, horseradish, watercress, cabbage, Chinese cabbage, broccoli, cauliflower, Brussels sprouts, kale, kohlrabi, or rutabaga
- Avocado, cinnamon, bay leaf, sassafras, cassia buds or bark
- Wheat, corn, rice, oats, barley, rye, wild rice, cane, millet, sorghum, or bamboo sprouts
- Vanilla
- Macadamia nuts, pine nuts, mushrooms, and yeast (brewer's, etc.)
- Milk products, such as butter, cheese, and yogurt; beef or lamb
- Any unsweetened juices from above

Bottom line: The triggers are going to be different for different people, so you have to do your own science experiment with you as the subject. Take your health in your own hands and figure out what's really going on. When you identify the foods that cause your symptoms—or contribute to them—it's one of the most liberating experiences you can imagine. You may feel better than you have in years—even more so because you took charge of your own health.

Specific Carbohydrate Diet
for Inflammatory Bowel Disease

CARLY MCNAUGHTON WAS an energetic twenty-year-old member of the Colgate University women's ice hockey team in the summer of 2004 when she experienced a rapid weight loss of thirty pounds. Her energy was gone, she had no appetite, and she couldn't keep food down. Three doctor evaluations later, an obstruction the size of a grapefruit was found in her abdomen. It was a massive bowel infection. She underwent surgery and had thirty centimeters of her small intestine removed. So were her right ovary and her appendix.

The diagnosis? Crohn's disease.

Though her fitness level made her recovery quicker than most, everyone agreed it would be a good idea for her to take a year off from playing competitively, especially since stress levels can aggravate the disease. But by January 2004 she began practicing with the team again, continued her strength and conditioning program, and played her first game since the surgery in October of 2005. She played in all thirty-four games as a cocaptain and was named USCHO.com National Offensive Player of the Week on October 29, 2006.

Carly is unusual. But her recovery—and her indomitable spirit—are an inspiration and proof that determination and strength can keep you from being a victim of your disease. If you have inflammatory bowel disease (IBD) you may not be a star hockey player, but you certainly don't have to surrender your capacity to have a full and joyful life.

What Is IBD?

IBD is the collective name for two diseases in which the intestines become deeply inflamed: Crohn's disease and ulcerative colitis. Unlike irritable bowel syndrome (IBS—see page 230), in both forms of inflammatory bowel disease there is active pathology in the tissues. If you have IBD, a biopsy of your tissue would come back with visible, active inflammation, which would not be the case in irritable bowel syndrome.

Though there are similarities between Crohn's and ulcerative colitis, there are also differences, mainly in the location of the

---

Natural Prescription for Inflammatory Bowel Disease

SPECIFIC CARBOHYDRATE DIET

Essential fatty acids: 2–4 g

L-glutamine: 3–6 g

Probiotics: 10–20 billion

Digestive enzymes: Taken as directed with each meal

Boswellia (optional): 1,200 mg, three times a day (extract standardized to 37.5 percent boswellic acids per dose)

Aloe vera: 800–1,600 mg (look for a product with high content of acemannan)

Vitamin D: 400–1,000 IU

Note: All dosages are daily dosages and in pill or capsule form unless otherwise noted.

---

inflammation. Crohn's can affect you anywhere, from the mouth through the anus, and usually causes sores along the length of the small and large intestines. Ulcerative colitis always begins in the rectum, extends for a bit, and then stops. There's a clear "line of demarcation" between the tissue that is affected and the tissue that's not. It's characteristic of ulcerative colitis that usually just the mucosa and submucosa are involved, whereas in Crohn's all layers of the bowel are involved. Crohn's has "skip spaces"— that is, unaffected areas interspersed between involved areas. Ulcerative colitis does not; it's one contiguous inflammation for however long it extends from the rectum (it is confined to the rectum in about 25 percent of cases). Crohn's usually "spares" the rectum, but not always.

According to William Shapiro, M.D., of the Scripps Clinic and Research Foundation, about 20 percent of patients have a clinical picture that falls somewhere between ulcerative colitis and Crohn's—they are said to have "indeterminate colitis." As of this writing, about 1 million people are thought to have IBD in the United States. Both can cause extreme bouts of watery (Crohn's) or bloody (ulcerative colitis) diarrhea and abdominal pain.

The exact cause of IBD is not known, but like most multifaceted, highly complex disorders, it probably has a genetic component and is certainly made worse by trigger foods, bad nutrition in general, and stress. It's more common among whites, and it's higher in Ashkenazi Jews than in other groups, and slightly higher rates are seen in females. Antibiotic exposure has been mentioned as a possible factor, as have food sensitivities (more on that in a moment).

It's unlikely that any one factor "causes" IBD, but it's *very* likely that there's an interaction among factors. That said, it makes sense to support the immune system and to remove as many potential triggers from the diet as possible. It also makes sense to reduce stress and to manage any secondary symptoms like depression.

The Specific Carbohydrate Diet

The Specific Carbohydrate Diet, or SCD, is a dietary intervention that has been used with success by thousands of people. Developed by Elaine Gottschall, it's based on the theory that a balance in intestinal flora (good and bad bacteria) is absolutely essential to the health of the digestive system, and that an overgrowth of the "bad" bacteria like yeast leads to an imbalance in the gut that can create havoc. These "bad" bacteria create their own waste products and toxins and interfere with digestion and absorption of carbohydrates, which in turn leaves undigested carbohydrates to remain in the gut and become food for the microbes we host. The microbes digest these unused carbohydrates through the process of fermentation, creating waste products and acids that irritate and damage the gut.

Gottschall believed that some individuals with intestinal disease can't digest certain carbohydrates known as *disaccharides* (a kind of sugar). She believed that some individuals have impaired ability to break down disaccharides and that certain bacteria and yeast thrive on these molecules, creating a "vicious cycle" that can only be broken by changing the diet. The SCD is based on the principle that "specifically selected carbohydrates requiring minimal digestive processes,are well absorbed and leave virtually none to be used for furthering microbial overgrowth in the intestine," she wrote.

The guidelines for the Specific Carbohydate Diet are, well, very specific. And they have to be followed for a year before adding in any other foods. But thousands of people swear by the diet's effectiveness. General guidelines are no grains (e.g., rice, wheat, corn, or oats); no processed foods; no starchy vegetables (e.g., potatoes and yams); no canned vegetables of any kind; no flour, sugar, or sweeteners other than honey and saccharin; and no milk products except for homemade yogurt fermented for 24 hours.

Other Dietary Interventions

The Specific Carbohydrate Diet is a very special version of a more generalized approach that has been used with some success for a number of digestive and gastrointestinal problems. Joe Brasco, M.D., a gastroenterologist with a decidedly holistic and nutritional bent, puts all his patients on a foundational program that is a basic "caveman"-type diet: lean meats, fish, poultry, vegetables and vegetable juices, stocks, and traditionally fermented foods like sauerkraut. He also recommends coconut oil because of its high content of lauric acid, a natural antimicrobial. The only dairy products he recommends are the highest-quality cultured dairy products from sheep or goats (yogurt).

"I wish I could tell you that I see people get completely off medications 100 percent of the time using this kind of dietary approach," Brasco says, "but I see it at least 10 percent of the time. And that tells me there's a significant subset of the population who responds unbelievably well to this intervention." Brasco uses the rule of thirds: "Using diet, lifestyle, and supplements, about one-third of patients will get off all medications. About one-third will be able to reduce their medications. And about one-third won't be helped. But a dietary plan like this doesn't cost anything. What's the downside of trying it?"

Alan Gaby, M.D., one of the leaders of the complementary medicine movement in America, is even more bullish about the success rate when treating patients with dietary modification and nutritional supplementation. "In my experience," he says, "at least half of the patients with Crohn's disease improve, and many become completely symptom-free."

A high-fiber diet is highly recommended for both types of inflammatory bowel disease, except when there is an active flare-up, during which you might have to go easy. The problem is that a lot of people associate high fiber with wheat, grains, and cereals, which may be exactly what you *don't* need. A good idea would be to increase fiber as much as possible from vegetables, seeds, nuts, and even fiber supplements like psyllium husks. (You might want to lightly steam or cook the vegetables if eating them raw is a problem.) Make sure to drink plenty of water—a good idea in any event, but especially important when you're increasing fiber in your diet.

"Dietary fiber has a profound effect on the intestinal environment," says Michael Murray, N.D., a noted naturopath and the author of *The Encyclopedia of Natural Medicine.*

Regardless of whether you buy the exact theory behind Gottschall's SCD, the balance in intestinal flora between "good" and "bad" bacteria is essential for good health and especially for good digestion and absorption of nutrients. A high-quality probiotic formula is just absolutely essential. Several research studies have significant improvement in people with inflammatory bowel disease who were put on probiotics. Vitamin D deficiency is common in people suffering from intestinal malabsorption. The Cedars-Sinai web-site gives vitamin D supplements a three-star rating (their highest) for Crohn's disease, meaning there is reliable and consistent scientific data showing a health benefit.

Turmeric
for Inflammation

PICKING THE ONE best thing that turmeric does for the body was difficult. If you read my previous book, *The 150 Healthiest Foods On Earth,* you know that I consider

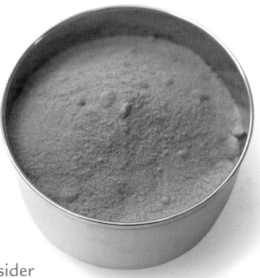

this spice a superfood. It has anticancer activity, it helps support liver health, and it's a powerful antioxidant. But the one property of turmeric that stands out—and that may even help support its other healthful activities—is its enormous power as an anti-inflammatory.

The family of compounds thought to be responsible for turmeric's medicinal effects are the curcuminoids, which are also responsible for giving turmeric its bright yellow color. The curcuminoids are believed to be responsible for turmeric's phenomenal anti-inflammatory properties. The most studied of the curcuminoids is *curcumin.* In one study, curcumin was found to be virtually as effective as the anti-inflammatory medication phenylbutazone.

In India, where 94 percent of the turmeric in the world originates, it's used to relieve arthritis. It can be useful for muscle pains as well as joint inflammation and even carpal tunnel syndrome. In a study published in the journal *Arthritis and Rheumatism,* researchers from the University of

Arizona in Tucson showed that turmeric extracts had positive effects on arthritis in animals. The researchers found that a turmeric extract prevented the activation of a protein called *NF-kappa B*, which controls the expression of genes that produce an inflammatory response. Other researchers believe that turmeric may exert its anti-inflammatory effect by lowering histamine. While the exact mechanism of its anti-inflammatory action isn't fully understood yet, in the long run it may not matter. Turmeric works as a powerful anti-inflammatory, and it does so without any toxic side effects. That's all that counts.

The Silent Killer

Understand this: Inflammation is not just limited to an occasional sore joint. It's serious stuff. Inflammation is now known to be a component of a baker's dozen of diseases, such as heart disease, diabetes, obesity, cancer, and Alzheimer's, not to mention the more obvious ones like arthritis, allergies, and asthma. Not long ago, a major national news magazine devoted a cover story to inflammation, calling it "the silent killer."

Newer blood tests are beginning to measure inflammatory markers like C-reactive protein and homocysteine in recognition that these are major risk factors for heart disease. Bottom line: The more natural anti-inflammatories we have in our diet, the better. Turmeric fits the bill perfectly.

WORTH KNOWING

The majority of the studies are done on curcumin since it's easy to isolate chemically and therefore study scientifically. But there's every reason to believe there are dozens of other healthy compounds in the turmeric spice itself that can benefit you in addition to the curcumin (which is only one of the many curcuminoids). Turmeric is easy to use and tastes great on everything. I use it on virtually everything I cook (well, almost). Try it on eggs!

Turmeric is also a powerful antioxidant, meaning it helps to protect both DNA and cells from the damage done by oxidation—damage that contributes to disease and that ultimately ages the body in a myriad of ways. In one rat study, for example, curcumin provided significant protection from cataract development. The unfortunate rats were exposed to a powerful oxidizing chemical that would normally produce cataracts as well as other damage. But one group of the rats was also treated with curcumin. The curcumin group not only had protection against the damage done by this chemical, but the transparency of the lenses in their little eyes was improved as well.

Other Health Benefits

The ability of turmeric to fight inflammation and also to serve as an antioxidant makes curcumin a very liver-friendly food. It's a great thing to use regularly if you have hepatitis. One study, in the journal *Toxicology*, demonstrated curcumin's significant liver protection in male rats largely through its antioxidant properties. Mark Stengler, N.D., recommends it for hepatitis and says that it is frequently used to lower elevated liver enzymes.

And then, to top it off, there's cancer. There are at least thirteen published studies indicating that curcumin reduced either the number or the size of tumors or the percentage of animals in the studies that developed them. Of course, these are mostly animal studies, but still, that's pretty promising. And not all the studies are on animals: One study, published in 2006 in the medical journal *Oncogene*, showed that curcumin inhibited the growth of human colon cancer cells. No one is claiming that turmeric is a natural cure for cancer; but between its antitumor effects, its antioxidant power, and its ability to reduce inflammation, there are plenty of reasons to believe that it is a really useful adjunct to the diet of everyone concerned with staying healthy.

PLANT CURES

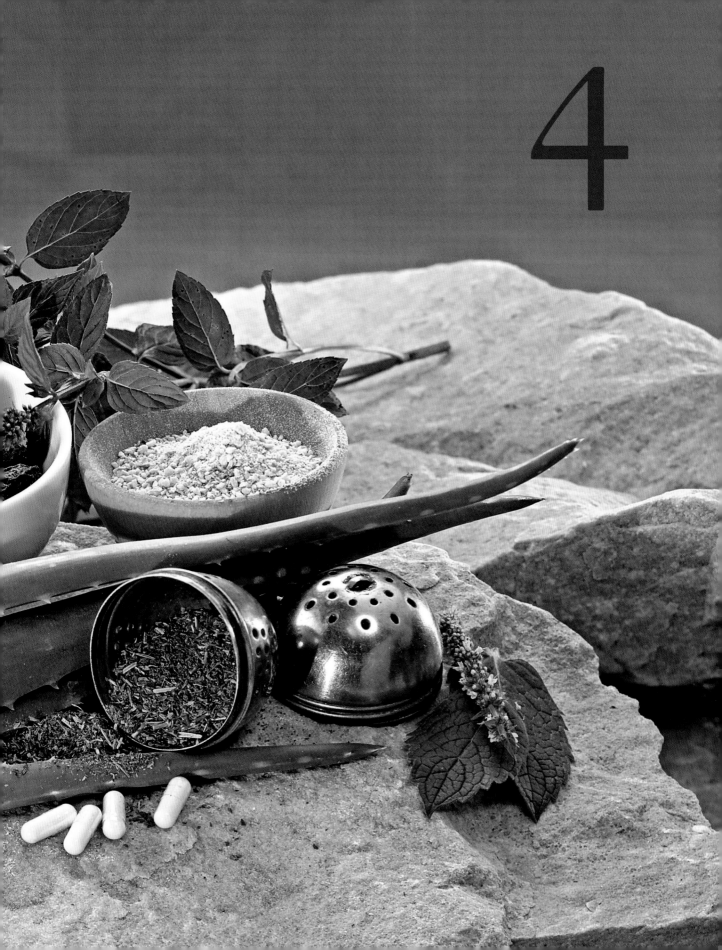

4

Aloe Vera

for Burns, Wounds, and Stomachaches

PICTURE THIS: You're a hunter-gatherer, living in the Arabian Peninsula a thousand years ago, and you've never seen anything that resembles modern civilization (think of the movie *The Gods Must Be Crazy*). While hunting one day, you brush up against a nasty bunch of thorns, leaving a red, inflamed patch of skin that burns and irritates. The big pharmacy chains are not on your radar—in fact, they're 900 years or so away from coming into existence. What to do, what to do? Simple: You reach for the nearest aloe vera plant.

For thousands of years, people have depended on the curative and healing powers of natural medicines found in the local plant kingdom. There's hardly a better example than the aloe vera plant. Does it cure cancer, herpes, diabetes, or heart disease? No. But if you've got a burn, a wound, or an irritation—either externally or internally—there are few substances on the planet that come in as handy and work as effectively as the aloe vera plant.

Aloe vera—and its juice—has been recognized for centuries for its remarkable health-enhancing and medicinal properties. Many people know that the gel of the aloe vera plant has a proven ability to soothe and heal the skin, but

truth be told it's darn good for healing and soothing a variety of conditions in the digestive tract, too. Virtually anywhere there's an irritation—on the skin or in the digestive tract—aloe vera can help.

The Healing Power of Glyconutrients

There are more than 240 species of aloe, which grows in Africa, the Near East, Asia, Europe, the southern Mediterranean, and the Americas. Although it's a member of the lily family, it looks like a cactus. In fact, it's the full, fat, cactus-y leaves that contain the healing gel, which you can get by just opening or breaking one of the leaves.

Of the many species of aloe vera, only four are recognized as having significant nutritional value, with *Aloe barbadensis miller* being the leader of the pack. The aloe leaf is a nutritional bonanza. It contains no fewer than 75 nutrients plus an astonishing 200 active compounds, including 20 minerals, 90 percent of the necessary amino acids, and twelve vitamins. According to H.R. McDaniel, M.D., a pathologist and researcher at the Dallas–Fort Worth Medical Center, who has spent the better part of two decades researching the therapeutic nature of aloe, its active ingredients are eight sugars that form the eight essential saccharides: glucose, galactose, mannose, fructose, xylose, N-acetylglucosamine, N-acetylgalactosamine, and N-acetylneuraminic acid. The mannose molecules join together to form a kind of starch that is known by different names: acemannan, acetylated polymannans, polymannose, or APM.

But don't confuse these natural, healing sugars with the white stuff you see on the table. These sugars—also called glyconutrients—don't taste sweet, don't raise blood sugar, and do provide many health benefits. (Glyconutrients are powerful compounds—ongoing research is looking at the value of glyconutrients in cancer treatment, but that's a whole other story.) The aloe vera gel has all the active medicinal sugars (glyconutrients) mentioned above.

Wound Care in a Gel

The gel reduces inflammation when applied to the skin. It also has antibacterial effects. It's great

WORTH KNOWING

Aloe vera is also excellent for constipation. You can try two or three 500 mg capsules as needed or 4 ounces of the juice; use just enough to maintain a soft stool.

as a skin salve, serving as a mild anesthetic and relieving pain, itching, and swelling.

A 1989 study in the *Journal of the American Podiatric Medical Association* found that both oral and topical aloe preparations speed wound healing. In this study, mice were given either aloe in their drinking water (100 mg/kg of body weight for two months), or a 25 percent aloe vera cream, which was applied directly to wounds for six days. The results were impressive. Both the oral and the topical gel worked well—the size of wounds decreased 11 percent more in the animals taking oral aloe vera (compared to a control group that didn't get aloe). In the group that had topical aloe vera gel applied to their wounds, the size of the wounds decreased 18 percent more than the wounds of a control group that healed without the help of aloe.

If you ever undergo dermabrasion—an increasingly popular cosmetic procedure used for smoothing the skin and removing acne scars—don't leave home without your aloe. Aloe decreases surgical recovery time, according to a report in the *Journal of Dermatologic Surgery and Oncology*. In this report, eighteen patients had facial dermabrasion to scrape away acne lesions. Dressings were applied to their faces, but half of each person's face was coated with standard surgical gel while the other half had additional aloe loaded into the mix. The half of the face treated with the aloe healed nearly three days faster than the other side.

Dermatologist James Fulton, M.D., of Newport Beach, California, says, "Any wound we treat, whether it's suturing a cut or removing a skin cancer, heals better with aloe vera on it."

Internal Inflammation

The benefits of aloe vera aren't limited to the gel. The juice of the plant is pretty potent stuff as well.

It works as an anti-inflammatory agent in the digestive system and is often used to ease heartburn and constipation. According to a study in the *Journal of Alternative Medicine*, aloe vera juice can be effective for treating inflammatory bowel disease. In this study, ten patients received 2 ounces of aloe vera juice three times a day for a week. After one week, 100 percent of them were cured of diarrhea. Four had improved bowel regularity. Approximately one-third of the patients reported feeling increased energy, probably because they were doing so much better.

Some research has pointed to the ability of aloe vera juice to rebalance the pH of the intestines, as well as its ability to possibly reduce the populations of certain microorganisms, including yeast. Other studies have shown that aloe vera juice helps detoxify the bowels, neutralize stomach acidity, and may help with gastric ulcers.

Natural Prescription for Burns or Digestive Upset

For mild burns or wounds: Apply aloe vera gel (as directed) for its soothing effect.

For digestive upset: Drink 4 oz of pure aloe vera juice as needed.

Note: All dosages are daily dosages and in pill or capsule form unless otherwise noted.

The juice is produced in much the same way as juice from any other fruit, like apples, for example. The gel-containing leaves are pressed, and concentrate is extracted and then diluted and reconstituted with water by the manufacturer, which then puts it on the shelves at better health food stores. Many people drink the juice as a way of getting the benefits of the aloe vera plant internally.

Though the juice is loaded with vitamins, minerals, and amino acids, according to Steve Meyerowitz, author of *Power Juices, Super Drinks,* the real healing wallop of aloe vera and aloe vera juice comes from the wealth of phytochemicals, such as the organic acids chrysophanic, salicylic, succinic, and uric, plus polysaccharides such as acemannan, enzymes such as glutathione peroxidase, and various resins. None of this, of course, was known to those hunter-gatherers a thousand years ago.

They just knew that it worked.

Arnica
for Muscle Pain and Inflammation

ARNICA IS PROBABLY best known in the United States for its anti-inflammatory properties and analgesic and antiseptic abilities. This makes it a good, all-around useful natural treatment for many aches and pains, including sports injuries, osteoarthritis, insect bites, and plastic surgery.

Arnica (*Arnica montana*), also known as leopard's bane, is a perennial herb native to the mountains and meadows of Europe and North America. Arnica flowers were used in German spiritual rituals dating back to the twelfth century. Arnica has been used as a topical medicine for more than four centuries to heal a variety of ailments, including bruises, sprains, muscle aches, wounds, inflammation from insect bites, and swelling because of fractures. It's available as a topical application, in a gel or cream, or as an oral homeopathic remedy (more on that in a moment).

What the Studies Show

Clinical trials have focused on the use of arnica for different conditions, ranging from pain management (women undergoing a total abdominal hysterectomy) to diabetic retinopathy to trauma.

The studies on arnica have been mixed—not all of them show it is beneficial—but enough of them show positive results to make this preparation worthy of inclusion as a natural cure.

You're likely to see the biggest benefits of arnica where there is pain and bruising. Many people report a decrease in overall pain and seem to heal quicker than normal.

Arnica is also popular with athletes for sports injuries and sprains. In one 2003 study, a homeopathic preparation called Arnica D30 had a positive effect on muscle soreness after marathon running. In a 1991 double-blind study, thirty-six marathoners who took five pills of Arnica twice daily for five days reported reduced stiffness. (Truth be told, other studies with athletes have not shown any measurable benefit—I told you the studies were mixed!)

How Arnica Works

Meanwhile, we now think we have an understanding of at least one of the mechanisms by which arnica may work. The *Arnicae flos*—the collective name for flower heads from *Arnica montana*—contain a number of active ingredients that have been identified, notably one called helenalin. Helenalin seems to be a powerful anti-inflammatory agent, and research from Germany published in the journal *Biological Chemistry* has shown that helenalin affects an immune chemical called NF-kappa B, which is involved in a number of processes in the body, especially inflammation.

Recently arnica has been shown to be equal to topical ibuprofen in treating osteoarthritis of the hands, a sometimes debilitating condition that produces potentially painful, nodule-like swellings on both sides of the joints.

Osteoarthritis is conventionally treated with the help of painkillers and nonsteroidal anti-inflammatory drugs, such as ibuprofen and diclofenac. But one study in particular proved that arnica might be even more effective than the traditional approach. Jörg Melzer, M.D., of the Institute of Complementary Medicine, Department of Internal Medicine, at the University of Zurich in Switzerland, took 204 patients and gently rubbed arnica or an ibuprofen gel over their affected joints three times a day for three weeks. The participants were asked not to wash their hands for one hour after application. At the end of the three weeks, the arnica group reported that they had less pain and better hand function

Natural Prescription for Muscle Pain and Inflammation

Homeopathic arnica is completely safe in any dosage and can be taken in a variety of ways from one tablet three times a day to three tablets (or more) three times a day. It can also be combined with the topically applied ointment. Following surgery, take three tablets every fifteen minutes for the first three hours after surgery, tapering off to three tablets per hour for the rest of the day and then nine tablets per day for the next five days.

than the ibuprofen group. Similar studies have shown that arnica is just as useful for knee osteoarthritis.

Arnica as Part of a Homeopathic Prescription

As for plastic surgery, it seems that arnica as a homeopathic remedy could provide relief for the bruising that is common after surgeries such as face-lifts. In 2006, thirty women who received face-lifts took an oral dose of arnica or a placebo. They started taking it the morning of surgery and repeated it every eight hours for four days. At the end of the eight days, the area of bruising was significantly smaller on the first and seventh days after surgery in those taking the arnica than in those taking the placebo.

You may also want to consider arnica after carpal tunnel surgery or a tooth extraction or as a preventive measure against heightened muscle soreness after extreme exercise (in particular, marathons).

I told you earlier that arnica was available as a gel or orally as a homeopathic medicine. Homeopathy is the practice of treating conditions by giving miniscule doses of compounds that would cause adverse effects in larger amounts, much like a vaccine does. And we're talking tiny amounts. Homeopathic doses are extremely diluted. They have no detectable amount of the plant in them and are generally considered safe for internal use when taken according to the directions on the product labeling. It's important to understand this because the only time arnica is safe when taken orally is in a legitimate homeopathic preparation. Taken orally in any other way it can cause some really nasty side effects. No kidding. (The *Physicians Desk Reference for Nutritional Supplements* lists nausea, vomiting, abdominal pain, diarrhea, coma, and death, if you really want to know.)

WORTH KNOWING

Don't take arnica when you're pregnant, and don't put the topical preparations on broken skin. People with a known sensitivity to members of the daisy family, such as chamomile, marigold, or yarrow, should avoid arnica preparations.

These side effects are not—repeat *not*—associated with the over-the-counter homeopathic arnica remedies you can buy in the store, and are certainly not associated with the topical application of arnica. The *Physicians Desk Reference for Herbal Medicines* says that when applied topically, arnica preparations have demonstrated "wound healing, antiseptic, and mild analgesic properties." Just don't ingest the whole plant—or parts of it—in some homemade version.

Enteric Coated Peppermint Oil

for Irritable Bowel Syndrome

IRRITABLE BOWEL SYNDROME (IBS) is characterized by a lot of symptoms most people don't love to talk about—abdominal cramping, lower abdominal pain, changes in bathroom behavior, gas, bloating, diarrhea, and constipation.

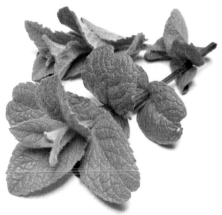

It's also known as spastic colon and is very common. An estimated 20 to 50 percent of visits to gastroenterologists are for IBS. Enteric-coated peppermint oil capsules have brought relief to many IBS sufferers, and quite a bit of research supports the positive effects of peppermint oil on IBS symptoms. In at least two studies, peppermint oil helped an impressive 75 percent of patients. In one randomized, double-blind, controlled study, forty-two children with IBS were given enteric-coated peppermint oil capsules or a placebo. After only two weeks, 75 percent of those who received the peppermint oil reported reduced severity of pain associated with IBS. And in another study conducted in Italy on fifty-seven adults, 75 percent of those treated with the oil showed a greater than 50 percent reduction in IBS symptoms.

Peppermint oil capsules can be so effective that one group of researchers concluded that it might be the "drug of first choice" for certain IBS sufferers.

What the Research Shows

The August 2005 issue of *Phytomedicine* published an analysis of sixteen clinical trials that investigated using 180 to 200 mg of enteric-coated peppermint oil in children with IBS or recurrent abdominal pain. Twelve of these trials were placebo controlled. Eight out of the twelve placebo-controlled studies showed statistically significant effects in favor of peppermint oil. The average response rate in terms of "overall success," meaning a reduction in symptoms, was 58 percent. The investigators stated: "Taking into account the currently available drug treatments for IBS, peppermint oil [one to two capsules three times daily over 24 weeks] may be the drug of first choice in IBS patients with non-serious constipation or diarrhea to alleviate general symptoms and improve quality of life."

Other researchers have suggested that the overall beneficial effect of peppermint oil might be due in part to its antimicrobial activity. Researchers have noted that bacterial overgrowth is associated with IBS (as well as a number of other disorders such as fibromyalgia and chronic fatigue syndrome), and one case study published in *Alternative Medicine Review* suggests that the antimicrobial activity of peppermint oil might be partly responsible for its positive effect in IBS. More research is needed, but this certainly passes the common-sense test.

Joe Brasco, M.D., a nutritionally minded gastroenterologist whose work I've admired for years, considers IBS "wholly a disease of diet and lifestyle." That's actually good news. IBS is one of those conditions where self-help really works, always an empowering scenario. There are countless tales of people living with this disease who "took the bull by the horns," empowered themselves to make changes to their diet and lifestyle, and are now living with minimal (or in some cases, significantly reduced) symptoms.

An IBS Myth Debunked

For years IBS was considered to be a psychological problem ("it's all in your mind"), but it's not. The American Gastroenterological Association considers IBS "a real medical condition."

Yet the psychological dismissal continues to endure, and rankles countless sufferers. One activist who maintains a wonderful website for IBS information and support (www.ibstales.com) puts it this way: "Some myths die hard and some just need killing." The next time you hear that IBS is "all in your head," consider the following statement from the International Foundation for Functional Gastrointestinal Disorders:

"IBS is not caused by stress. It is not a psychological or psychiatric disorder. It is not 'all in the mind.' Because of the connection between the brain and the gut, symptoms in some individuals can be exacerbated or triggered by stress. Dietary and hormonal factors can affect symptoms of IBS."

This is an important point. Though stress will not cause a person to develop IBS, it can trigger symptoms, just as it can trigger symptoms of asthma, herpes, and probably countless other conditions. The bowel is a sensitive organ and can react to all manner of things from stress hormones to food. (More on the stress connection below.)

Food for Thought

The connection between food sensitivities and IBS is an important one, and most nutritionally minded health practitioners will recommend cutting out certain foods as a good starting place. Though trigger foods can be different for different people, some seem to crop up consistently and should be considered a good starting point. These usual suspects include:

- Wheat
- Gluten (a component of grains, especially wheat barley and rye and to a lesser extent, oats)
- Caffeine
- Alcohol
- Dairy products
- Citrus fruits
- Red meat
- Fried foods

"As the controversy about food intolerance and IBS goes on, we continue to treat this common condition with a high degree of success, while conventional doctors continue to struggle. It would be amusing, were it not sad, to describe some of our patients' long journeys that included thousands of dollars spent on doctors, tests, and ineffective treatments, years of suffering, and frustration at being told their problems were purely emotional. Many of these patients, after discovering that their bowel problems could be cured simply by avoiding wheat, corn, or dairy products, experienced alternating joy and anger [at their previous doctors]—a significant improvement, one would suspect, over alternating constipation and diarrhea."

—Alan Gaby, M.D.

Past President, American Holistic Association

Dairy and grains appear to be the most common items linked to food sensitivities for those suffering with IBS (and, come to think of it, in the general population as well). These food groups don't necessarily cause classic food allergies, which is why conventional allergists tend to pooh-pooh their impact. That's because conventional allergy tests investigate a particular kind of immune response called IgE immunoglobulins, which will show up as a rash or otherwise make itself obvious almost immediately.

However, there are many *other* kinds of immune responses that can produce symptoms (such as those caused by IgG immunoglobulins, like bloating or fatigue) and, while not being true allergies, these immune responses nonetheless cause a lot of problems for a lot of people. Functional medicine tends to refer to these as "food sensitivities" or "food intolerances" rather than true allergies. Whatever. They

cause problems. And they seem to cause a lot of problems for IBS sufferers, which is why eliminating them often brings relief.

Then there is the sugar connection. People with IBS don't absorb lactose, fructose, and sorbitol particularly well and have more symptoms of gastrointestinal distress than healthy people do when they consume high concentrations of lactose or the combination of fructose and sorbitol. In one study, cutting out these foods resulted in symptom reduction for 40 percent of people with IBS-like symptoms. It's not surprising that many people report benefits when they eliminate milk, and even concentrated sources of fructose like fruit juice and dried fruit.

Whether it's sugar, dairy, or wheat, the best way to identify trigger foods is to simply cut out all the usual suspects and then see what happens. If you add them back slowly, one at a time, you'll soon know which ones are problematic for you.

Natural Prescription for Irritable Bowel Syndrome

Enteric-coated peppermint oil capsules: One or two 200 mg capsules, three times a day

GOES WELL WITH:

Fiber: 35–50 g

Glutamine: 1–20 g

Probiotics: 10–30 billion

Zinc: 15–30 mg

Calcium and/or magnesium as needed: Calcium, 1,000 mg; magnesium, 400–800 mg

Elimination diet: Get rid of gluten, dairy, and sugar. For some people, also eliminate caffeine, alcohol, red meat, and citrus.

Stress reduction: Hypnotherapy program by Michael Mahoney (see Recommended Reading and Resources, page 335), yoga, or acupuncture

Note: The above dosages are daily and in pill or capsule form unless otherwise noted.

A food diary is a great idea for IBS sufferers (come to think of it, it's a great idea for a lot of people, for a whole host of reasons). Those who choose to use a food diary have decided to take positive action aimed at uncovering exactly what triggers their symptoms so that they can take the necessary steps to remove those triggers. Keeping a food diary can be an empowering experience for IBS sufferers (and for many people in general).

Eliminating the Other Trigger—Stress

As noted above, though stress alone does not cause IBS, it certainly can aggravate it. In fact, IBS and asthma, while being very different conditions, are alike in that stress can be a huge trigger for symptoms. For this reason, it's always a good thing to identify "triggers"—situations that are particularly stressful or even emotionally toxic—and eliminate them. By paying close attention to the body and listening to its messages, IBS sufferers can often head off symptoms at the pass. So any kind of stress reduction program is a great thing for those with IBS. Remember that the intestines are like a second brain in that most of the serotonin made in the body is manufactured in the gut. Doesn't it make sense that the bowels would respond with great sensitivity to any emotional situations?

Yoga, acupuncture, and hypnotherapy have all been found to be helpful to people with IBS, with different folks responding differently to the various modalities.

The Hope in Hypnotherapy

One stress reduction method stands out: Hypnotherapy, particularly the program developed by a British practitioner of hypnotherapy named Michael Mahoney, the best-known expert on the use of clinical hypnotherapy for IBS. Mahoney, held in very high esteem by the IBS community, was originally asked by gastroenterologists at his local medical center in Cheshire, England, to see whether he could help their IBS patients, whom they had little or no success treating.

"I had to learn about IBS from scratch ... by interviewing patient after patient and learning about their fears, anxieties, horrible episodes of 'emergency' diarrhea, panic attacks for the 'loo,' and public accidents of untold embarrassment. I learned about the heartache and frustration of a patient population that had little or no recourse for relief," he says.

Mahoney has said that many of the IBS sufferers he saw had to deal with doctors who didn't recognize or fully appreciate the emotional impact of IBS. "IBS is far from a purely physical condition," he says, pointing out that it can take an enormous emotional toll, which involves anxiety, weepiness, depression, resignation, and disheartenment. None of this is helped by doctors who dismiss it as not being a "real" condition.

Mahoney, a member of the Primary Care Society for Gastroenterology, developed an IBS hypnotherapy program on CD called the *IBS Audio Program 100*. The program also includes a bonus CD that explains IBS to nonsuffering family and friends. A program booklet provides a symptom checklist, progress log, listening schedule, and essential information for IBS sufferers. It's relatively inexpensive, there's absolutely no downside to using it, and it's highly recommended. You can order it at www.ibscds.com.

Other Helpful Hints

In addition to stress reduction, fiber seems to have a good effect on IBS symptoms for a lot of people. One problem you might find is that most people associate high-fiber foods with cereal grains and breads, which are also loaded with wheat, one of the foods you want to avoid for a while. Get your fiber from vegetables or limited, gluten-free grains. Some people can tolerate oatmeal even though it has a bit of gluten; you might also try rye. (Flaxseeds can be sprinkled on anything for additional fiber.) Consider fiber supplements like PaleoFiber (found on my website, www.jonnybowden.com) or ordinary psyllium husks. One fiber that enjoys an excellent reputation among IBS sufferers is acacia fiber, the best known of which is Tummy Fiber. Make sure to accompany the extra fiber with plenty of water.

Other supplements make a nice addition to a regimen built around enteric-coated peppermint oil. Calcium can be used as a "constipating" agent and magnesium as a diarrheal. Sophie Lee, an IBS activist who maintains one of the best IBS resource sites on the Internet (www.irritable-bowel-syndrome.ws) wrote to me to say that "the number of people I hear from who have successfully used calcium carbonate to control their diarrhea is astonishing, and lots of people use magnesium for constipation as well."

Ginkgo

for Memory Enhancement

OKAY, NOW THAT I've got your attention, let me add the requisite and boring disclaimers: If you're healthy, young, and have no particular health issues or memory problems, taking ginkgo isn't going to help you ace an exam that you would have otherwise failed, or suddenly start remembering what you had for breakfast four days ago. But that doesn't mean ginkgo doesn't have profound and important effects on the brain and other aspects of your health. It does.

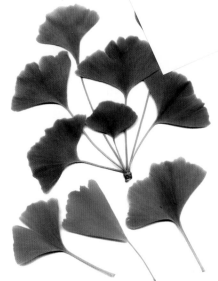

The overwhelming majority of research studies have demonstrated that ginkgo supplementation has a positive effect on cognition. There have been numerous double-blind, placebo-controlled studies that show ginkgo extract is effective in reducing either the progress of dementia or the severity of its symptoms. The results are not always dramatic, but they are significant.

A number of studies have shown that ginkgo modestly improves both memory and the speed of cognitive functioning, as well as the symptoms of Alzheimer's and vascular or mixed dementia. Some studies even show that ginkgo leaf extract can stabilize or improve some measures of cognitive and social functioning in patients with multiple types of dementia.

In one major U.S. trial published in the prestigious *Journal of the American Medical Association* (*JAMA*), 300 participants with Alzheimer's or dementia received either 40 mg of ginkgo biloba extract or a placebo three times a day. Compared to the placebo group, almost twice as many of the patients in the ginkgo group showed significant improvement on a rating scale that evaluates the severity of Alzheimer's disease. In Germany, physicians are so sure of ginkgo's benefits that it's hard to get them to perform scientific studies of the herb.

"To them, it is unethical to give a placebo to people with Alzheimer's when they could be taking ginkgo instead and have additional months of useful life ahead", says Steven Bratman, M.D., author of *The Natural Health Encyclopedia*.

Other studies that examined the effects of ginkgo on men and women who didn't suffer from any mental impairment have also demonstrated improvements in mental functioning.

The Key May Be in Circulation

How exactly does ginkgo improve mental functioning? We don't exactly know, but we have some suspicions. For one thing, it's a great circulation enhancer. Ginkgo may get more blood to the brain, helping it function better. It may also stimulate the activity of nerve cells and protect them from injury.

There's also the fact that ginkgo is a powerful antioxidant. Through its many components—notably the flavonoid glycosides and the terpenoids (ginkgolides and bilobalides)—it helps prevent the cellular damage from free radicals that can damage tissue and cause vascular harm and the loss of neurons, all of which can lead to dementia.

Ginkgo's reputation took a big hit when a study published in *JAMA* concluded that there were no differences in the memory abilities of people treated with ginkgo and people who weren't. But there were a lot of problems with this study, not least of which was the fact that it only went on for six weeks (many researchers believe the effects don't show up until after at least twelve weeks of taking it). Only participants with no previous memory problems participated, and it's hard to demonstrate improved memory with people who don't have memory issues to begin with! This study also doesn't negate the possibility that ginkgo could be effective for people with memory problems or other forms of dementia. And of course the *JAMA* study doesn't address the many other benefits of ginkgo—as an antioxidant and anti-inflammatory, for example. (Interesting FYI: *JAMA* also published the above-mentioned study showing the benefit of ginkgo for patients with dementia and Alzheimer's!)

"The value of any dietary supplement cannot be determined on the basis of one study alone," says Mark Blumenthal, executive director of the American Botanical Council. You need to consider the entire body of evidence that supports ginkgo's beneficial use.

Natural Prescription for Memory Enhancement

Standardized ginkgo extract: 40 mg, three times a day (total 120 mg)

You can also take 60 mg, twice a day, or double up with 120 mg, twice a day.

★ **FOR ADDED EFFECTIVENESS:**

Vinpocetine: 10–20 mg

Acetyl-L-carnitine: 500 mg, twice a day

Phosphatidylserine: 200 mg

GPC (glycerophosphocholine): 1,200 mg

Huperzine A: 50–100 mcg

Note: All dosages are daily dosages and in pill or capsule form unless otherwise noted.

Physician Steven Bratman, M.D., author of the excellent *Natural Health Bible*, says that "The scientific record for ginkgo is extensive and impressive."

Ginkgo is by far the most widely prescribed herb in Germany, reaching more than $200 million in sales (for 1996). There are at least two proprietary ginkgo medicines (Tebonin and Rokan) on the market in Germany, and German docs consider it to be as good as any available drug treatment for Alzheimer's disease as well as other severe forms of mental function decline.

Ginkgo's Other Benefits

Ginkgo's positive effect on circulation doesn't end with the brain. A 1991 study in the *Journal of Sex Education and Therapy* evaluated the effect of ginkgo on erectile dysfunction caused by poor circulation and found about a 50 percent success rate. Ginkgo is often used to counter the sexual side effects of antidepressants, a little-known use that is deserving of much more attention.

Ginkgo is also recommended by the prestigious German Commission E for the treatment of intermittent claudication—the restricted circulation in the legs due to hardening of the arteries. One small study also suggested that ginkgo may be helpful in relieving some of the symptoms of premenstrual syndrome.

My friend Daniel Amen, M.D., whom I consider to be one of the world's foremost experts on the brain, pioneered the SPECT method of brain scanning imagery and has a

WORTH KNOWING

The most studied form of ginkgo biloba is an extract called EGB 761. Try to find a brand that has been standardized for that extract. (One such brand in the United States is Ginkgold by Nature's Way.) According to the Herb Research Foundation, you can also look for standardized extracts that have been standardized for 24 percent ginkgo flavone glycosides.

Some researchers suggest that the combination of ginkgo and Panax ginseng might be even more effective than either used alone.

You should give ginkgo at least a twelve-week trial, the length of time used in many studies.

database of thousands of pictures of brains in every state imaginable. Brains on alcohol, brains on drugs, healthy brains, sick brains, brains with attention deficit disorder, you name it. Amen says ginkgo enhances circulation, memory, and concentration. "The [best-looking] brains I have seen are those on ginkgo," he says. That's a pretty ringing endorsement.

Amen, who is a distinguished fellow of the American Psychiatric Association, assistant clinical professor of psychiatry and human behavior at the University of California–Irvine School of Medicine, and the author of more than nineteen books, says that ginkgo "enhances circulation, memory, and concentration."

Ginseng

Boost your Immune System and Give Yourself an Energy Lift

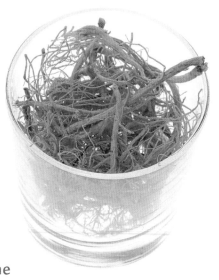

NEXT TIME YOU adjust the thermostat on your central heating, think about ginseng. When you set a thermostat in your home, you're basically telling the unit to figure out what the temperature currently is and then to bring it in line with what you decide is comfortable. If the temperature is 80°F and you set the thermostat to 70°F, the unit will gradually cool the air. If the temperature is 60°F and you set the thermostat to 70°F, it will gradually warm it.

Ginseng works in a similar way. It basically helps you adjust to physical stressors, like cold or heat, or to nonphysical stressors, like the demands of modern life. It raises your resistance to stress. That's why it's known as an *adaptogen*—it can adapt to any circumstances, depending on what's needed.

An adaptogen is defined as any compound that has a *normalizing* influence on physiology, regardless of the direction of change caused by the stressor; in other words, it works exactly like your thermostat.

The idea that ginseng is an adaptogen was first introduced by Israel Brekhman, Ph.D., a Russian scientist who wanted to promote a ginseng look-alike that grows in Siberia. Real ginseng takes a long time to grow and is ridiculously expensive. The Siberian variety, which is not really ginseng, was promoted as being just as good, and Brekhman touted it as the perfect answer to stress. In Chinese medicine, where ginseng has a long and distinguished history of use, it is used for entirely different purposes, not the least of which is supporting the immune system.

The Many Uses of Ginseng

But there's little doubt that ginseng, when used properly, can give you a boost. It seems to help the immune system. In one multicenter, placebo-controlled, randomized, double-blind study, a standardized ginseng extract was given over twelve weeks; at week four, all volunteers also received a flu vaccination. The ginseng group had significantly fewer cases of flu or the common cold, as well as significantly higher levels of antibodies.

The Complete German Commission E Monographs—an authoritative guide to herbal medicine, translated by the American Botanical Council—approves ginseng to help fight lack of stamina. The monograph notes research supporting ginseng's ability to improve the quality of life in persons subjected to high stress as well as its use in the treatment of functional fatigue. It's been investigated for dozens of other applications as well, including its ability to improve blood sugar, cerebral blood flow, and cognitive function.

There are two basic kinds of ginseng: American ginseng (*Panax quinquefolius*) and Asian or Korean ginseng (Panax ginseng). Siberian ginseng (*Eleutherococcus senticosus*) is a poor relative of ginseng and may or may not have medicinal properties; its chemical makeup is quite different from Panax ginseng. Ginseng root that's dried and unprocessed is called "white ginseng," whereas "red ginseng" refers to root that has been steamed and heat-dried.

A review in the *Annals of the Academy of Medicine Singapore* in 2000, titled "Panax (Ginseng)—Panacea or Placebo?" concluded that compounds in ginseng (*saponins*) had "positive anti-mutagenic, anti-cancer, anti-inflammatory, anti-diabetes and neurovascular effects." None of this is new information.

A 1992 article published in the *Journal of Ethnopharmacology* called "Recent Advances on Ginseng Research in China" stated that ginseng "has a wide range of pharmacological and therapeutical actions; it acts on the central nervous system, cardiovascular system and endocrine secretion, promotes immune function and metabolism, possesses biomodulation action, anti-stress and anti-aging activities, and so on." Hardly an undistinguished résumé. China has approved many preparations of ginseng for clinical application.

Ginseng and Blood Sugar

Recently several studies have shown that ginseng can lower blood sugar in people with or without diabetes. In three different studies, a dose of ginseng given before drinking a sugar solution lowered participants' blood sugar significantly more than a placebo. These studies, performed jointly by researchers at the University of Toronto, St. Michael's Hospital in Toronto, and the University of Ottawa, demonstrated that doses as small as

Natural Prescription for Boosting Immunity

Panax or American ginseng: 100 mg–1g

★ **FOR ADDED EFFECTIVENESS:**

Zinc: 15-30 mg

Vitamin C: 500-1,000 mg

Note: All dosages are daily dosages and in pill or capsule form unless otherwise noted.

1 g of American ginseng can lower the blood sugar response after eating carbohydrates in people with or without diabetes.

In the first study, researchers gave subjects either 3 g of American ginseng or a placebo. Nine of the subjects had type 2 diabetes; ten did not. Compared to the placebo group, all of the ginseng takers experienced an 18 to 22 percent lower level of blood sugar after drinking a sugar solution. In the second study, researchers compared three different doses of American ginseng with diabetic subjects and found that any one of the doses—3 g, 6 g, or 9 g—worked equally well to lower blood sugar after drinking a sugar solution. The third study also tested three different doses—this time 1 g, 2 g, and 3 g—and found that there wasn't much difference. Even 1 g did the trick.

The evidence was a little mixed on when it was best to take the ginseng. Two of the studies showed that it only worked if it was taken about 40 minutes prior to drinking the sugar solution.

In another study, however, it worked when taken between 0 minutes or 2 hours before drinking the solution. To be on the safe side, if you're using ginseng to modulate your blood sugar response, take it about 40 minutes before eating. In any event, ginseng's ability to lower blood sugar, by anywhere from 10 percent to 22 percent, is good news indeed for people with or without diabetes.

Horny Goat Weed

for Impotence

EVER HEAR OF *Epimedium sagittatum?* Me, either. But this herb, found throughout Asia and the Mediterranean, goes by another name in the United States, one you might recognize if you've thumbed through the ads in men's magazines in the last few years: horny goat weed.

Legend has it that this plant got its nickname from a goat herder who happened to notice that his flock would graze on this herb and then get noticeably more, well, *frisky*. Also known as yin yang huo, epimedium has a long history in Chinese medicine as a tonic for the liver, joints, and kidneys. But in the United States, its principal use is as an aphrodisiac.

What Do the Chinese Know That We Don't?

Horny goat weed is loaded with flavonoids, polysaccharides, sterols, and an alkaloid called magnaflorine, according to herbal medicine expert Chris Kilham, author of the *Hot Plants: Nature's Proven Sex Boosters for Men and Women.* This time-tested aphrodisiac "increases libido in men and women, and improves erectile function in men," Kilham says.

He went to China to interview traditional Chinese medicine practitioners for the Discovery Channel, and was told by Diao Yuan Kuang, M.D., that horny goat weed "… gives you back your sexual strength." Chinese doctors use it to treat erectile problems, boost libido, and recapture the sexual vitality of youth. Herb traders in China estimate that they sell more than 100 tons of the stuff every year.

Little research has been done on horny goat weed and libido, but it has a long history of successful use, and many health practitioners, not only in Asia, but over here, endorse it. "Epimedium is, in fact, likely to make you horny. Most users will notice a mild to moderate effect on the third or fourth day of use," says Ray Sahelian, M.D., author of *Natural Sex Boosters.*

Kilham, who's my go-to guy for exotic herbal products, recommends supplements that are standardized to a flavonoid called *icarlin.* Two to four 500 mg capsules per day should be enough to help with libido and heat up your sex life.

Peruvian Ginseng

Maca, also known as "Peruvian ginseng," has been used for sex enhancement since the time of the Incas. It's actually a radish-shaped vegetable that grows well in the Andes Mountains. I first heard about maca when I interviewed a researcher on my New York radio show who found that feeding maca to rodents increased their spontaneous erections. (This study was published in the April 2000 issue of the medical journal *Urology*.) Maca root contains a chemical called p-methoxybenzyl isothiocyanate, which is reputed to have aphrodisiac qualities. It also contains a bunch of chemicals found in other plants from the Brassica family (broccoli, cabbage, etc.), which are documented to be cancer preventive.

Other research has demonstrated increased sexual activity in mice that are fed maca, though some of this research has been criticized because it was performed and sponsored by people marketing maca. But there's been some human research as well, notably by G.F. Gonzales et al., published in the *Asian Journal of Andrology*. Men aged twenty-one to fifty-six received either a placebo, 1,500 mg of maca, or 3,000 mg of maca. Sperm count and semen volume were increased with maca at either dose.

Why the effects? Who knows? Maca contains two novel groups of compounds—macamides and macaenes, which may be responsible for its effects. Maca also contains the amino acid L-arginine (see below), which has been shown to increase sperm production and motility and is necessary for the creation of nitric oxide, a molecule that is necessary for erections.

"For the Sex, of Course!"

An interesting theory on maca and sexual activity has to do with the fact that maca contains high amounts of an amino acid called *histidine*. Histidine plays an often-overlooked role in both ejaculation and orgasm. It gets tricky here, but stay with me. The body uses histidine to produce *histamine*. High levels of histamine are often found in men who have premature ejaculation. (That's one reason why a side effect of *anti*histamines is difficulty in achieving orgasm.) According to the Tropical Plant Database website, a *pro*histamine like maca might have exactly the opposite effect of an *anti*histamine. It might make it easier for men and women who have trouble reaching orgasm to achieve it.

Natural Prescription for Impotence (Libido)

Horny goat weed, standardized to 10 percent icarlin: 2–4 500 mg capsules

Maca: 1,800–2,500 mg

L-arginine: 1,000–2,000 mg

Zinc: 25 mg

Note: All dosages are daily dosages and come in pill or capsule form unless otherwise noted.

Regardless of the science, the proof is in the pudding. Kilham, investigating maca in Peru on one of his frequent "Medicine Hunter" expeditions, asked a number of people why they used maca. "One woman stands out in my mind," he says. "She smiled at my question and replied, 'Well, for the sex, of course.'"

Then there's L-arginine. While no cure for impotence, L-arginine has a documented role in the body as a vasodilator, benefiting circulation and helping with endothelial dysfunction, a dysfunction of cells that line the inner surface of blood vessels. (Endothelial dysfunction is often a predictor of later vascular events like heart attacks and strokes.) What's the connection to sexual performance? Simple: circulation.

"I've almost never seen a case of erectile dysfunction that didn't also have a component of the *other* ED—endothelial dysfunction," says Mark Houston, M.D. "They frequently go together."

Let's be clear. Impotence has multiple causes. If you're not turned on by your partner, if you're depressed, or if you've got a ton of things on your mind, you may not be in the mood for love. It's unlikely that horny goat weed, even

WORTH KNOWING

Chris Kilham points out that many people in this country think of herbs as drugs and figure that a little amount will do some good. He believes, as I do, and as many people in our field do, that consumers often take far too little of most herbs to get the real benefits that are available.

"Rare is the herb that works in small doses," Kilham says. To use maca as the Peruvians do, for example, you'd have to take about 3,000 to 5,000 mg a day or more. Since some products are purer than others, this is variable, but the small doses aren't likely to cut it. Kilham recommends that 4 or 5 capsules a day (between 1,800 and 2,250 mg each) is the right range.

with maca and L-arginine, are going to make you suddenly fall in lust with Miss Anderson in accounting, particularly if you can't stand her to begin with. But if circulation or blood flow is an issue, this "natural cure" may indeed give your sex life a boost.

Horse Chestnut

Banish Varicose Veins or Prevent Them in the First Place

NO ONE THINKS varicose veins are pretty, but truth be told they're pretty harmless. Because they're rarely seen in parts of the world where high-fiber diets are the norm, it's been hypothesized that the typical Western diet—high in junk carbs and fats and low in fiber—is partly to blame.

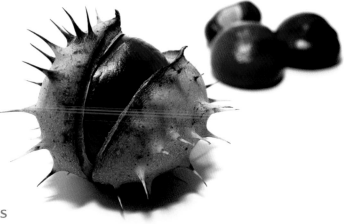

One theory is that low-fiber diets produce constipation and straining on the toilet. People eating low-fiber diets pass smaller and harder stools, and the straining increases pressure in veins. The standardized American diet also increases the risk of obesity, which, while it doesn't technically "cause" varicose veins, can definitely raise the risk for them, especially if you have a genetic tendency toward them in the first place. Interestingly, the list of risk factors for varicose veins in general is pretty similar to the list of risk factors for heart disease.

Women are more than twice as likely to develop varicose veins as men, and female hormones may play a part as well as genetics. Obese people of either sex are prone to them as well (see above). Standing and sitting for long periods of time doesn't help, nor does a lack of exercise.

The risk increases with age as the walls of the veins can become weaker, causing blood that ought to be moving toward your heart to flow backward. Yet varicose veins are clearly not a "natural" part of aging, since they're practically nonexistent in third world countries. Prevention beats the heck out of treatment, but there are still plenty of things you can do if you already have them.

Horse chestnut seems to be the number-one compound of choice for treating varicose veins. The horse chestnut tree gets its name from horseshoe markings that appear on the branches that are in actuality scars from where leaves previously grew. The tree itself is native to the Balkan Peninsula (Greece and Bulgaria, for example) and is grown for ornamental purposes in towns, private gardens, parks, and the like.

A fluid extract is made from the bark and the fruit of the tree, and this is what's commonly called "horse chestnut" or "horse chestnut extract" and is used for medicinal purposes.

The bark, seed, twigs, and leaves from the horse chestnut trees are used in traditional Chinese medicine. Horse chestnut extract is helpful for improving circulation, which makes it also useful for relieving leg cramps. The German Commission E, which is responsible for testing herbs and supplements, approves horse chestnut for "venous insufficiency," meaning lack of blood flow through the veins.

Those Delicate Veins

Varicose veins are almost always related to a weakness in the walls of the veins, which are fairly delicate structures to begin with. The veins contain valves that prevent blood from flowing back down due to gravity, but when these valves get weak, blood pools in the veins and causes them to bulge and/or become purplish.

The active ingredient in horse chestnut—*escin*—helps strengthen vein valves, walls, and capillaries.

Lack of good circulation can be another factor in causing varicose veins. Standing and sitting for long periods of time, as well as being obese, can increase the likelihood of getting them. So can pregnancy (though the condition usually gets better after delivery). If you've got varicose veins, try to avoid sitting or standing for long periods of time, and walk on a regular basis. Anything to get the circulation going is a good thing.

Natural Prescription for Varicose Veins

Horse chestnut (standardized for escin): 600 mg

High-fiber diet (and/or fiber supplements): 35–50 g fiber

Grape seed extract: 100 mg, three times daily, or Pycnogenol capsules (use as directed)

Vitamin C with bioflavonoids: 1,000–3,000 mg

Vitamin E: 400–800 IU

Coenzyme Q10: 50–150 mg

Plenty of berries, cherries, grapes, and tea

Exercise: Especially walking, jogging, stair climbing, hiking, and bike riding

Note: All dosages are daily dosages and in pill or capsule form unless otherwise noted.

Horse chestnut—standardized for its content of the active ingredient escin—has been found to be just as effective as compression stockings, which are expensive, annoying to put on, and a pain in the neck.

In addition to horse chestnut, a number of supplements, herbs, and lifestyle modifications can make a big difference. Key among them are the following.

1. **Exercise.** Exercise contracts the leg muscles, which pushes blood back into circulation. When you walk, run, or ride a bike, the leg muscles squeeze and the

venous pump—the mechanism that sends blood back to the heart—works well. When you do nothing, that blood doesn't have much help in circulating through the body. Instead, gravity will work against you, and pooling in the lower extremities is far more likely. In general, anything that increases circulation and gets the blood pumping, such as exercise, is going to help prevent varicose veins.

2. **High-fiber diet.** Low-fiber diets increase the risk of getting varicose veins and probably make them worse. The relationship is probably due to the connection between low-fiber diets and constipation (see above), but there are so many benefits—and no downsides to a high fiber diet in general—that it's hard to not recommend it as one of the top "natural cures" for varicose veins. Don't rule out fiber supplements, like psyllium husks (cheap and available at all health food stores). Every major health organization recommends that we consume between 25 and 35 g of fiber a day; our Paleolithic ancestors got well over 50. The average American gets between 8 and 11 g. Enough said.

3. **Flavonoids, grape seed extract, and Pycnogenol.** Plant compounds called flavonoids, proanthocyanidins, and anthocyanidins are all helpful in the treatment of varicose veins. All seem to help strengthen the delicate walls of the veins and capillaries. Foods richest in these substances include berries (blueberries and blackberries) as well as cherries, grapes, and tea. Add these foods to your diet and take a supplement of grape seed extract, which is rich in these compounds.

4. **Vitamin C.** Vitamin C in combination with a bioflavonoid called hesperidin has been used in research (often with butcher's broom) with good effect. It helps promote better circulation and strengthens the walls of the veins. Lack of these nutrients has also been shown in research to increase pain in the limbs and fragility in the capillaries.

Huperzine A
for Dementia and Alzheimer's

LET'S BE CLEAR about one thing: There's no known cure for Alzheimer's disease at this time. I'm truly sorry. I wish it were different. And one day it may well be. But that doesn't mean there isn't anything we can do to protect the brain, and with it, our ability to think clearly, for as long as possible.

The more we understand about the causes of dementia and Alzheimer's, the more we find that at least some of the mechanisms that contribute to these devastating conditions respond to things we can actually choose to *do*. Foods we can eat that are rich in anti-inflammatories (and foods we can *avoid* that create chronic high blood sugar, an emerging risk factor for Alzheimer's). Aerobic exercise that gets oxygen into our brain. Antioxidants, like ginkgo and vitamin E, which protect neurons from damage. And other, less well known supplements we can take.

Like huperzine A, for example.

Huperzine A is a naturally occurring alkaloid that's found in the plant *Huperzia serrata*, also known as the Chinese club moss plant. For centuries, it's been used in Chinese medicine, mostly for things like fevers and inflammation. But in the past decade or so, research has shown that huperzine A works in the brain to prevent the breakdown of an important neurotransmitter needed for memory and cognition. It's pretty exciting stuff.

As of this writing, there is an ongoing phase 2 clinical trial to evaluate huperzine A in the treatment of Alzheimer's disease. The trials, conducted by the National Institute on Aging (NIA), are taking place at no fewer than twenty-nine different medical centers and universities across the United States. The results of the trial, "A Multi-Center, Double-Blind, Placebo-Controlled Therapeutic Trial to Determine Whether Natural Huperzine A Improves Cognitive Function," should be available soon.

We don't know the exact cause of Alzheimer's disease. We *do* know that it's a progressive disease of the brain that's characterized by impairment of memory and a disturbance in at least one other thinking function—like language, for example, or perception of reality. The Alzheimer's Association points out that although scientists know that Alzheimer's involves progressive brain failure, they've not been able to identify any one reason why cells fail. There are a number of risk factors for Alzheimer's, including age, family history, and genetics.

Alzheimer's patients have *plaques*—buildups of protein called *beta-amyloid*—that are toxic to nerve cells. They also typically have neurofibrillary tangles, pathological proteins first described by Alois Alzheimer himself when he discovered them in one of his patients suffering from the disorder that now bears his name.

The Role of Acetylcholine

Though the complete story of what causes what in Alzheimer's may remain unclear for a while, many scientists suspect that at least *part* of the picture has to do with an important chemical called *acetylcholine*. Deficiencies in acetylcholine can affect memory and thinking, and researchers suspect that at the very least, this is a contributing factor in dementia, and possibly even ordinary memory loss.

Acetylcholine is what's called a *neurotransmitter*—a chemical produced in the brain that transmits information. Acetylcholine is absolutely essential for memory, attention, and thought. The cells that produce acetylcholine are among the first to die off in Alzheimer's disease. Parkinson's disease, dementia that results from multiple strokes, multiple sclerosis, and schizophrenia, are all, like Alzheimer's, associated with lower levels of acetylcholine in the brain.

Acetylcholine is broken down in the brain by an enzyme called *acetylcholinesterase*. If you could somehow inhibit the action of this enzyme—making it perform its job less efficiently—you'd have more acetylcholine hanging around in the brain. Some Alzheimer's medicines—notably Aricept—work in just this way.

Can Huperzine A Help? Maybe!

Enter huperzine A, a natural acetylcholinesterase inhibitor. By blocking the breakdown of acetylcholine it essentially increases the levels of acetylcholine hanging around your neurons. And while that doesn't "cure" Alzheimer's or address some of the other myriad issues in the Alzheimer's brain (like the plaques and tangles), it's still a very good thing indeed. Huperzine A has been shown to improve memory, thinking, and behavioral function in people with Alzheimer's disease, dementia caused by multiple strokes, and senile dementia.

Natural Prescription for Cognitive Decline

Huperzine A: 60–200 mcg

★ **FOR ADDED EFFECTIVENESS:**

Vitamin E (mixed tocopherols): 1,000–2,000 IU daily

A daily antioxidant or vitamin supplement: taken as directed on package label

Ginkgo biloba: 120–480 mg in divided doses

Omega-3 fatty acids (or an essential fatty acid supplement): 1–3 g per day

(see also cognitive decline on page 109)

Note: All dosages are daily dosages and come in pill or capsule form unless otherwise noted.

H.Y. Zhang, of the Chinese Academy of Sciences in Shanghai, has studied huperzine A for more than a decade, and published multiple papers on its effects on senile memory disorders. In one recent paper, he stated that huperzine A has neuroprotective effects that "go beyond the inhibition of acetylcholinesterase."

Huperzine A can potentially ameliorate the learning and memory deficiency in both animals and Alzheimer's patients through a number of mechanisms that include reducing oxidative stress and protecting against neuronal cell death, according to Zhang. In one of Zhang's earlier studies (1991), he injected huperzine A into 56 patients with multi-infarct dementia or senile dementia and 104 patients with senile and pre-senile simple memory disorders. He then tested them on the Wechsler Memory Scale. Huperzine A produced significant positive effects.

Research at the Weizmann Institute of Science in Israel used x-ray crystallography to reveal exactly how huperzine A blocks acetyl-cholinesterase. It seems to bind specifically to the sites where acetylcholinesterase is broken down, closing off the enzyme's "cutting" action and protecting acetylcholine from danger. "HupA could be a potent drug, even when used in small quantities, so that the risk of side effects would be minimal," says professor Israel Silman of the institute.

Other research out of China has shown that huperzine A is as effective as at least two other drugs used in Alzheimer's disease.

Various types of huperzine A are available, and the natural form is about three times stronger and more potent than the synthetic kind. Doses of natural huperzine A used in the studies ranges from 60 mcg to 200 mcg daily. The *Physicians' Desk Reference* recommends that it be used with a physician's recommendation and monitoring.

Rhodiola

for Stress-Induced Fatigue, Memory, and Concentration

IF YOU'RE LOOKING for a natural lift of energy because you've had a rough day, put down the coffee and read on.

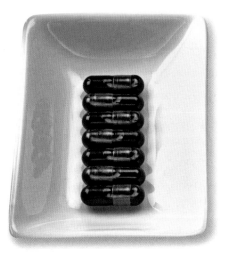

Rhodiola is an herb steeped deep in history and tradition. Traditionally in Eastern Europe and in Asia, rhodiola has been used to stimulate the nervous system, enhance performance, improve sleep, and reduce fatigue. The herb has been included as an official Russian medicine since 1969 and as a Swedish medicine since 1985. Of the 200 Rhodiola species, *R. rosea* has been studied most extensively, but its properties are not well known in the West since most publications are in Slavic and Scandinavian languages.

Grown primarily in arctic areas of Europe and Asia, rhodiola is categorized as an adaptogen. An adaptogen doesn't necessarily move things in one direction; it senses the needs of the system and acts accordingly. Much like the thermostat on your central air conditioning that makes the room warmer if it's too cold and colder if it's too warm, an adaptogen helps protect you by helping your body adapt to physiological stressors. And if you're looking for a natural stress buster, this might be just the ticket.

Firsthand Field Studies

Richard P. Brown, M.D., associate professor of clinical psychiatry at Columbia University College of Physicians and Surgeons in New York, experienced the benefits of *R. rosea* firsthand when he went with a colleague to northern Mongolia to gather wild *R. rosea*. They were interested in testing the wild form of *R. rosea* against domestically grown *R. rosea*. Brown decided to start taking the herb himself and almost immediately noticed that his mind was sharper, he felt less stressed, and he had more energy.

His wife, Patricia Gerbarg, M.D., also experienced the restorative benefits of *R. rosea*. Suffering from chronic and debilitating pain and fatigue after being treated for Lyme disease, she started taking *R. rosea* for its energy-boosting properties. After ten days, her mind was clearer, her concentration was sharper, and her memory was improving.

So from Siberia to Mongolia to Columbia University, the reputation of rhodiola's benefits spread. And there are plenty of studies to back up the folklore. In one study, physicians on night duty received a low dose of *R. rosea* over two weeks. At the end of the two weeks there was a significant improvement in the doctors' ability to counteract the effects of fatigue: The tests showed positive results on mental fatigue, involving associative thinking, short-term memory, calculation, ability to concentrate, and speed of audiovisual perception. How cool would it have been if the cast of *Grey's Anatomy* could have had access to rhodiola while they were interns at Seattle Grace? The show might not have been as interesting, but they sure would have been less stressed.

A Cold War Casualty—Almost

Another study examined *R. rosea's* effect on the fatigue of Russian students caused by stress during examination periods. One group was given *R. rosea* for twenty days during an examination period, while the other group received a placebo. Their physical and mental performances

were assessed before and after the time period, using both objective and subjective criteria. The results? Significant improvement in physical fitness, mental fatigue, and motor skills. The group taking rhodiola also rated their own subjective, general well-being significantly better than the placebo group rated theirs.

During the Cold War, the Soviets looked for a medicine that could boost energy, improve memory, and enhance performance so they could give their military an edge and improve the stamina and performance of their cosmonauts. Soviet scientists documented a wide range of benefits associated with *R. rosea* from calming the stress response and increasing energy to enhancing physical and mental performance under stress. According to author Peter Jaret, this "superherb" was very nearly lost to Cold War politics.

Protecting the Brain

Because it is an adaptogen, *R. rosea* may also protect against all sorts of stressors. A number of studies have shown that *R. rosea* increases

Natural Prescription for Stress-Induced Fatigue

Rhodiola rosea: 100–170 mg. Make sure it's an extract of the *R. rosea* root. This is the most effective and has significant animal and human studies.

Note: All dosages are daily dosages and in pill or capsule form unless otherwise noted.

physical work capacity and dramatically shortens the recovery time between periods of high-intensity exercise. Admittedly, some controversy exists over its power to increase physical stamina; more clinical trials are needed, but it's looking promising. And speaking of stressors, it's worth noting that in Middle Asia, *R. rosea* tea was an effective treatment for cold and flu during severe Asian winters.

Stress, over time, can interfere with memory systems and ultimately cause shrinkage of an important area of the brain called the hippocampus, which is intimately involved with memory.

R. rosea's protective effect on neurotransmitters (chemical messengers) in the brain helps to enhance thinking, analyzing, evaluating, calculating, planning, and remembering.

But wait, there's more! *R. rosea* has effects on the endocrine and reproductive systems. In mountain villages of Siberia, a bouquet of rhodiola roots is still given to couples prior to marriage to enhance fertility and assure the birth of healthy children. Studies have shown that *R. rosea* improves amenorrhea (loss of menstrual cycle) in women and sexual dysfunction in men. That alone makes it worth the price of admission!

St. Johns Wort
for Mild Depression

LET'S BE VERY CLEAR, in case there was any doubt in your mind: Depression is no picnic. Not only is depression one of the greatest problems of our time, it's also potentially life-threatening.

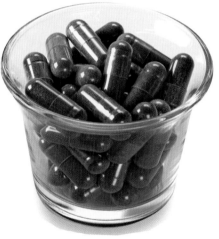

According to the Australian government—whose statistics are comparable to those of the United States and Britain—every single person will, at some time or another in their life, be affected by depression, either their own or someone else's. It's serious stuff. And in case you

get the idea that I'm wholly against the use of pharmaceuticals here, let me disabuse you of that notion: there's no doubt in my mind that antidepressant medications have saved lives. But for some people, with some forms of depression, there may be other options.

St. John's Wort is one of them.

Back in 2002, the media gave a ton of attention to a study that was published in the *Journal of the American Medical Association* (*JAMA*). Typical headline: "St. John's Wort Proved Ineffective for Depression." (You could practically see the anti-supplement brigade gloating over the latest "evidence" that we shouldn't bother with "natural" cures and instead stick with good old pharmaceuticals.)

As usual, the truth was far more nuanced.

The Types of Depression

Like the spicy sauces in a taco restaurant, depression actually comes in three "flavors." The National Institute of Mental Health breaks depression down into three categories (major depression, dysthymia, and bipolar disorder), but there are wide variations within each category, and the severity of symptoms varies with individuals and also over time. In everyday terms, depression is often ranked in terms of severity—mild, moderate, or severe. The 2002 study tested people with moderately severe major depression. We're not talking slight feelings of sadness or the "blues" here; we're talking real disability. Many of these people are completely non-responsive to drugs.

And guess what? St. John's Wort didn't help them very much. (What a lot of the media stories buried inches deep in the text was the fact that sertraline, a.k.a. Zoloft, didn't help them either.)

So what should you conclude from this one study? Does it mean you shouldn't try St. John's Wort if you are mildly depressed? Not at all. While it's true that in the *JAMA* study, St. John's Wort didn't show much effect on the most intractable and difficult of depressions, dozens of other studies—and the experience of an enormous number of people—suggest that St. John's Wort may be very effective for some of the lighter varieties of depression, which afflict untold numbers of people.

An Historic and Helpful Herb

St. John's Wort is actually a perennial herb with many flowers that can be found growing wild in much of the world (the word "wort" just means plant). It's got a long and honorable history of use, probably dating back to the ancient Greeks, who believed that the fragrance of St. John's Wort caused evil spirits to simply fly, fly away. (Okay, maybe these days, not so much.) But it does have a 2,400-year history of folk use for everything from anxiety to sleep disturbances. St. John's Wort was officially recognized as an antidepressant drug in Germany in 1998, is

> *"Natural medications such as St. John's Wort, SAMe, and omega-3 fatty acids eventually may prove to be valuable additions to the psychiatrist's pharmacologic armamentarium, both as monotherapy and as adjunctive therapy for mood disorders. Current research data are compelling, from a standpoint of both efficacy and safety...."*
>
> —David Mischoulon, M.D., Ph.D.,
> *Harvard University Department of Psychiatry Depression and Research Program, Massachusetts General Hospital*

covered by the country's national health care system, and in fact is the number one prescribed antidepressant in Germany and most of Europe.

According to noted expert Steven Bratman, M.D., author of the excellent reference book The *Natural Pharmacy*, St. John's Wort has a scientific record approaching that of many prescription drugs, and is effective in about 55 percent of cases. Bratman also points out that there is good evidence that it's at least as effective as fluoxetine (Prozac) and sertraline (Zoloft). If you're feeling mild symptoms of depression, St. John's Wort is definitely worth a try.

Supported by Studies

A meta-analysis published in the *British Medical Journal* in 1996 reviewed 23 published trials on St. John's Wort involving more than 1,700 patients. The researchers, lead by Klaus Linde, M.D., reported findings that extracts of St. John's Wort were more effective than a placebo for the treatment of mild to moderately severe depression. The authors emphasized that it's not yet known whether the extracts are more effective for some types of depression than others, but that certainly looks to be the case. It's worth noting that overall, only about 10 percent of the patients in the studies had side effects with St. John's Wort (like dry mouth, allergic reactions, and some gastrointestinal upset), compared with about 35 percent of patients who reported side effects from prescription antidepressants. Only about 5 percent of the patients stopped taking it because of side effects, a low number indeed.

Many other studies have shown St. John's Wort to be effective, and with virtually no significant side effects (more on that in a moment). Another 1999 study, also published in the *British Medical Journal*, tested hypericum extract—one of the active ingredients in St. John's Wort—against both a placebo and a standard antidepressant (imipramine) in a randomized multi-center study involving 263 patients with moderate depression. Hypercium was more effective than the placebo at reducing depression (as measured by the Hamilton depression scores and, even more dramatically, by the Zung self-rating depression scale), and performed just as well as the drug, with notably fewer side effects. The researchers noted that while both the drug and St. John's Wort improved the mental component scale of Short Form-36 (a widely used standardized test), only St. John's Wort improved the physical component scale. "The rate of adverse events with the hypericum extract was in the range of the placebo group but lower than that of the (drug) group," researchers noted.

A Rich Cast of Plant Chemicals

There are many active ingredients in St. John's Wort, but for a long time the one believed to be responsible for the herb's antidepressant action was *hypericum*. But the plant actually contains dozens of active components (including chlorogenic acid, flavonoids, and xanthones). More recently, researchers have focused on *hyperforin*, another active ingredient in St. John's Wort. "Hyperforin, rather than hypericin as originally thought, has emerged as one of the major constituents for antidepressant activity," one 2001 article in the *Journal of Pharmacy and Pharmacology* pointed out.

The rich cast of active plant chemicals is undoubtedly why St. John's Wort has been found useful for such a wide variety of conditions besides depression. In fact, the *Physician's Desk Reference for Herbal Medicine* lists positive results in clinical trials for anxiety, cognitive function, fatigue, ear pain in children, dermatitis, and PMS, in addition to depression. And in addition to depression, the German Commission E

WORTH KNOWING

The best preparation seems to be the St. John's Wort extract standardized to contain 0.3 percent hypericin, and the recommended dosage of this as an antidepressant is 300 mg, taken three times a day, close to meals. You can also drink it as a tea (boiling water poured onto one to two teaspoons of the dried herb, infused for 10–15 minutes).

St. John's Wort interacts with a lot of medications, so if you're on meds, check with a health professional knowledgeable about both St. John's Wort and pharmaceuticals before beginning to take it. It also is known to make you more sensitive to the sun, so if you like to spend time at the beach, be careful if you're on St. John's Wort.

approves it for anxiety, inflammation of the skin, blunt injuries, wounds, and burns. The U.S. National Institutes of Health (NIH) funded a $4.4 million grant for research into St. John's Wort's anti-inflammatory, anti-viral, and analgesic properties.

St. John's Wort is no cure for major, crippling depression, and I don't for a moment want to give the impression that it is. But for many people suffering with mild forms of this debilitating condition, it may indeed be helpful. Like most treatments for depression, it takes a while to work. The PDR recommends that you try it for four to six weeks; if no improvement is apparent, try something different.

Saw Palmetto

May Ease Acne and Female Hair Loss

RECENTLY, SARAH HINER of *Bottom Line Health*— one of my favorite editors in the world—told me about a letter from a reader, a thirty-year-old woman named Jessie. Jessie had suffered with adult acne for years and recently started using a product (Usana's Palmetto Plus) that is a formula featuring a well-known herb called saw palmetto. (Saw palmetto is best known for use in treating a male condition called benign prostate hyperplasia; see page 260.)

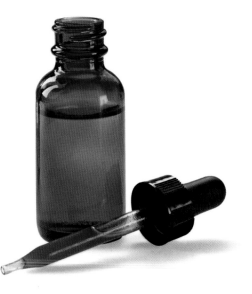

"I've been looking in the mirror and seeing clear and healthy skin that I haven't seen for years," wrote Jessie. Obviously she was thrilled, but she was also concerned because saw palmetto is marketed as a "man's supplement." Specifically, she wanted to know whether saw palmetto can have any adverse effects if and when she wants to conceive. (The short answer: Don't take it if you're pregnant.)

So what's the deal? Could saw palmetto indeed be a natural "cure" for acne? And if so, why?

The Causes of Acne

Besides Usana's Palmetto Plus, there are a number of other high-quality saw palmetto products on the market. (I use Prostate Supreme, available on my website, www.jonnybowden.com.)

There's also one special saw palmetto-based product called Clearogen that offers a high-octane version of saw palmetto and is applied topically. (More on that later.) But other than Clearogen, saw palmetto products are marketed for a well-known male problem known as benign prostate hyperplasia, as mentioned above. However, there's a growing buzz about saw palmetto—it's beginning to get a reputation as being very good for clearing up acne. Though as of this writing there aren't any solid research studies on acne and saw palmetto, there's quite a lot of anecdotal evidence from a growing number of people who've had good luck with it. To understand why saw palmetto is getting so much attention as a possible treatment for acne, you need to understand a bit about what causes acne in the first place.

Two events conspire to create or aggravate most forms of acne. One is blockage, two is infection. Here's how it works: Keratin is a fibrous protein that's the main component of the outermost layer of the skin. Sebum is part of the oil found on the surface of the skin and is produced by the sebaceous glands, most of which open into a hair follicle. When either too much keratin or too much sebum is produced, they can block the skin pores. Those overstuffed pores then can become infected by bacteria, which literally eat up the sebum and thrive.

One of the main things that drives the overproduction of either sebum or keratin is hormones. According to Michael Murray, N.D., acne is considered a "male hormone dependent condition" because the male hormone testosterone fuels the growth of keratin and causes the sebaceous glands to enlarge and overproduce sebum. (Don't forget—females also have testosterone, just not as much as we guys.) But it's not just the amount of testosterone you have that causes the problem. It's how your body metabolizes it. In response to an enzyme called 5-alpha reductase, testosterone converts in the body to a nasty little compound called DHT—dihydrotestosterone—which stimulates the sebaceous glands to produce even higher levels of sebum. (DHT is also partially responsible for male pattern baldness and for benign prostate hyperplasia.) Point is, it's not the friend of anyone with acne. To complicate things further, a high glycemic (high-sugar) diet accelerates the conversion of testosterone to DHT. (See the Paleo Diet for acne, page 203.)

Enter saw palmetto.

The Testosterone Connection

Saw palmetto is an herb with a documented ability to prevent some of that conversion of testosterone to DHT. The question is, what role exactly does DHT play in acne? We know it

Natural Prescription for Acne

Clearogen as directed (www.clearogen.com) or saw palmetto (make sure to get a high-quality formula from a reputable company): 320 mg

An antioxidant supplement containing vitamin C and E: Take as directed.

Zinc: 30 mg, two to three times a day; taper off to 30 mg as maintenance

Essential fatty acid supplement or fish oil: 1–2 g

GLA: 320 mg

Topical tea tree oil (antiseptic): Apply as needed.

Azelic acid (anti-inflammatory): Use as directed.

FOR BEST RESULTS, FOLLOW:

Paleo Diet, which contains no grains, dairy, beans, or soy but is high in proteins such as fish and grass-fed meats, as well as vegetables, fruits (especially berries), nuts, and omega fats (see page 203).

Note: The above dosages are daily and in pill or capsule form unless otherwise noted.

plays a big role in male pattern baldness, it probably plays an even bigger role in female hair loss, and it definitely plays a starring role in benign prostate hyperplasia. How much of hormone-driven acne is due to testosterone and how much is due to its metabolite DHT (which I like to call "son of testosterone") no one is quite sure. But it's very possible that DHT plays a substantial role, and if so, limiting the conversion of testosterone to DHT—which saw palmetto can clearly do—would be a boon for acne sufferers.

Richard Fried, M.D., Ph.D., the author of *Healing Adult Acne* and one of my "go-to" guys for skin problems, explains it this way: "There are people who, through God, bad luck, or genes, are just susceptible to the effects of testosterone and DHT. The cells that line the hair follicle over-respond to this hormonal stimulation."

When this happens, the oil glands produce too much oil, which in turn clogs the follicles and creates a welcome environment for bacteria. "The immune system mounts an attack against that bacteria, which leads to inflammation, which is why a pimple can turn into a nasty, red cyst that can scar both physically and emotionally," Fried says. The theory—and it remains a theory—is that by downsizing the conversion of testosterone to DHT, saw palmetto can make a big difference.

The Proof is in the Profile

Opinion is divided on saw palmetto as a natural cure for acne, but only because there aren't any good solid research studies on using it for acne. But it passes the smell test and it makes good

common sense that it might be a terrific adjunct to the Paleolithic diet in a natural prescription for acne.

Alex Khadavi, M.D., a dermatologist in California, is one of the people banking on the likelihood that down-regulating the conversion of testosterone to DHT will make a big difference to acne sufferers. His company has developed a product called Clearogen that is based on saw palmetto plus a few other active ingredients.

"Saw palmetto is a good ingredient, but it's gotten more credit than it deserves," says Khadavi. He believes that most capsules of saw palmetto contain a small amount of the active ingredients that block androgen receptors. Clearogen contains high concentrations of the active ingredients in the saw palmetto plant—specifically, beta-sitosterol, phytol, and ethyl laurate—added to a formula that also contains omega-3s (alpha linolenic acid), omega-6s (gamma linolenic acid and linoleic acid), and omega-9s (oleic acid). The omegas help block the conversion, plus they act as powerful anti-inflammatories. To top it off, Clearogen is administered topically. "Orally, you would need very high amounts of these ingredients," Khadavi told me.

Fried feels that saw palmetto holds quite a bit of promise, though he won't go so far as to call it a cure for acne. "We know DHT is a main player in hair loss—the question is, how much of a player is it in acne?"

Fried told me that there are no convincing studies that oral (or topical) saw palmetto decreases acne, but nonetheless he didn't want to dismiss the possibility that it might help a number of people, especially because, as he pointed out, individuals with acne respond differently to different interventions.

"A cynic might say that the reason that there are no clinical published studies is that it's not a patentable medicine," he wryly says. "My feeling is that anything that decreases androgen stimulation of the hair follicle has the potential to decrease acne."

The Supporting Players in the Acne Fight

In addition to saw palmetto (either in conventional form or as the product Clearogen), a number of other supplements and herbs have been found helpful for acne. Tea tree oil has remarkable antibacterial and antiseptic activity and is great for cleaning the skin. One study showed that a 5 percent tea tree oil solution worked as well as a similar solution of benzoyl peroxide but with much fewer side effects.

Azelaic acid kills bacteria associated with acne and acts as an anti-inflammatory. It's recommended by my good friend Alan Gaby, M.D., considered by many to be among the most respected sources for information on natural and nutritional medicine (along with his teaching partner Jonathan Wright, M.D.). Azelaic acid can be applied topically as a cream and has been shown to be about as effective as .05 percent Retin-A, erythromycin ointment, benzoyl peroxide, or oral tetracycline. Gaby says that a combination of azelaic acid cream twice daily along with 100 mg of oral minocycline daily (a tetracycline derivative) is even more effective. Because on rare occasions azelaic acid has been associated with a loss of skin pigmentation, Gaby recommends that a doctor monitor its use. Discontinue after maximum improvement is obtained.

Finally, there's zinc, which many people have used with success. Some studies have shown a lot of improvement, though others have not. Gaby prescribes a well-absorbed form of zinc such as zinc picolinate or zinc citrate, at a dose of about 90 mg a day (30 mg, two to three times a day). He cautions that because large doses of zinc can promote copper deficiency, you should take a copper supplement of about 2 to 4 mg per day (depending on zinc dosage) as well.

Saw Palmetto

for Benign Prostatic Hyperplasia

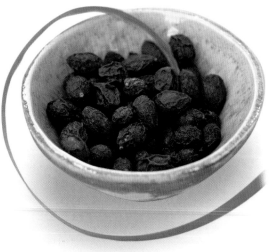

DOES WAKING UP in the middle of the night to go to the bathroom sound familiar? If you're a man over forty, chances are you've experienced the all-too-common symptoms of benign prostatic hyperplasia (BPH). Frequent urination, especially in the middle of the night, is the signature of this annoying but essentially harmless condition. So are a hesitant, interrupted, or weak stream of urine, a pressing urgency to urinate, leaking, or dribbling.

Annoying as it is, BPH is not usually dangerous. However, you need to be aware of two things. One, urine retention and strain on the bladder can lead to more serious problems, including bladder damage, kidney damage, bladder stones, urinary tract infection, and the inability to control urination. If you catch BPH early, there's a much lower risk of such complications. And fortunately, there are some easy and natural ways to bring relief (more on that in a moment).

Saw palmetto is the "go-to" herb when it comes to taming the urge to pee every few hours. A three-year study in Germany found that 160 mg of saw palmetto extract taken twice daily reduced nighttime urination in 73 percent of people and improved urinary flow rates significantly. Another multicenter study showed that a similar amount treated BPH as well as the drug Proscar, but without the side effects.

Though we don't know the exact cause of BPH, it's widely believed that it's fueled by hormones, specifically testosterone and even more specifically the metabolism of testosterone. But what's even more important is what happens to the testosterone that we do make. Some testosterone is converted in the body to a nasty little metabolite called DHT (dihydrotestosterone). DHT is thought to be partly responsible for male baldness, and a high conversion of testosterone to DHT in women is thought to be connected to a host of "male" symptoms like hair loss (on the head) and hair growth (on the face). This conversion—in both men and women—is fueled by an enzyme called 5-alpha-reductase. Saw palmetto helps to down-regulate this enzyme, meaning a reduction in the amount of DHT. Saw palmetto also contains compounds that act as anti-inflammatories.

Note: It's always good to rule out cancer as a cause of the urinary symptoms. A blood test called a PSA (for prostate-specific antigen) is a good idea. Though the test is hardly conclusive for cancer, PSA is frequently elevated in the blood of men with prostate cancer.

Other Helpful Supplements

Although saw palmetto is the superstar nutrient for "curing" all-night bathroom breaks, four other supplements have also been found to be helpful. Pygeum is an extract from the bark of an African tree and is approved in at least three countries in Europe as a BPH remedy. It relieves symptoms of BPH and contains at least three types of compounds that help the prostate.

Beta-sitosterol is a plant sterol found in almost all plants, especially in rice bran, wheat germ, corn oils, and soybeans. In clinical research it's been shown to help lower blood cholesterol, but more to the point, it's also been shown to reduce the symptoms of BPH. Four double-blind, placebo-controlled studies including 519 men and lasting from 4 to 26 weeks concluded that beta-sitosterol significantly improved urological symptoms and flow measures.

Nettles (stinging nettles) are frequently combined with other "prostate herbs" like saw palmetto and have long been believed to have a beneficial effect on prostate health. One recent double-blind, placebo-controlled study in a 2005 issue of the *Journal of Herb Pharmacotherapy* found that it had beneficial effects, and other studies have also been encouraging.

Pumpkin seeds have a well-deserved reputation as a prostate-friendly food and are an approved "therapy" for men with BPH in Germany. In a few studies, pumpkin-seed oil has been shown to have a good effect on BPH symptoms, but no good research shows that they work by themselves. You may use pumpkin extract in combination with saw palmetto in supplements for prostate health.

Although the research on zinc for BPH is spotty, most complementary and holistic health practitioners recommend it. Zinc is absolutely essential to prostate health. Prostatic secretions contain a high concentration of zinc. Zinc also tones down the activity of the 5-alpha-reductase enzyme, which, you may recall, fuels the conver-

> ## Natural Prescription for Benign Prostate Hyperplasia
>
> **Saw palmetto:** 320 mg (160 mg, twice a day)
>
> **CAN BE COMBINED WITH (APPROXIMATE VALUES):**
>
> **Pygeum:** 100–200 mg (50–100 mg, twice a day)
>
> **Stinging nettles:** 300 mg (150 mg, twice a day)
>
> **Beta-sitosterol:** 100–300 mg (150 mg, twice a day)
>
> **Zinc:** 50 mg to start; reduce to 30 mg after a few months
>
> **Note:** All dosages are daily dosages and in pill or capsule form unless otherwise noted.

sion of testosterone to dihydrotestosterone. (And let's not forget that stress depletes zinc like crazy, so many individuals may be low to begin with.)

"Whatever you do, if you have an enlarged prostate along with the usual symptoms, don't reach for that saw palmetto without picking up the zinc and essential fatty acids too," says the noted teacher of nutritional medicine Alan Gaby, M.D. Gaby and others usually recommend beginning with a large amount of zinc (typically 50–100 mg a day). Since that dose of zinc can conceivably lead to an imbalance in copper, Gaby and others also add 2–4 mg of copper. "After several months, the dose is typically reduced to 30 mg once or twice a day, depending on the patient's response," says Gaby. The best-absorbed forms of zinc are zinc picolinate and zinc citrate.

Tea Tree Oil
for Wound Healing

SUPPOSE YOU'RE AN Australian aborigine, and you've never seen a drugstore. In fact, suppose you're an Australian aborigine a couple of hundred years ago when there weren't any drugstores to see, even if you *could* get into a city, which you couldn't anyway because you're an Australian aborigine and you live in the forest.

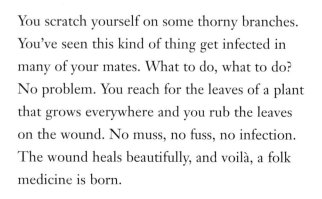

You scratch yourself on some thorny branches. You've seen this kind of thing get infected in many of your mates. What to do, what to do? No problem. You reach for the leaves of a plant that grows everywhere and you rub the leaves on the wound. No muss, no fuss, no infection. The wound heals beautifully, and voilà, a folk medicine is born.

Now it probably took a bit of trial and error for the aborigines to figure out which tree leaves had this amazing property, but think of those hit-and-miss tests as the primitive version of what we now call clinical trials. But figure it out they did, and the plant they used—not just for scratches and infection and wound healing but for all manner of things that required what we now know as an antibiotic—was the tea tree.

Legend has it that the tree that produced those healing leaves was named the "tea tree" by none other than British explorer Captain James Cook, who made a drink from the leaves and discovered it made an excellent tea. (Some authorities actually think he also discovered it could cure scurvy, which was killing more than a few of his sailors at the time.) About 150 years later, an Australian scientist named Arthur Penford rediscovered the tea tree's curative properties, and it's been a staple in Australia for the treatment of wounds and infections ever since. It was considered so essential in Australia that during World War ll, the government allowed producers of the oil to be exempt from military service.

What It's Good For

Whoever gets credit for discovering it, we now know that the oil of this tree—which comes from the melaleuca tree and is native to New South Wales, Australia—is rich with healing properties. Though its traditional use for treating infected wounds remains its claim to fame, it's also effective against a host of fungi and bacteria, making it a terrific antiseptic. According to the Kevala Center for Holistic Health, it's quite effective for cuts, burns, and insect bites, and it's a powerful antiviral agent as well and may even be useful in helping fight off infectious diseases such as flu and colds. The center recommends putting a couple of drops of the oil in a bowl of steaming water, covering your head, and inhaling for five to ten minutes to relieve congestion and fight infection.

WORTH KNOWING

Tea tree oil shouldn't be applied to broken skin or rashes that aren't from fungus. It may irritate the skin, so start with a small amount to see whether it works for you. It's not believed to be effective orally, so don't take it internally.

Besides its traditional uses, tea tree oil has actually been studied scientifically for its ability to reduce the symptoms of athlete's foot, an area in which it performs admirably. In one study it didn't cure the infection 100 percent of the time (what treatment does?), but it cured many cases and performed significantly better than a placebo. Since it is an effective natural antibiotic when used topically, it may be of help when applied to the skin in cases of acne. For acne, the typical strength of preparations is 5 to 15 percent tea tree oil, while 70 to 100 percent strength is usually used for fungal infections. You can also put it on your gums as a preventive against periodontal disease.

The active ingredient appears to be a compound called terpinen-4-ol, and good tea tree oil should be standardized to contain at *least* 30 percent of this compound. You also want to make sure it's standardized to contain no more than 10 percent cineole (preferably much less), which is an irritant. According to experts, the finest tea tree products come from the oil of the *Alternifolia* species of the melaleuca plant.

NATURAL
TREATMENTS

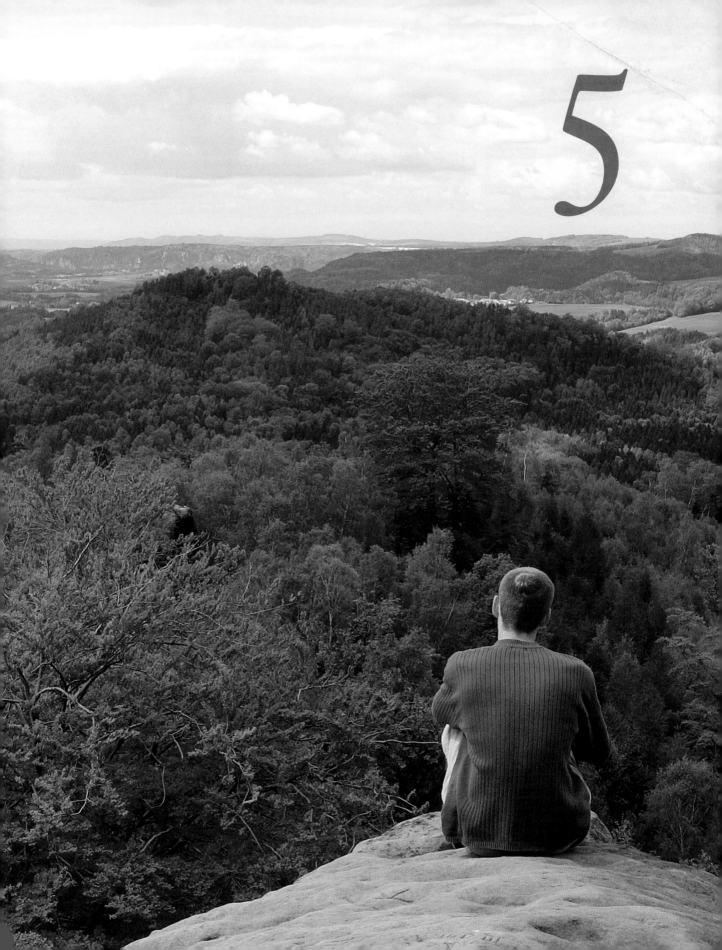

5

Acupuncture
for Infertility

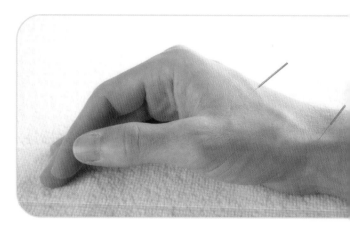

HAVING TROUBLE getting pregnant?
You might want to consider acupuncture.
Acupuncture might not be the first thing
you think of if you're having a problem
with infertility, but maybe it should be.
Studies—and a great deal of clinical experience—suggest that it might
help, even if you're already undergoing standard therapies like in vitro
fertilization or intrauterine insemination.

Acupuncture is actually one of the oldest medical practices in the world. Although it originated in China more than two millennia ago, it first gained popularity in the United States when a well-known and respected *New York Times* reporter named James Reston wrote glowingly about it after it helped ease his postsurgical pain. As of this writing, more than eight million American adults have had acupuncture treatment. As practiced by licensed practitioners who undergo extensive training and are often trained in traditional Chinese medicine (TCM) as well, it is completely safe and quite effective for a number of conditions.

One of those conditions is infertility.

The Yin, the Yang, and Baby Makes Three

Acupuncture, like TCM, is based on a concept of the body as a balance of forces—yin (the cold, the slow, and the passive) and yang (the hot, the excited, and the active). The general theory of acupuncture is based on the premise that vital energy (known as *qi* or *chi*) flows along pathways in the body, that there are patterns of this energy flow that are essential for health, and that disruptions of this flow are responsible for disease. Optimal health is achieved when energy is in balance, flowing effortlessly through the body. Qi travels twenty major pathways, which TCM calls meridians. They're accessible through 400 different acupuncture points. By stimulating these meridians at carefully chosen points and in carefully chosen combinations, the acupuncturist can overcome blocks, help balance energy, and promote health.

One of the reasons conventional Western medicine has trouble wrapping its mind around acupuncture is that it's hard to subject it to the kind of specific scientific study that Western scientists are used to. In a standard scientific study, one group is given a drug (the experimental group) and the other group (the placebo group) is given a sugar pill. No one knows who gets what, including the researchers measuring the results (hence the description double blind). The researchers then observe whether there's a difference in some variable of interest (cholesterol, blood pressure, and so on), and if the difference is great enough, they attribute it to the pill. But how do you give the "sugar pill" equivalent of acupuncture? You can put the needles in neutral places (called a "sham" treatment) and compare it to the "real" treatment, but this isn't a perfect solution and there's a lot of disagreement about how to do it.

In addition, Western medicine doesn't really have a concept that's equivalent to "energy." For left-brained Western doctors, you either see something or you don't. If it's not measurable and observable, they're usually not interested. Acupuncture—for many conservative, rigid thinkers trained conventionally in Western medicine—is just plain weird. But that's changing. In 1997, a blue ribbon panel at the National Institutes of Health issued a statement on acupuncture that said, in part: "[P]romising results have emerged, for example, showing efficacy of acupuncture in adult postoperative and

chemotherapy nausea and vomiting and in postoperative dental pain. There are other situations such as addiction, stroke rehabilitation, headache, menstrual cramps, tennis elbow, fibromyalgia, myofascial pain, osteoarthritis, low back pain, carpal tunnel syndrome, and asthma, in which acupuncture may be useful as an adjunct treatment or an acceptable alternative or be included in a comprehensive management program. Further research is likely to uncover additional areas where acupuncture interventions will be useful."

Indeed, one of those areas of "further research" has been infertility. And the results have been hard to argue with.

The Causes of Infertility

Two basic types of problems can interfere with fertility: structural problems (e.g., damaged fallopian tubes) or functional problems (e.g., an irregular menstrual cycle).

"By needling certain points on the meridians you can influence and rebalance the endocrine and hormonal system," says Cindy Lawrence, LAc, a licensed acupuncturist who also holds a master's degree in oriental medicine. "Regulating the menstrual cycle is very important—maybe the patient is not ovulating or [her] luteal phase is too short." Lawrence points out that together with the traditional Chinese herbs often used by acupuncturists as complements to the treatment, acupuncture can increase blood flow to the uterus, further increasing the chances of successful implantation.

Then, of course, there's the stress connection.

A running theme throughout this book is the effect stress can have on many health conditions. Stress hormones wreak havoc with virtually every metabolic process, influencing everything from weight to brain function. And acupuncture really shines when it comes to reducing stress.

"If energy is stagnated or out of balance in certain meridians or organs it can result in stress and anxiety," Lawrence explains. Patients typically report an almost otherworldly, completely pleasant feeling of relaxation after a session. (For what it's worth, that's been my experience the dozen or so times I've tried acupuncture. You literally can fall asleep on the table, and invariably sleep like a baby afterward.)

Then there's the research, and it's pretty impressive.

One study in Germany compared a group of eighty women undergoing in vitro fertilization with eighty women undergoing the same treatment *plus* acupuncture. Only twenty-one of the women who received only in vitro fertilization became pregnant (26.3 percent), but thirty-four of the women who *also* received acupuncture conceived (42.5 percent). An American study produced equally impressive results. Fifty-one percent of those who had the additional acupuncture treatment became pregnant, while only 36 percent of those receiving only in vitro fertilization did. In addition, fewer than half as many who received acupuncture miscarried.

Yet another study, done at Women's Hospital at the University of Heidelberg, Germany, involved forty-five infertile women.

Following a complete gynecological and endocrinologic exam, they were treated with acupuncture. Their results compared with those of a matched sample of forty-five women of the same age and history who had been treated with conventional hormones. The women treated with hormones had twenty pregnancies (and a number of side effects). The women treated with acupuncture? Twenty-two pregnancies (and no side effects).

Finally, a study at the Fertility Clinic Trianglen in Denmark concluded that "acupuncture … significantly improves the reproductive outcome of IVF (in vitro fertilization) and ICSI (intracytoplasmic sperm injection) compared to no acupuncture."

Best of all, acupuncture for infertility is truly a "whole person" treatment that looks at the woman as much more than just a dysfunctional reproductive system. "People come into my office and they're completely unprepared for conception," Lawrence told me. "They're overworked, sleep deprived, not happy, overweight, and stressed out, which is not the best environment for a conception or a pregnancy."

Lawrence spends considerable time with the women who come to see her, making sure they take time to relax, eat the right foods, and manage their stress and sleep. She prescribes herbs on a completely individual basis to strengthen the areas of the patient's body that are not in balance. "It's very important in Chinese medicine to prepare the body—you don't plant a seed in infertile ground," she says.

Oh, one more thing in case you're wondering—acupuncture doesn't hurt a bit. If you closed your eyes during the treatment, you'd never even know that there were needles actually sticking out of you. I know this for a fact because I've had it done. Obviously it didn't make me pregnant—but it definitely felt good afterward.

Chiropractic
for Back Pain

YEARS AGO, when I was in charge of the curriculum at the Equinox Fitness Training Institute in New York City, I had a lot of occasion to work with chiropractors. One thing I noticed was that, as a group, they seemed way more interested and knowledgeable about nutrition than most of the medical doctors I knew.

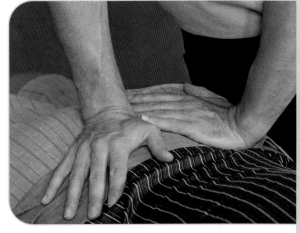

Maybe because chiropractors do not prescribe drugs, their orientation always seemed to be toward maximizing the body's natural ability to heal. The guiding philosophy behind chiropractic is the belief that the structure and condition of the body influences how the body functions as well as its ability to heal itself. Chiropractic philosophy has also long held that the mind-body relationship is instrumental in both health and healing.

Effective Back Pain Relief

Though chiropractors, like acupuncturists, can address a wide variety of health needs, the one they're best known for—and the one in which they excel—is healing back pain. A study in the October 2005 *Journal of Manipulative and Physiological Therapeutics* showed that when it comes to lower back pain, chiropractic care provided significantly better outcomes than standard medical care. Patients with chronic lower back pain who underwent chiropractic treatment had higher levels of satisfaction with the care, lower disability scores, and higher pain relief than those who underwent medical treatment. To top it off, chiropractic care was more cost effective overall.

If you've never experienced bad back pain, you're one of the lucky ones. Back pain is the second most frequent problem that brings people to a doctor's office (the common cold is the first). Back pain is also one of the most common reasons for missed work. Experts estimate that 80 percent of the world population will experience back pain at some point in their life. According to the American College of Rheumatology, lower back pain disables 5.4 million Americans and costs at least 90 billion—read that again, *billion*—dollars in medical and nonmedical expenses.

So What's a Subluxation, Anyway?

So how does chiropractic work its magic on back pain?

It all starts with what chiropractors call a *subluxation*. "In layman's terms, it's a misalignment," says my friend, Matthew Mannino, D.C., an Arizona holistic chiropractor. Best described as "not quite a dislocation," which is a complete separation of a joint, a subluxation is actually a degenerative condition in which one or more of the spinal vertebrae are out of place. In other words, it's lost its proper juxtaposition with one, or both, of its neighboring vertebrae.

"Over time, damage and stress occur, resulting in pain," says Mannino. "This kind of mis-

alignment always has a price—deteriorating tissue, ligaments, and tendons, accompanied by inflammation."

Mannino likens the deterioration to that of tooth decay. "You don't feel the bone in a tooth decaying," he says. "It's only when the nerve gets irritated or inflamed that the pain comes and you run to the dentist. But that deterioration has been going on for a while."

Management of Misalignment

Because the majority of back pain complaints are mechanical in nature, chiropractic is the number-one conservative approach for back pain. No surgery, no drugs, but plenty of pain relief. Why? Because chiropractic adjustment treats the root cause—a misalignment of the body's structure that ultimately produces a painful inflammatory response. By realigning the vertebrae and other bones, the cause of the inflammation is removed. Back pain is gone—not because its symptoms were suppressed with drugs, but because the body no longer needs to send a message to your brain saying "Pay attention! Something is deeply wrong down here!"

Electrical impulses that begin in the brain and travel through the cords of the spinal cord out through to specific nerve roots pass through an area between every vertebrae called the intervertebral foramin, or IBF, Mannino says. The nerve travels through this hole to get out of the spinal column. But because of the subluxation—that displacement of the surrounding vertebrae—there's now an electromagnetic field around the nerve impulse.

"When the nerve travels through it's like walking through a security gate at the airport," Mannino explains. "Frequency and amplitude are changed, and the signal is altered all because of the subluxation." Nerve impulses, according to chiropractic theory, are messenger systems for the innate wisdom of the body. They tell the lungs to breathe, the liver to detox, and the heart to beat.

"If the signal is altered because of the subluxation," Mannino told me, "the tissues have no other choice than to respond. If it's asthma, they overrespond. If it's a nerve going to the stomach, the digestive process is slowed. If cells aren't instructed to break down food, you're going to have a toxic buildup. In other words, every organ in the body is susceptible to the effects of subluxation."

What Inflamation and Spasms Mean

When you're feeling back pain, it's a good bet that you're feeling the results of either inflammation or muscle spasm. Conventional medicine treats this either with a muscle relaxant or a painkiller. Both give relief but are akin to taking the battery out of the smoke alarm because you don't like that high-pitched sound emanating from the ceiling. In the case of your back, the fire's still burning, but you're just not smelling the smoke.

"Spasm is the body's natural protective action," Mannino says. "If there's harm to the nerve, the body says, 'Muscles, I'm locking you up so you can't hurt the nerve anymore.' The muscle spasm is actually the body's way

of protecting its most valuable asset—the nervous system."

Chiropractic's way of dealing with muscle spasms is to remove its reason for spasming in the first place. By adjusting your spine and realigning your vertebrae, the chiropractor removes the pressure on your nerve. The brain says, "Okay, pressure's off, let's party!" and sends a signal to the muscles that essentially says "You can relax now, the danger's gone!" Though chiropractors will typically use other modalities besides adjustment—ice, muscle stimulation, and other physical therapies—the corrective series of chiropractic adjustments remains their number-one tool with a bullet.

Fixing the Problem, Not the Symptom

Besides "fixing" the pain, chiropractors also focus on rehabilitative exercise, stabilization, and flexibility.

"Remember the subluxation happens in a complex system—there's a bone, a nerve, and a soft tissue component. So while the adjustment removes pressure on the nerve, we also have our patients do some specific movements in the form of stretching, flexibility, strengthening, and range-of-motion exercise to rehabilitate the soft tissue," Mannino says.

Finally, chiropractors focus on what they call activities of daily living; Mannino calls it spinal hygiene. "We help people learn how to lift, bend, sit, and stand in a way that helps them be cognizant of their body so they don't injure it again," he told me.

Remember, pain is not in your tissue, it's in your brain. A conventional medical approach to back pain will simply give a chemical to stop the pain signal from damaged tissue from ever getting to the brain in the first place.

"But that's a two-way street," says Mannino. "The drug is blocking the pain signals, but it's also blocking the healing information, and that's the price you pay. Sure, the brain can't get the pain signal, but it also doesn't get to know there's something wrong. After all, the body tightened up for a reason."

Chiropractic works because instead of blocking that signal from the brain that there's a problem, it treats the cause of the problem in the first place.

And when you think about it, that's the ultimate definition of a natural cure.

EFT

for Emotional Relief

EFT STANDS FOR Emotional Freedom Technique. Described by its founder, Gary Craig, as an emotional version of acupuncture, EFT is a technique that people use to liberate themselves from the energetic blocks caused by anger, grief, negative self-image, self-defeating beliefs, and even disease.

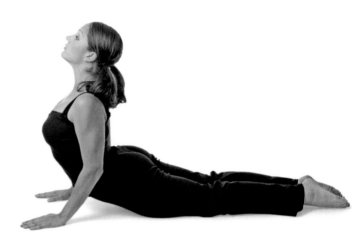

I decided to include it in this book because it's endorsed by a number of people for whom I have great respect, such as my friend Joe Mercola, D.O., who has made it an integral part of his practice for years. Candace Pert, Ph.D., author of the groundbreaking book *Molecules of Emotion*, says that "EFT is at the forefront of the new healing movement," and Deepak Chopra has said "EFT offers great healing benefits."

The premise of EFT is based on the idea that there are energy pathways throughout the body (similar to the *meridians* in acupuncture) and that if this energy is not flowing well, health is negatively affected. In this way it does indeed share a similar philosophical underpinning with acupuncture. In EFT, you stimulate these meridians (or energy pathways) with fingertips instead of needles. Specifically, you simply tap with the fingertips on nine specific meridian spots while stating an affirmation related to the issue you want to address (more on that in a moment).

Tapping Pain Away

There are nine "tapping points" on the body, one located on the top of the head, five located on various parts of the face and chin, two on the body, and one on the wrists. It doesn't matter in what order you do them, just so long as you hit them all (though it makes it a snap to remember if you go from top to bottom), Mercola says. The classic technique taught by founder Gary Craig relies on using just two fingers of one hand for the tapping, but Mercola's version uses four fingers of both hands.

"There are a number of acupuncture meridians on your fingertips, and when you tap with your fingertips you are likely using not only the meridians you are tapping on, but also the ones on your fingers," he says.

The affirmations that you say while tapping have to do with creating a sense of self-acceptance that includes accepting the issue you are addressing. So, for example, if you're addressing migraine headaches, you might say something like, "Even though I have this blinding headache, I deeply and completely accept myself." (It doesn't seem to matter whether you believe the affirmation or not. What's important

is that you say it anyway.) You repeat the statement, tuning in to "the problem" while tapping the meridians. It's that simple.

The idea is that thinking about the problem while doing the tapping—what Mercola calls "tuning in"—will bring about the very energy disruptions involved in the problem. (You know this is true for yourself if you've ever started thinking about an anxiety-producing situation in your life and noticed your heart racing, even though you didn't get off the couch. Thoughts have power.) The tapping (and the affirmation) creates a correction that will then balance the disrupted energy.

"Without tuning in to the problem, thereby creating those energy disruptions, EFT does nothing," says Mercola.

Curing the Incurable

EFT falls squarely into the camp of what might be called "energy medicine" or "energy healing." "The body will tend to heal itself if its energy is allowed to flow," says urologist Eric Robins, M.D., a huge EFT proponent. "The biggest thing that blocks that flow of energy is how emotional issues and past traumas are held in the body."

NATURAL TREATMENTS

Whether the positive results that people report from EFT are due to the actual tapping of the meridians, the focus on acceptance, or some unspecified neurobiological change that may ensue when performing the tapping is hard to say. What's pretty clear is that there is a huge emotional component to most physical problems, and the power of neurochemicals in the brain is nearly as great as that of any pharmacy. I don't know whether those neurochemicals can heal every disease on earth—or even all the conditions that EFT proponents claim to be able to improve. What I do know is that it has dramatic results for many people. Even the *Wall Street Journal*, in a 2007 article called "The Unmedicated Mind," quoted people who had tried EFT and found relief that they had been unable to get through conventional routes.

"It's possible to clear emotional issues at a deep enough level that physical healing results," says Robins. "I see EFT 'cure' things that are incurable all the time."

EMDR

for Post-Traumatic Stress and Trauma

I FIRST HEARD about EMDR therapy back in the 90s when I was doing my daily radio show on the (sadly) now-defunct Eyada.com. I interviewed someone who practiced it, and frankly, I thought it was a little kooky. Well, it's not.

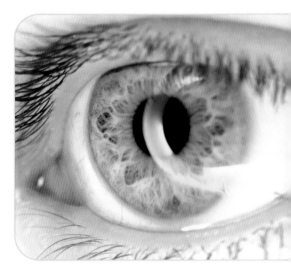

More than ten years later, EMDR, or eye movement desensitization and reprocessing, is a highly regarded, well-researched form of therapy for trauma and post-traumatic stress disorder that has gained the respect of the American Psychiatric Association, which found it to have "robust empirical support and demonstrated effectiveness." In its 2004 edition of *Practice Guideline for the Treatment of Patients with Acute Stress Disorder and Post-Traumatic Stress Disorder*

(PTSD), the association gave EMDR therapy its "highest level of recommendation" for the treatment of trauma. And if that's not enough, the Department of Veterans Affairs' and the Department of Defense's 2004 *Clinical Practice Guideline for the Management of Post-Traumatic Stress* placed EMDR in the "A" category as "strongly recommended" for the treatment of trauma.

The Theory behind EMDR

The originator and developer of the therapy is Francine Shapiro, Ph.D., a senior research fellow at the Mental Research Institute in Palo Alto, California, and a recipient of the Distinguished Scientific Achievement in Psychology Award presented by the California Psychological Association. Back in 1987, while walking in the park and thinking about some personal distressing memories, she happened to notice that eye movements appeared to decrease the negative emotions associated with them. Like many great innovators in healing (or in science, for that matter), she expanded on what was essentially a fortuitous personal discovery, began experimenting, developed a theory, put it to the test, and eventually developed the treatment approach that is now EMDR.

So what the heck is it?

As noted above, EMDR stands for eye movement desensitization and reprocessing, and it's based on a theory about the way we process information. The theory, simplified, is this: We humans all have a built-in "data processing" system that takes all the multiple elements of

experience and integrates them. These "memory networks" contain thoughts, images, associations, emotions, and sensations. So, for example, you might have an experience of learning to ride a bicycle that involves visual information, sensory information, data (time, place, and year), and emotions (it was thrilling, it was scary, I felt powerful, I felt helpless, etc.).

Shapiro sees the brain's information processing network as analogous to other body systems like digestion, where food goes in and gets "processed," and the gut extracts nutrients for health and survival. If something interferes with food being wholly "processed" in your body, any number of things can result, from an upset stomach to a food sensitivity to—in a severe case of allergy—anaphylactic shock.

The strong negative feelings may very well interfere with the normal information processing that would otherwise take place when trauma occurs, according to Shapiro. And if the information related to a distressing or traumatic experience isn't fully processed by the brain's central processing mechanism, the initial perceptions, emotions, and distorted thoughts will be "undigested"—they'll be stored exactly as they were first experienced at the time of the event, and you may well relive them every time a memory is triggered.

So let's take, for example, a rape victim. A rape survivor may very well know intellectually that the attack wasn't her fault, but this information may not override or connect with her feeling that she somehow brought the attack on herself. The memory is then stored "dysfunctionally," without the appropriate connections, much like food that hasn't been processed by the right digestive enzymes. When she thinks about the trauma—or when a memory of it is triggered by some situation or image or thought—she may feel like she is reliving it. This is pretty much a definition of what happens in post-traumatic stress disorder (PTSD).

How EMDR Therapy Helps

So what happens in therapy? At the heart of EMDR is what's called *dual attention stimulus*. Most commonly, the therapist will ask you to mentally focus on the distressing (or desired) experience while at the same time directing your attention to an external stimulus (most commonly eye movements, though auditory tones or even tapping can be used as well). It's believed that this dual attention phenomena helps facilitate information processing and helps the trauma survivor integrate the elements of the experience in order to deal with them.

While the various theories that have been proposed to explain why EMDR works are dense and laden with terminology from neurobiology, a simple version is that humans have what's called an orienting response hardwired into our brains. We pay attention to what moves: It served us well from an evolutionary perspective, else our caveman ancestors would not have recognized danger in the woods. (The orienting response could also be seen as a kind of investigatory reflex, the brain's way of saying, "What the heck is this?" You can see a

WORTH KNOWING

The EMDR Humanitarian Assistance Program (HAP) is a nonprofit organization that has been described as a kind of mental health equivalent of Doctors Without Borders. It's a global network of clinicians who travel anywhere there is a need to stop suffering and prevent the aftereffects of trauma and violence. Its trauma recovery network coordinates clinicians to treat victims and emergency service workers after such crises as Hurricane Katrina and the 9/11 attacks. (See Recommended Resources, page 333.)

demonstration of this phenomenon by playing peek-a-boo with any infant!)

It's been suggested that the orienting response somehow disrupts the traumatic memory network and interrupts previous associations to negative emotions. It's also been suggested that the investigatory reflex itself is like a psychic deep breathing in that it results in a basic relaxation response. None of these theories are mutually exclusive.

Whatever the underlying neurobiology, the treatment works. An enormous amount of research has validated its ability to help people with trauma and PTSD deal with their issues so that previously disturbing memories (and present situations that trigger them) are no longer debilitating and new healthy responses can emerge. Two separate studies have indicated an elimination of the diagnosis of PTSD in

83 to 90 percent of civilian participants after four to seven sessions, and many others have found a significant decrease in a wide range of symptoms after three or four sessions. My friend Daniel Amen, M.D., a psychiatrist, brain imaging specialist, and professor of psychiatry at the University of California, has been taking SPECT scans (brain pictures) of his patients and using EMDR with post-traumatic stress patients. He's reported a decrease in the activity of the anterior cingulate, basal ganglia, and deep limbic areas, all sections of the brain deeply involved in emotions, trauma, and memories.

By the way, it's not just major traumatic events—or what EMDR therapists call "large-T traumas"—that can cause psychological distress. It can even be a (relatively) small event like being bullied or teased. As we all know, even these seemingly small experiences can leave lasting imprints and still have the power to elicit powerful emotions years or even decades later. EMDR can help with these as well.

EMDR is not a one-session "cure," but rather an eight-phase process in which the EMDR-trained psychiatrist or psychotherapist may integrate other effective psychotherapy protocols ranging from cognitive behavioral therapies to body-centered approaches. It's not necessarily effective for every condition, nor does it claim to be. But it positively shines in the area of trauma and PTSD. At a recent seminar I attended on the brain given by Amen and largely attended by therapists, I met more than one practitioner who said to me, "I'd never recommend a therapist for post traumatic stress disorder who didn't incorporate EMDR in [his or her] treatment."

Image Therapy
for Asthma

THE OTHER DAY a friend of mine, Carole Jackson, the editor of *Bottom Line Daily Health News,* told me about Jeffrey, the son of a friend of hers who has suffered from asthma for a long time. He's been hospitalized several times because of it.

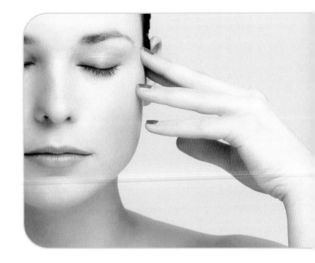

Jeffrey's mom was raving about a new therapy they've been trying called image therapy, according to Carole. The image therapist they've been going to specializes in people with asthma, and the treatment has been phenomenal. Jeffrey's mom says it's completely changed the severity and treatment of his asthma.

Anything that can help an asthmatic child is worth looking into. If you've ever seen a child—or an adult for that matter—in the throes of a full-blown asthma attack, you know what I mean.

Asthma is a chronic disease in which the airways are constantly inflamed and swollen, making them very sensitive and likely to react strongly to things your body finds irritating, such as a substance to which you're allergic. The symptoms are wheezing, coughing, and difficulty breathing. But during an attack, the muscles around the airways tighten up and less air flows through. The results can be devastating. A severe asthma attack can be so bad that not enough oxygen gets to vital organs. You feel like you can't breathe—which you can't, really—and you panic. It's a medical condition that people can—and have—died from.

The Mind-Body Connection

Conventional treatment for asthma is a mix of common sense, e.g., avoiding things that bring on symptoms, long-term control medicines taken as a preventive measure, and emergency "rescue" medicines like bronchodilators (inhalers) that act quickly to relax tight muscles so you can breathe. Image therapy doesn't replace any of those things; rather, it complements them by addressing the emotional and psychological components that even conventional doctors now admit can worsen the condition and bring on an attack.

Kathryn Shafer, Ph.D., is an image therapist who has suffered from asthma all her life. "Mental imagery is a technique that's based on addressing the thoughts that go on in the mind in the form of an image," she told me. She explained that an image therapist asks those suffering from the discomfort to describe what the image of their discomfort looks like and then work on changing that image.

"For example, we might ask the [person with asthma], 'If you could give your asthma an image, what would it look like?' We then work on changing that image through a technique called 'healing visualizations.'"

Here's an example of how an actual session with a person with asthma might proceed: "We'll tell the person to close their eyes, sit with their hands on the tops of their thighs, sit up straight, feet flat on the floor. Then we'll have them take a nice, deep breath into the nose and out through the mouth, three times, slowly," Shafer says. She informs patients that the purpose of this exercise is to breathe freely and notice what they sense and feel as they perform the exercise.

Shafer tells patients on the next breath in, "Imagine that you're inhaling a blue golden light, like the image you see when you look up to the sun and sky. Then, as you exhale through your mouth, imagine that you're exhaling gray smoke." This technique trains the mind to associate inhaling with what's healthy and needed for your body and exhaling what's unhealthy.

A Psychologist Designs Her Own Treatment

Shafer's own asthma, diagnosed when she was only fifteen months old, was the impetus for her exploration of complementary healing techniques. Over time she began exploring alternatives to the prescribed steroids, inhalers, and medications that had been staples of her life. She found that few practitioners were interested in complementary and alternative techniques, so she decided to make it her life's work.

"The most I'd hear from conventional doctors was that maybe 'the asthma attacks are psychosomatic, but here, take your medicine,'" she told me. Shafer acknowledges that asthma has both psychological and physical components. For example, a psychological irritant, such as stress, can trigger an attack as much as a physical cause, she says, which is why image therapy can be so beneficial.

She herself has been asthma-free for some time. "It becomes very important to think about what you're doing every second," she told me. Shafer believes that visualizing and imagining healthy lungs breathing in clean air can help calm inflammation and accelerate the healing process.

"Einstein said that imagination is more important than knowledge," she says. "If you open the imagination to what's possible, then everything is limitless."

Image therapy is an amazingly effective adjunct in the healing arsenal for asthma, Shafer told me. For many people, herself included, it's significantly reduced their symptoms and overall need for medication. But she was also quick to point out that image therapy doesn't replace conventional treatment.

"When I'm in the middle of not being able to breathe, I'm not interested in exploring the mind-body connection and the psychological components," she says. "All I want is a shot to open up my lungs and save my life. But once stabilized, I'd like to explore the psychological and emotional components."

This exploration is done in the hope of preventing future attacks.

Exercise

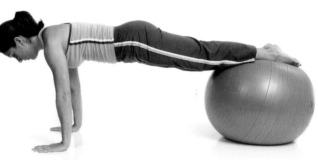

WHAT WOULD YOU think of a natural cure for arthritis, osteoporosis, heart disease, dementia, depression, and diabetes? Pretty good, right? Well, exercise won't cure every one of those conditions 100 percent of the time, but it will cure many of them, make a high percentage of the rest considerably better, and it may prevent most of them from happening in the first place. Sound like a great deal? It gets better.

Exercise is the ultimate natural cure. It's free, you can do it just about anywhere, it doesn't require any equipment, and you can do it at any age. Here's a list of the things that exercise has been shown in countless research studies to actually accomplish:

- Make your heart healthier
- Make your brain larger
- Improve your mood
- Strengthen your bones

- Decrease or eliminate depression
- Decrease the risk of diabetes
- Help maintain a healthy weight
- Reduce the effects of aging
- Lower blood pressure
- Relieve anxiety and stress
- Increase energy and endurance
- Improve sleep
- Keep joints healthy and mobile
- Lower the risk for some types of cancer

But how exactly does exercise do all these amazing things?

The Heart of the Matter

It begins with your heart, which is, after all, a muscle. By exercising at even moderate intensity, your heart is forced to pump a little faster and ultimately performs more efficiently.

Asking your heart to pump a little harder not only strengthens the heart itself but also improves the overall circulatory system. Blood flows easier, and blood pressure is lowered. Red blood cells deliver nourishing nutrients and oxygen to the tissues, including the brain, helping to keep all systems active and firing. Continuous exercise at an elevated heart rate also boosts chemicals in the brain called catecholamines, which improve mood and help fight depression. After exercise, many "feel-good" neurotransmitters are elevated, including dopamine, serotonin, and norepinephrine.

Harvard psychiatrist John Ratey, M.D., says that having a workout will help you focus better, calm you down, and reduce impulsivity. "It's like taking a little bit of Prozac and a little bit of Ritalin," he says.

Exercise can also reduce levels of the stress hormone cortisol, elevated levels of which ultimately age the brain by shrinking the hippocampus. Thus exercise improves both heart and brain function. It's the ultimate antiaging drug.

Pump Iron, Live Longer!

And that's just aerobic exercise, which is defined as exercise that's dependent on a steady flow of oxygen, e.g., walking, biking, stair-climbing, and the like. Add weight training to the mix and you get even more benefits. Weight training—or any weight-bearing exercise (e.g., body weight exercises like push-ups)—forces your muscles to work hard against resistance. This ultimately causes them to grow (or at the very least, not to atrophy). And that's a very good thing indeed.

Most older people wind up in nursing homes largely because they are no longer mobile or strong enough to take care of themselves. Their muscles and bones become too weak to perform everyday tasks that require a degree of strength most of us take for granted until it's not there anymore. Lift weights on a regular basis and you strongly improve the odds that the day will never come when you can't open a jar or move a box of books.

Weight-bearing exercise keeps muscles strong and toned; it also strengthens the bones, helping to ward off osteoporosis. The increased muscle you have on your body gives you the ability to burn more calories (since most fat is burned in the muscle cells). This makes it far easier to maintain a healthy weight.

But wait, there's more. Thirty-five percent of all cancer deaths may be related to a lack of activity and/or to being overweight, according to one study. Overweight people also frequently struggle with elevated levels of the hormone insulin, which can not only make you fat, but can raise blood pressure and even promote the growth of tumors.

If you're already diabetic, exercise may lower your requirement for insulin and help you manage blood sugar naturally. Exercise also promotes a healthy pregnancy; women who are fit and exercise before and during pregnancy tend to have a much easier time of both pregnancy and childbirth, and get back in shape a lot faster after the baby is born.

Exercise and Sex

Then there's sex. If nothing so far has motivated you to get off the couch and use exercise as the ultimate natural cure, consider this: Exercise can and does improve your sex life. Think about the popular term for male sexual performance problems—erectile dysfunction, or ED. Coincidentally, ED also stands for *endothelial dysfunction*—a condition that involves circulatory problems. The two are intimately connected.

"I've never seen a case of erectile dysfunction where there wasn't also endothelial dysfunction," says Mark Houston, M.D., director of the Hypertension Institute in Nashville.

Endothelial dysfunction happens when the inner cells of the blood vessels don't behave properly. It almost always involves problems in circulation and is a great predictor of strokes and heart attacks. Whether in the inner part of the arteries (endothelium) or in the sex organs, poor circulation and impaired blood flow show up as dysfunction—and both are helped greatly by getting your heart pumping and your tissues flooded with blood and nutrients. Plus the improved mood, outlook, and physical appearance that go with regular exercise never hurt anyone in the bedroom department. It's hard to feel sexy (and to perform) if you're feeling crummy all the time. And exercise is one of the best ways we know to feel good.

Train Your Body, Save Your Brain

Most baby boomers I know worry about losing their minds. Not literally, of course. But all too many of us have had the heartbreaking experience of caring for aging parents who no longer recognize them, no longer know where or who they are, and suffer from either vascular dementia or full-blown Alzheimer's disease. It's a fate many of my boomer friends fear more than almost any other—the gradual and inexorable loss of the ability to think, feel, and act as the person they've always been. Exercise may not cure Alzheimer's—but it's looking more and more like it might prevent it. Or at the very least delay it by a significant period of time. And that's a natural cure we'd all want to know about.

The key to the whole thing seems to be in an area of the brain called the hippocampus, which is responsible for memory. One of the first targets of Alzheimer's disease is the hippocampus, the same area of the brain that shrinks when under constant deluge from the stress hormone cortisol. Recent research shows that exercise makes new brain cells grow, and they seem to be created in an area of the hippocampus that controls memory and learning (the denate gyrus).

Exercise releases chemicals like IGF-1, which in turn ramps up production of another chemical called brain-derived neurotrophic factor (BDNF). Ratey calls BDNF the

"Miracle-Gro for the brain." The hippocampus is particularly responsive to the effects of BDNF, and exercise seems to act as the ultimate antiaging drug for this critical brain area. People who exercise a few times a week seem to develop Alzheimer's later than those who don't, and sometimes not at all.

How Much Exercise Do I Really Need?

So if exercise is really such incredible medicine, what exactly is the dose?

Well, it depends.

Thirty minutes a day of aerobic exercise—running, bicycling, swimming, walking, hiking, etc.—for most of the days in the week will do you just fine if you're trying to improve either cardiovascular health or the health of your brain. One study by Arthur Kramer, Ph.D., and his group found that healthy but sedentary folks 60 to 80 years of age who began a relatively easy aerobic program and worked up to 45 to 60 minutes of aerobic exercise three times a week actually grew bigger brains.

"Both the gray matter and the white matter showed increased volume," he told me.

"And the level of exercise needed to do this was pretty moderate."

If you're trying to lose weight, or more properly, body fat, you'll probably need to work out longer or harder (or both). You can increase the intensity of exercise either by doing it for a longer period of time or by doing it harder. A good place to start: Subtract your age from the number 220. Then calculate 50 percent of that number and 70 percent of that number. Keep your heart in that "target range" between the two percentages. You can always up the ante and go higher for a more intense workout later on, but there are striking benefits even at the 50 percent level.

There are dozens of books and videos and hundreds of references on exercise and how to do it (see the Recommended Reading and Resources section on page 329). Just keep in mind that while most of the research has been done on aerobic exercise, most health professionals now think weight training is equally important. If you want to get the full benefits of exercise as the outstanding natural cure that it is, you'll want to do both.

Interval Training
for Fat Loss

HOLD ON TO your seats because I'm about to burst one of the biggest bubbles in exercise mythology. The "fat-burning zone" is an urban legend.

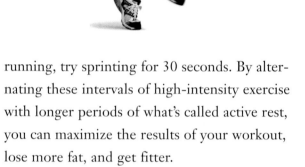

Like most urban legends, slaying it is easier said than done. Treadmill manufacturers continue to insist on putting "fat-burning" programs on their machines, and legions of aerobic teachers continue to teach people that they must achieve some mythical heart rate zone during exercise to lose weight and burn fat.

The result is that millions of people exercise with long, slow cardio programs in the hope that they will eventually slim down their thighs or lose their love handles. That may happen for a few lucky souls, but it's an obsolete way to attack fat.

Far better—and far more effective—is something called interval training.

The Best Workout for Burning Fat

Interval training is nothing more than the incorporation of short bursts of high-intensity exercise (intervals) into your regular workout. The Swedes have a term for this that's made it into the vocabulary of trainers and coaches everywhere—fartlek training (meaning "speed play"). Simply translated, it means, for example, if you're walking for an hour, try running for 30 seconds every few minutes. If you're already

running, try sprinting for 30 seconds. By alternating these intervals of high-intensity exercise with longer periods of what's called active rest, you can maximize the results of your workout, lose more fat, and get fitter.

Research on interval training and its benefits for both aerobic fitness and fat loss have been going on for decades, but one of the most recent studies was done by an exercise physiologist at the University of Guelph in Ontario, Canada, named Jason Talanian.

"We've always assumed that if you're not too fit you should just get on the bike and go for an hour," Talanian told me in an interview. "But our research has shown really powerful improvements in overall fitness and in fat burning when you increase the intensity for specific intervals."

Doing these spurts of high-intensity exercise leads to physiological adaptations that literally help us burn fat. Specific enzymes in the mitochondria—the powerhouse energy-burning factory in the cell nucleus—become more active through this kind of training. These enzymes—specifically, citrate cynthase and beta-hydroxyacyl-CoA dehydrogenase—break larger fatty acids down into smaller ones.

"This makes it easier to actually burn fat," Talanian says. Besides actual fat burning, measures of cardiovascular fitness—such as maximum oxygen capacity (known as VO_2 max)—also improve significantly with this kind of training.

The Research Doesn't Lie!

In Talanian's study, published in the April 2007 *Journal of Applied Physiology*, eight university-age women worked out in his laboratory every other day for two weeks, for a total of seven sessions. During each workout, they performed ten high-intensity intervals of four minutes each. In between each interval they would have two minutes of rest time.

The women were all over the map when it came to fitness levels. Some were completely sedentary, but one was a triathlete and another was a competitive soccer player. The rest were of average fitness and had been exercising in a conventional manner prior to the study (three times a week or so, moderate intensity, kind of what I normally see at the local gym).

"Regardless of their beginning fitness level, all were able to complete at least seven of the ten intervals," Talanian told me. "It was completely doable. And in all subjects we saw increases in the transporters (called fatty acid binding protein and fatty acid translocase/CD36) that escort the fat into the mitochondria where [it] can be burned for energy."

Talanian's study was unusual in that the "high-intensity" intervals were quite long at four minutes each. In previous studies, they were typically thirty seconds, followed by a lower-intensity, active rest period of two to three minutes. So, for example, if you were walking, you'd speed walk (or run) for your thirty-second interval, and then continue walking (active rest) for two to three minutes while your heart rate slowed a bit. You could repeat that sequence up to ten times per workout.

Talanian hypothesized that one of the reasons for the impressive results in his study was indeed the longer interval of high-intensity work. "I think it's possible that the aerobic component—the last two minutes of the interval—has a lot to do with why we're seeing such adaptations in fat burning."

If four-minute intervals of high intensity seem daunting to you, don't despair. You can get the benefits of interval training with much shorter intervals. One earlier study at McMaster University in Ontario, Canada, found that only four to seven "all-out" bouts of thirty seconds each, alternating with a full, four-minute "recovery" period, still doubled the endurance capacity of the subjects in a mere two weeks of training.

Talanian suggests starting your interval training by computing your maximum heart rate (220 minus your age) and then shooting for a high-intensity interval of 80 percent of that maximum. (You can, of course, work up to that, and you can also start with shorter intervals and increase to longer ones as you improve.)

Urban Legend: The Fat-Burning Zone

You can understand why the whole concept of a "fat-burning zone" is bogus if you understand what fat burning really means. "Fat burning" is actually a vernacular expression, shorthand for what exercise professionals refer to as "the beta oxidation of fatty acids."

Here's where part of the confusion arises. When we regular people talk about "fat burning," we have in our minds some vague concept of cellulite literally melting in a furnace of exercise-induced body heat. In fact, what happens is a little different.

At any given moment in time, you are "burning" (or technically, "oxidizing") fuel (food), breaking it down for energy. The body takes apart the food you eat—carbohydrates, fats, and proteins—and breaks it down into its smallest components (fatty acids, amino acids, and glucose, respectively) that provide energy for the body to do anything and everything that it needs to do. That means providing energy to grow nails and hair, breathe, make enzymes, digest food, exercise, think, sit at the computer, garden, run for the bus, and even sleep. The particular *mix* of fuel that it uses depends on a number of things.

And therein lies the rub.

See, at rest, the greatest *proportion* of your fuel comes from fat. So in theory, if you wanted to "burn" the highest percentage fat, you would simply stay in bed. The "fuel split" then would be, theoretically, about 70 percent "fat" and 30 percent "carbohydrates." (Let's leave protein out of the equation for the moment. The body

prefers to use protein for other things, and won't ordinarily use it for energy unless it has to.) Why then don't you lose any weight just staying in bed?

Because even though the lion's share of the calories burned by just staying in bed does indeed come from fat, the *total amount of calories burned* is tiny. In other words, you're burning a *high percentage* of a very small number (about 1 calorie a minute in the "average" person).

The Fat-Burning Game

Now, what happens when you begin to exercise?

Well, the minute you start to move from a resting position, the "fuel split" changes: Carbohydrates start to contribute a slightly higher percentage of the mix, and fat a slightly smaller one. The greater the intensity of the exercise, the greater the *proportion* of calories from carbohydrates and the smaller the *proportion* of calories from fat. But—and this is a big, important but—the harder the exercise, the greater the total number of calories per minute. So although your *percentage* from fat goes down, your *total number* increases.

When I demolish the concept of the "fat-burning zone" in lectures and workshops, I often use the example of Donald Trump. I ask the audience the following question: Would you guys rather have 90 percent of however much money I happen to have in my pocket right now or 10 percent of the total Trump fortune?

Most people—if they're not on drugs—pick a smaller percentage of the Trump fortune. At which point I innocently ask, "But why? 90 percent is such a bigger percent!"

Then they usually get it.

See, if you "burned" 300 calories during a low-intensity exercise session (walking for an hour) and 70 percent of them came from fat, you'd "burn" 210 fat calories. Great. But let's say you worked at a *higher* intensity and burned 600 calories during that same hour. Even if your percentage of calories from fat dropped to 50 percent you'd still be burning 300 fat calories and be ahead of the game!

Most people can't sustain high-intensity exercise for long periods of time. However, we can sustain it for thirty seconds to four minutes. By mixing those "high-intensity" intervals into the workout, we're increasing the number of calories burned for the same amount of time.

And here's the real joke: It doesn't matter where your calories come from when you're working out. There's absolutely no evidence that the actual fuel your body uses during a workout, whether fatty acids or glucose, has anything to do with whether fat comes off your hips and thighs. What matters is what happens in the body afterward.

The PACE Program

One of my favorite docs in the country, Al Sears, M.D., C.N.S., has written and trademarked an entire program based on fat loss through interval training. It's called PACE (Progressively Accelerating Cardiopulmonary Exertion—a fancy way of saying interval training). Sears—a bit of a contrarian, but a brilliant one—goes so far as to call what most people call "cardio" exercise a waste of time. He believes that forced, continuous endurance exercise induces your heart and lungs to "downsize" because *smaller* organs allow you to go further, more efficiently, with less rest and less fuel. What's wrong with that, you might ask?

"Instead of building heart strength, (long, slow endurance exercise) robs (the heart) of vital reserve capacity. Heart attacks don't occur because of a lack of endurance. They occur when there is a sudden increase in cardiac demand that exceeds your heart's capacity," he says. Sears believes that short bursts of high-intensity exercise create not just a reserve for your heart, but a hormonal environment conducive to fat loss.

If you still doubt this, ask yourself when you last saw a flabby sprinter. Flabby marathoner? Maybe. Sprinter? Never.

You can start PACE with an easy, ten-minute program. After warming up, spend one minute working hard enough to break a sweat and give your heart and lungs a challenge. Then slow down and let your heart rate recover for another minute. Repeat. Alternate one minute of exertion with one minute of recovery five times, for a total of 10 minutes. It's a great way to start interval training and really begin to lose the fat.

And your heart will thank you for it at the same time.

Reflexology
for PMS

IF YOU SQUINT and don't look very carefully, you might mistake a reflexology treatment for a plain old garden-variety foot massage. But it's not.

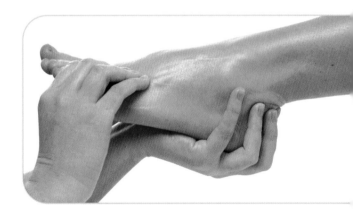

"Reflexology is a powerful natural health science that studies the relationship of areas in the feet, hands, and ears to the rest of the body," explains Bill Flocco, one of the leading practitioners of reflexology in America. "When you apply a nurturing touch to a particular part of the hands, feet, or ears, the nerve pathways go directly to the brain and then outward to a specific part of the body that corresponds to that area on the hands, feet, or ears."

If someone has stress in the heart, for example, a message goes to the brain, which then in turn goes to "reflex areas" for the heart, which are located in the hands, feet, and ears. "We work on these reflexes by applying attentive, nurturing pressure with our thumbs and fingers," he says.

What the Research on Reflexology Says

If Flocco is any example, reflexologists can be some of the most caring, nurturing practitioners in complementary health care. And they're interested in seeing their techniques, which they believe to be effective for a variety of conditions that have stress as a component, validated through research.

One particular 1993 research study that's received a lot of attention was published in the prestigious journal *Obstetrics and Gynecology*. The study investigated reflexology for PMS and found that it had a noticeable and significant effect on symptoms. In this study, thirty-five women who complained of previous distress with PMS were randomly assigned to be treated either by "real" reflexology or by a sham, placebo treatment. This is an interesting study because of an inherent dilemma—how do you do a "placebo" test of something that looks like massage? Unlike a drug test, where you can give an empty sugar pill as a placebo to compare the results with the real drug, a placebo for a touching treatment would still have to involve, well, touching. In this case, the placebo group actually got massages—like treatment, but it was uneven, tactile stimulation to areas of the ears, hands, and feet that would not be considered good "reflex points" or appropriate targets for real reflexology treatment for PMS. In this case, all the placebo subjects reported finding the treatment relaxing and pleasant, though a few complained that the manual pressure was too light. They all thought they were getting "real" reflexology treatment.

The results were pretty interesting. The placebo group had a 19 percent reduction in severity of PMS symptoms; but the reflexology group had a 46 percent reduction, a 58 percent difference that is statistically significant. You might argue that any relaxing, touching treatment might help reduce the stress and symptoms of PMS, which would explain why almost 20 percent of the subjects felt better after the phony treatment, but if there was nothing special about reflexology, you'd have to explain why more than twice as many felt better after receiving the real treatment. The researchers concluded that their clinical findings "support the use of ear, hand, and foot reflexology for the treatment of PMS."

Navigating a Map of the Body

Flocco is quick to point out that though reflexologists respect what massage therapists do, reflexology is completely different from conventional massage.

"The theory of reflexology is based on a kind of 'map' of the human body," he says. "Imagine dividing the body into ten wide vertical strips—one for the thumb and big toe, all the way over to one for the small toe and small fingers. Then imagine a similar division into horizontal zones. The reflexologist determines where the stress in the body is and then goes to work on the corresponding zone for the hands, feet, or ears. The concept is that the work we do on those areas that correspond to the stress areas in the body significantly relieve the problem stress."

ffers some examples. "The ball and foot and the big knuckles of the hand the chest." he says. "The soft sole of the foot and the soft palm of the hand relate to the upper abdomen." When the reflexologist applies a particular kind of nurturing touch and pressure to these areas, it results in a cascade of chemical events that winds up making you feel great, he says.

"When reflexologists work on those areas, they break down chemicals such as substance P, which is related to pain. The nerves become soothed. As nerves become soothed, muscles relax. As muscles relax, circulation improves, capillaries open up, and more blood is carried to the cells of the body. More oxygen and nutrition are taken to the cells, and as the cells get more oxygen and nutrition they're better able to produce the thousands of chemicals—like endorphins—that are carried around the body and that support the healing process," he says.

So who is reflexology particularly suited for? Flocco says that there are four types of people who benefit: person who just wants to experience profound relaxation and a safe, nurturing touch; a high-stress person who wants to minimize the effects of stress to operate optimally at home and work; a person who has sciatica or muscular discomfort in the lower jaw, lower back, neck, or shoulders; or a person with severe medical problems who is looking for a complementary adjunct approach to his or her conventional medical treatment.

Cathy Wong, N.D., says that reflexology promotes relaxation, improves circulation, reduces pain, soothes tired feet, and encourages overall healing. I agree. It's certainly worth a try as an adjunct natural "cure" for PMS and would go particularly well with the PMS Cocktail (page 162) and/or 3 g a day of Neptune Krill Oil.

The Relaxation Response

for Stress Management

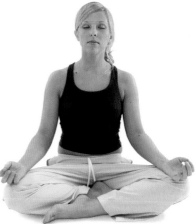

IT WOULD BE hard to find a better candidate for "hot topic of the moment" than stress. We now know that stress is more than just a mild feeling of being under the gun—it's a whole complicated series of biochemical and hormonal processes in the body that can significantly contribute to everything from sleep disorders to obesity, from hypertension to heart disease. No wonder stress management is not only a major health goal for the twenty-first century, but big business as well: witness the mushrooming of high-end spas, yoga classes, relaxation techniques, and spiritual retreats.

The research on stress and its damaging effects is hardly new, and there's no deficit of techniques for dealing with it. But in the rush to try the latest, hippest technique for stress busting, let's not forget that the basics have been around for eons. And one of the best-researched, most respected, most effective techniques has been around since 1968: It's called the Relaxation Response. Pioneered in 1968 by Harvard professor Herbert Benson, M.D., this simple-to-do technique now has an impressive résumé of research showing it can improve a baker's dozen of parameters from blood pressure to school performance.

The Results are in the Repetition

"The Relaxation Response is the exact opposite of the bodily response to stressors," Benson told me. That stress response—also known as the fight-or-flight response—involves the release of stress hormones like cortisol and adrenaline. While cortisol is needed by every cell in the body, high levels of cortisol and adrenaline were meant to serve as emergency fuel generators in times of existential danger, such as when our forefathers were being chased by a wooly mammoth. The cortisol/adrenaline stress-hormone lever was not meant to be permanently frozen in the "on" position, a condition of modern life in which we frequently find ourselves. High levels of cortisol have been shown experimentally to shrink a part of the brain called the *hippocampus*, which is central to memory and thinking. High levels of cortisol also contribute to abdominal fat.

"The fact that, for most of us, these stress hormones are constantly in the 'on' position has significant health consequences," Benson says.

The Relaxation Response basically builds on a general technique that virtually every religion and meditative practice has used for eons, but without the religious trappings.

"All the major religions use prayer, generally repetitive words in a singsong, or almost chant-like rhythm," Benson says. In fact, the early research on the Relaxation Response used repetitive phrases like *Hail Mary, full of grace* for Roman Catholic research subjects and *Shalom* or *Echad* for Jewish ones. Benson uses the word *one* as a basic, nondenominational phrase that could elicit the healing response he was looking for in the widest variety of subjects, regardless of religious affiliation or lack thereof.

Research continues to confirm the effects of this kind of practice, whether it's called meditation, prayer, or the Relaxation Response. Recently my friends Dharma Singh Khalsa, M.D., and Daniel Amen, M.D. (along with Nisha Money, M.D.) teamed up to study a simple, twelve-minute form of kundalini yoga called Kriya Kirtan that's based on five primal sounds that are chanted consecutively. They performed SPECT scans—a type of brain imaging—on subjects at rest one day and then after meditation the next.

"We saw marked decreases in the left parietal lobes (decreasing awareness of time and space) and significant increases in the prefrontal cortex (which showed that meditation helped to tune people in, not out)," Amen says. They also observed increased activity in an area of the brain associated with both spirituality and sex—the right temporal lobe. So if decreasing stress isn't enough motivation for you to do the Relaxation Response, maybe improving your sex life is!

Lowering Your Blood Pressure, Not Your Bank Account

So how is the Relaxation Response different from meditation? Truth be told, there may not be a lot of difference, at least from a physiological point of view.

"There's one common physiology to all techniques that use different words, or sounds, or postures," Benson explains. "All these techniques—meditation, the Relaxation Response—produce decreased metabolism, lowered heart rate, and decreased blood pressure." In fact, the Relaxation Response has often been compared to Transcendental Meditation, the technique taught by Maharishi Mahesh Yogi and popularized in this country by the Beatles in the mid-1960s. Transcendental Meditation is great, but last time I looked, learning Transcendental Meditation from an authorized instructor cost thousands of dollars; doing the Relaxation Response technique is free.

Indeed, research on the benefits of the Relaxation Response is more than a little impressive. Heart rate slows down, muscles relax, breathing becomes more measured, and blood

How to Do It: Eliciting the Relaxation Response

Set aside 10 to 20 minutes to try this technique:

- Sit quietly in a comfortable position.

- Close your eyes.

- Deeply relax all your muscles beginning at your feet and progressing up to your face. Keep them relaxed.

- Breathe through your nose. Become aware of your breathing. As you breathe out, say the word *one* silently to yourself. For example, breathe in ... out, (one), in ... out (one), etc. Breathe easily and naturally.

- Continue for 10 to 20 minutes.

- You may open your eyes to check the time, but don't use an alarm. When you finish, sit quietly for several minutes at first with your eyes closed and later with your eyes open. Don't stand for a few minutes.

- Don't worry about whether you are successful in achieving a deep level of relaxation. Maintain a passive attitude and permit relaxation to occur at its own pace. When distracting thoughts occur, try to ignore them by not dwelling upon them and return to repeating one.

—From *The Relaxation Response* by Herbert Benson, M.D., used with permission.

Note: Benson points out that with practice, the response should come with very little effort. He suggests practicing the technique once or twice a day but also suggests not doing it within a couple of hours of eating, as the digestive process seems to interfere with eliciting the Relaxation Response.

pressure is lowered. Levels of an important biochemical called *nitric oxide*—a molecule that is important for circulation and the improvement of blood flow—increases. And research since the 1990s in the school system (grades K–12 and college) shows that teaching the Relaxation Response and incorporating it into the curriculum leads to higher grade point averages, increased self-esteem, decreased psychological distress, better attendance, and less aggression.

According to the Benson-Henry Institute for Mind Body Medicine at Massachusetts General Hospital, between 60 and 90 percent of all doctor visits are for complaints related to, or impacted by, stress.

"Scores of diseases and conditions are either caused or made worse by stress," Benson explained. "These include anxiety, mild or moderate depression, anger, hostility, hot flashes of menopause, infertility, PMS, high blood pressure, and heart attacks. Every one can be caused by stress or exacerbated by it. And to the extent that that's the case, the relaxation response is helpful."

DESERT ISLAND CURES

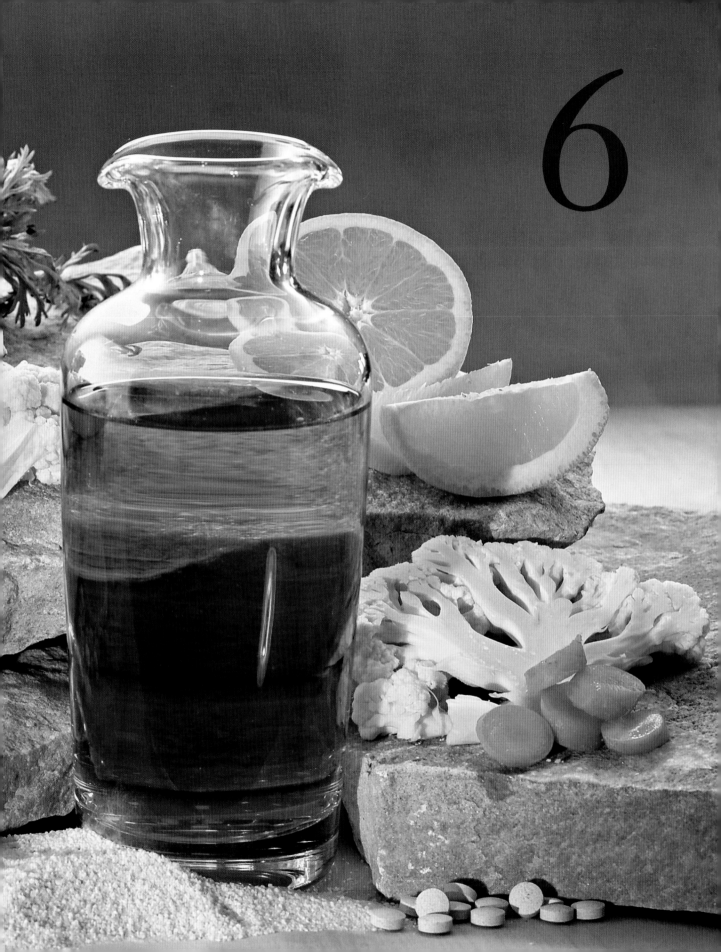

6

Apple Cider Vinegar

LET ME COME CLEAN: I have a checkered history with apple cider vinegar. The scientist in me wants to see some hard research supporting its health claims. But the adventurer/maverick in me acknowledges the fact that apple cider vinegar has been used as a folk remedy for more years than I've been alive, that people swear by it to help myriad conditions, that it has a long and honorable tradition in folk medicine, and that all that has got to count for something.

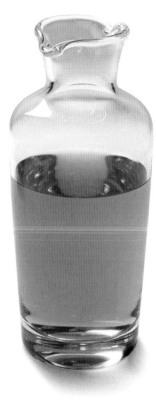

Remember, the absence of proof is not the proof of absence, and apple cider vinegar would hardly be the first—or last—substance whose benefits were familiar to your grandmother well in advance of being demonstrated in peer-reviewed research on www.pubmedcentral.nih.gov. As they used to say back in the day, "fifty thousand Elvis fans can't be wrong." If apple cider vinegar doesn't do any of the things thousands of people believe it does, it would be the biggest placebo hoax in history.

A Folk Remedy for the Ages

So what is apple cider vinegar anyway? And why do all these people sing its praises?

Vinegar itself is a terrific food. It can actually be made from any fruit as long as it's fermented to less than 18 percent ethyl alcohol. The kind made from apples, however, has some

special properties. It's a virtual infusion of amino acids, vitamins, and minerals. Unpasteurized vinegar can contain as many as fifty different nutrients, especially if the "starting" material is as rich in nutrition as apples. (Note well the reference to unpasteurized: Pasteurization destroys microorganisms, sure, but it's a little like throwing out the baby with the bath water. Pasteurization also destroys valuable heat-sensitive vitamins, enzymes, and organic acids like malic acid and tartaric acid, which are important in fighting body toxins and inhibiting unfriendly bacteria, and are some of the main reasons apple cider vinegar is a desert island cure in the first place.)

Apple cider vinegar is believed to have anti-fungal, antibacterial, and antiviral properties. There are entire websites devoted to uses for apple cider vinegar, which is one reason I'd like a few bottles with me if I were stranded on an island. Folk wisdom says it's useful for heartburn, arthritis, lowering blood pressure, aiding digestion, fighting yeast infections, detoxification, allergies, and even for weight loss. Proponents claim it helps boost immunity. Does it do all these things? Maybe. There's good reason to believe it is highly alkalizing to the system, and since most of us are way too "acidic," this alkalizing (balancing) effect alone could be responsible for some of the many health effects people observe. (For an explanation of those terms, see sidebar at right.)

On one nonprofit website, Apple Cider Vinegar Cure Research (www.curezone.com/blogs/f.asp?f=179&p=1), people from all over the world have posted messages about the benefits they've received from apple cider vinegar. I've read credible reports of apple cider vinegar in warm water helping to cure morning sickness, sinus infections, brain fog (due to the potassium content), and acid reflux. One of the most impressive postings I read was from a thirty-six-year-old in Greece who suffered from acne all his life and claimed that he was acne-free for the first time in his life after a few weeks of drinking apple cider vinegar three times a day. Apple cider vinegar also has a huge reputation with animal lovers as being great for dogs and cats, especially for treating arthritis. In fact, oxymel—a combination of apple cider vinegar and honey—has been widely used to dissolve painful calcium deposits in the body, and for other problems like hay fever.

Acid and Alkaline

My trusted associate, nutritionist Suzanne Copp, M.S., suggested I explain the terms "acid" and "alkaline" in case they're new to you.

You've probably heard of pH, as in the pH of water; if you have a garden you might have measured the pH of your soil. What pH stands for is *potential of hydrogen*—it's a measure of the acidity or alkalinity of a solution. It is measured on a scale of 0 to 14—the lower the pH the more acidic the solution, the higher the pH the more alkaline (or base) the solution. (Remember that from high school chemistry? Don't worry, neither did I.)

When a solution is neither acid nor alkaline it has a pH of 7, which is neutral. Distilled water is completely neutral at about 7. Battery acid is around 1, drain cleaners are around 14. All your bodily fluids—blood, urine, and saliva—and your tissues have optimal ranges for balance between acid and alkaline.

When foods are "burned" in the body (i.e., digested), they leave an ash that can be acid, alkaline, or neutral, depending on the food itself. *Acidosis* results when there is a depletion of the alkali reserve in the blood and tissues. One theory that has been around forever is that imbalances between the acid and alkaline are associated with ill health and disease. The standard Westernized diet is highly acidic. The thinking is that anything that can help restore balance by alkalizing an overly acid system is a good thing. Vegetables qualify, as does apple cider vinegar.

What About the Research?

Earlier I mentioned some "hard-core" research, and here it is: A recent study in Diabetes Care demonstrated that apple cider vinegar improved insulin sensitivity in insulin-resistant subjects. Let me tell you how important this is: If you've read my other books—especially *Living the Low Carb Life*—you remember that insulin is an important hormone with multiple purposes that's made by the pancreas. Your body releases insulin when blood sugar goes up, as it does when you eat food, especially carbohydrates.

Insulin's jobs include escorting excess sugar in the bloodstream to the cells where it can be burned for energy. But in *at least* 25 percent of the population, this metabolic pathway doesn't work properly. Blood sugar goes up, insulin goes up, the cells refuse to allow either of them in, and you're left with the enormous health risks of high blood sugar and high insulin, a sure path to either metabolic syndrome or diabetes. We call this condition *insulin resistance*; its opposite is insulin *sensitivity*, which is what you want. Research demonstrates that vinegar makes the cells more "sensitive" to insulin, a desirable effect indeed. This makes apple cider vinegar a powerful natural weapon, along with cinnamon and chromium, in the fight to control blood sugar and help get carbohydrate metabolism on track.

Respected nutritional researcher Jeff Volek, Ph.D., R.D., suggests a salad with vinegar at the beginning of every meal for its potential in managing blood sugar. Make it apple cider vinegar and get not only the sugar-busting benefits, but the all the other benefits that come with this great natural cure as well.

Remember to get apple cider vinegar that is traditionally made. Look for products that say "unpasteurized," "traditionally fermented," or "aged in wood." One of the best on the market is made by Patricia Bragg, N.D., Ph.D. (Bragg Live Foods Apple Cider Vinegar, www.bragg.com), but there are others as well. You'll be getting a cornucopia of nutrients, including minerals like calcium, magnesium, phosphorus, sulfur, copper, silicon, trace minerals, and pectin as well as many other nutrients and enzymes. It's a real natural cure bonanza.

Fish Oil and Essential Fatty Acids

IF THERE WERE one thing you could do right now, besides diet and exercise, that would probably make the most profound difference to your physical health, it would be to consume fish oil on a regular basis.

The fatty acids in fish oil are members of a family of fats called omega-3s, which have been found to be helpful in so many clinical conditions that at least six books have been written touting their benefits and uses. I've been preaching about the importance of taking omega-3s for a long time. Andrew Stoll, M.D., director of the Psychopharmacology Research Lab at McLean Hospital in Belmont, Massachusetts, and a faculty member at Harvard Medical School, aptly named them "wellness molecules." If there was one supplement I could mandate for the entire population of the world—with the possible exception of those who live in Greenland and eat salmon all day—it would unquestionably be omega-3s (or a related supplement called essential fatty acids).

A Primer on Fats

The terms describing fats—saturated, unsaturated, omega-3, omega-6, and the like—simply have to do with their molecular arrangements. Other fats have important functions in our bodies, including omega-6s, omega-9s, and even, believe it or not, saturated fats. The body needs them all for various purposes. But two important facts distinguish omega-3s from all the rest.

First, their health benefits are simply enormous. Second, we don't get nearly enough of them in our diet.

Omega-3 fats protect the heart and the brain, support circulation, boost mood, and lower blood pressure. They've been studied for their effects on depression, cardiovascular health, skin, joints, and diabetes. Virtually every study of behavioral and mood problems (from aggression to depression) has demonstrated a correlation to extremely low levels of omega-3s. Large doses of these fatty acids are currently being studied at Harvard University for their role in combating some forms of depression. And a great deal of research has shown that omega-3s are great for the heart.

For all these reasons, omega-3s are number one with a bullet on the list of Desert Island Supplements.

How Omega-3s Help the Heart

An important risk factor for heart disease—some might say even more important than cholesterol—is having high triglycerides. *Triglycerides* are the main form of fat found in the body and are nearly always measured on a standard blood test.

Fish oil supplements reduce triglyceride levels by up to 40 percent in some research, an astonishingly high amount. The Agency for Healthcare Research and Quality (the research arm of the U.S. Department of Health and Human Services) analyzed 123 studies on omega-3 fatty acids and concluded that "omega-3 fatty acids demonstrated a consistently large, significant effect on triglycerides—a net decrease of 10 to 33 percent." The effect is most pronounced in those with high triglycerides to begin with. Even the extremely conservative American Heart Association recommends 2 to 4 g of the two omega-3 fats found in fish oil (EPA and DHA) for patients who need to lower triglycerides.

Another major risk factor for heart disease is hypertension, or high blood pressure. Fish oil lowers blood pressure, albeit modestly. But its effect on cardiovascular disease overall is anything but modest. Study after study has shown that the omega-3 fatty acids found in fish reduce the risk of death, heart attack, stroke, and abnormal heart rhythms (arrhythmias). It's been estimated that proper omega-3 fatty acid intake could reduce the rate of fatal arrhythmias by 30 percent. More than 70,000 lives could be saved each year if Americans had sufficient omega-3s in their bodies, estimates Stoll.

Natural Prescription for Vibrant Health

Fish oil: 1 to 4 grams every day in capsules or oil

Note: All dosages are daily dosages and in pill or capsule form unless otherwise noted.

Omega-3 blood levels are one of the best predictors of sudden heart attack. Those with the highest risk for heart attacks have the lowest levels of omega-3s. In Britain, heart attack survivors are now prescribed fish oil supplements for life in keeping with the guidelines of the British National Institute for Health and Clinical Excellence. Many physicians also consider supplementation with omega-3 fatty acids an important part of nutritional treatment for diabetes and metabolic syndrome.

Fish Oil for the Gray Cells

Fish oil actually contains two specific types of omega-3 fatty acids, one called eicosapentaenoic acid (EPA) and the other called docosahexaenoic acid (DHA). Both are important, though they have slightly different (and overlapping) actions.

Remember when your grandmother used to tell you fish was brain food? She was right. DHA forms an important part of cell membranes in the brain and in the retina of the eye and is considered extremely important in child development. My friend, the great nutritionist Robert Crayhon, once said that if there was one thing he could wish for to improve the health of the children of America it would be for every pregnant woman to take DHA (or fish oil) supplements. The last trimester of pregnancy is especially important for the accumulation of DHA in the brain. I can't think of a more important supplement to take during pregnancy and breast-feeding than fish oil or even straight DHA.

But the importance of omega-3s for the brain hardly stops after infancy. Too little omega-3s have been linked to both attention deficit disorder (ADD) and depression. Research at Harvard has shown significant improvement in bipolar depression with large doses of omega-3 supplements. And studies have strongly suggested that increased fish oil intake could reduce anger and hostility in alcoholics, troubled teenagers, and violence-prone prisoners.

"Clearly omega-3 fatty acids are essential to good brain health," says my friend Daniel Amen, M.D., professor of psychiatry at University of California–Irvine and the author of *Healing ADD* and *Change Your Brain, Change Your Life*.

One More Benefit

Another one of the many benefits of omega-3s is that they are anti-inflammatory. The full importance of inflammation as a factor in disease is only just now beginning to be fully appreciated. *Time* magazine recently ran a cover story aptly named "Inflammation: The Silent Killer."

Since inflammation is a component of every major degenerative disease from Alzheimer's to diabetes, the importance of foods and supplements that are anti-inflammatory can't be overstated. Fish oil, because of its omega-3 content, is one of the most potent anti-inflammatories on the planet. The anti-inflammatory action of the omega-3 fats found in fish oil has been proven in dozens of research studies, including the ongoing ATTICA study in Athens, Greece, that demonstrated direct evidence showing that omega-3s reduce blood markers of inflammation like C-reactive protein, which are increasingly accepted as key risk factors for heart disease. The anti-inflammatory action of fish oil makes it a terrific supplement for arthritis, for aging and aching joints, and for the inflamed airways of those suffering with asthma.

The Cell-Membrane Connection

No one's ever actually counted the number of cells in the human body, but the estimates generally given are between 60 and 100 trillion. Every one of those cells has a membrane, which surrounds and protects all the myriad of tiny structures inside the cell that do the metabolic factory work of the body. Inside that cell is a whole city of industry, with each little structure having a specific job or jobs to do. Nutrients have to get in, waste has to get out. That cell is literally a humming, buzzing factory of metabolic work. And if the cell membrane is not healthy and robust, that work doesn't get done, at least not well. The membrane has to be sturdy enough to protect the cell yet porous enough to allow information and material to get in and out as needed. It can't be too "leaky" and it can't be too "hard." Enter omega-3s.

The cell membrane is largely made up of fats. Omega-3s are among the best fats in the world for the cell membrane. When there are enough omega-3s in the body to create healthy cell membranes, everything works well. For instance, feel-good neurotransmitters like serotonin and dopamine can enter the brain cells (neurons) and make you feel good. (No wonder fish oil is good for depression.) Insulin, the hormone that escorts sugar into the cells, can do its job better because the cell membrane is more receptive. (No surprise that fish oil is one of the top supplements given to people with diabetes.) And because fish oil improves circulation, it can be helpful for those with an aging brain, suffering from vascular dementia.

It's hard to think of a condition that would not be improved by a healthy dose of fish oil on a daily basis. It's truly my number-one choice for a desert island cure.

Magnesium

IF YOU SCAN through the contents of this book, you'll find magnesium as a primary ingredient in no fewer than seven combo cures. Any natural prescription for almost any kind of heart disease is going to contain magnesium. Magnesium is a top nutrient for diabetes and blood sugar control. It's in my special combo cure for PMS. It's necessary for bone health and to prevent osteoporosis (as important as calcium and less publicized).

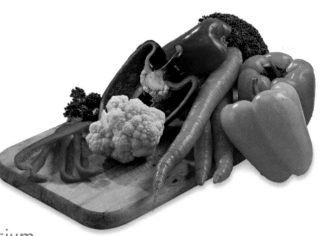

If you want to have the most restful sleep you've ever had and you happen to have access to an M.D. who believes in nutrition and uses vitamin drips in his or her practice, get that doc to give you a magnesium infusion and you'll sleep like a baby. Atkins used to call magnesium "a natural calcium channel blocker." (Calcium channel blockers are a major class of drugs used to treat high blood pressure and abnormal heart rhythms.) It's at the top of the list of the supplements used at the Hypertension Institute in Nashville for high blood pressure.

Necessary but Neglected

Magnesium earned its place here on the proverbial desert island because so many functions that are essential to life depend on its adequate levels. But here's the disturbing part: Almost three out of every four Americans fail to get the recommended intake of magnesium per day.

Sixty-eight percent of Americans consumed less than the recommended daily allowance of this critical mineral, according to a study in the June 2005 *Journal of the American College of Nutrition*.

Think that's no big deal? Consider this: Magnesium deficiency can affect virtually every single organ system in the body. It's involved in more than 300 enzyme reactions in the body including fat, protein, and glucose metabolism, muscle and membrane transport, and energy production.

In a classic article called *The Importance of Magnesium to Human Nutrition*, Michael Schachter, M.D., devotes a full four paragraphs to the possible symptoms and problems associated with getting too little magnesium—they range from salt and carbohydrate cravings to panic attacks, PMS, mitral valve prolapse, palpitations, cramps, muscle tensions, and insomnia.

And though the National Institutes of Health tends to be more sanguine, pointing out that symptoms of real magnesium deficiency are rarely seen in the United States, it does point out that "there is concern about the prevalence of sub-optimal magnesium stores in the body," and that "dietary intake may not be high enough to promote an optimal magnesium status, which may be protective against disorders such as cardiovascular disease and immune dysfunction."

The excellent magnesium website www.mgwater.com maintains a research database of more than 300 articles discussing magnesium and magnesium deficiency and lists no fewer than fifty conditions that can be either treated or prevented with magnesium.

Beginning to understand why magnesium is one of my "Desert Island Cures"?

Natural Prescription for Magnesium

Food sources: Dark green leafy vegetables, nuts (almonds, cashews), and certain fish (halibut) are my personal favorites, but a wide variety of fruits, vegetables, nuts, seeds, and even soybeans are all good sources.

Best way to take it: 400–800 mg day as a supplement (either alone or as part of a bone formula).

Try an Epsom salts bath. It's relaxing, and you absorb magnesium through the skin.

Magnesium is the fourth most abundant mineral in the body and is absolutely essential to good health. There's almost nothing I can think of that it isn't good for. (Okay, maybe it's useless for getting a date on a Saturday night or increasing the return on your 401k.) About half of your body's total magnesium is found in bones, and the rest is found mainly inside cells of body tissues and organs, with the highest magnesium concentrations found in those that are also the most metabolically active: the brain, liver, kidney, and heart. Only 1 percent of it is in the blood, so a blood test for magnesium deficiency is pretty useless.

Stress and Cardiovascular Health

Too much stress causes magnesium to be depleted, which can lead to hypertension, coronary artery constriction, arrhythmias, and heart attack. Here's how it works: When you're under too much stress your body overproduces substances called catecholamines. While some act as neurotransmitters and make us feel good (dopamine), catecholamines also act as hormones in the blood, and too high a level of them will cause magnesium to be released from cells into the blood and then excreted in urine. A low magnesium level in the cells causes heart tissue destruction. End result: heart attack.

There's a circular relationship between stress and magnesium. Stress causes low magnesium levels, low magnesium levels cause stress, and the circle continues downward. Both stress and magnesium deficiency set you up for cardiovascular disease. In animal studies, giving animals magnesium has been shown to prevent this process from happening, protecting heart tissue from destruction.

When you consume magnesium in optimal amounts it improves myriad heart conditions, including angina, arrhythmia, cardiomyopathy, mitral valve prolapse, intermittent claudication, and low HDL (the "good" cholesterol). It improves energy production within the heart, dilating the arteries and helping blood do its job of delivering oxygen to the heart more effectively. Studies have shown that people dying of a heart attack have lower magnesium levels than people of the same age dying from other causes.

Don't Water It Down

The relationship of magnesium to heart health has been noted for decades, interestingly by the discovery that there's an inverse relationship between water hardness (water high in magnesium) and mortality from cardiovascular disease.

"According to the U.S. National Academy of Sciences (1977), there have been more than 50 studies in nine countries that have indicated … that people who drink water that is deficient in magnesium and calcium appear more susceptible (to cardiovascular disease)," writes Harold D. Foster, Ph.D., in a paper entitled *Groundwater and Human Health*. The U.S. National Academy of Sciences has estimated that a nationwide initiative to add calcium and magnesium to soft water (low magnesium) might reduce the annual cardiovascular death rate by 150,000 people in the United States alone.

WORTH KNOWING

In dietary supplements, you're likely to see magnesium in many forms or "salts," such as magnesium citrate, magnesium glycinate, magnesium malate, magnesium ascorbate (bound to vitamin C), and magnesium oxide. Magnesium oxide is the cheapest form and has a reputation for not being as well absorbed as the others. Magnesium glycinate is considered very high quality.

In some cases, high doses of magnesium—especially magnesium citrate—can lead to a loosening of the stools. Interestingly, some health practitioners capitalize on this little "side effect" and have found magnesium citrate to be the supplement of choice for people suffering from constipation and an excellent alternative to over-the-counter milk of magnesia (magnesium hydroxide).

Jean Durlach, M.D., president of the International Society for the Development of Magnesium Research, has also noted that heart disease is less prevalent in areas where the water has a high magnesium content.

Studies also show that a high magnesium intake is associated with lower blood pressure. Simply put, blood pressure is lower when magnesium levels are optimal. One of magnesium's many functions is to help maintain the critical balance between sodium and potassium in a cell. (High sodium intake coupled with low potassium intake is an absolute disaster from the point of view of your heart.) Classic research on the

Paleolithic diet by Boyd Eaton shows that our hunter-gatherer ancestors got about ten times more potassium than sodium in their diet, but that the ratio has been completely reversed in our modern lives, setting us up for all sorts of heart problems. (See page 40 to find out more about why potassium is so important for heart health.)

Remember that the heart is, after all, a muscle. And magnesium—with the help of calcium—helps to maintain adequate muscle contractions. It also helps to send energy in the form of the "energy molecule" (adenosine triphosphate or ATP) to heart muscle tissues. At the University of Southern California Coronary Care Unit, researchers examined 100 consecutive admissions and found that 53 of them had low magnesium levels.

Diabetes and Blood Sugar Control

Magnesium plays a crucial role in carbohydrate metabolism. It also plays a critical role in the secretion and action of insulin, thereby helping to control blood sugar. Magnesium supplements are absolutely essential for anyone with type 2 diabetes or anyone at risk for it.

The Nurses' Health Study and the Health Professionals Follow-Up Study are two of the most respected, long-range studies of health ever done. More than 170,000 health professionals were followed in these studies for between twelve years (men) and eighteen years (women). As part of these studies, more than 125,000 participants with no history of the big three—diabetes, cardiovascular disease, or cancer—were investigated specifically for the purpose of examining risk factors for type 2 diabetes. Over time, the risk for developing type 2 diabetes was significantly greater in both men and women with a lower intake of magnesium.

Other studies have confirmed the relationship of magnesium and diabetes. In the Women's Health Study, researchers looked at the association between magnesium intake and the incidence of type 2 diabetes over an average of six years. Among overweight women, the risk of developing the disease was significantly greater among those with lower intakes of magnesium.

The Iowa Women's Study followed 40,000 women for more than six years and also examined the relationship between diabetes and magnesium. The findings suggest that a greater intake of whole grains, dietary fiber, and yes, magnesium, decreased the risk of developing type 2 diabetes in older women.

And a number of studies have looked at the potential benefits of magnesium supplements for helping to control type 2 diabetes. In one study, sixty-three subjects with below normal blood levels of magnesium received either 300 mg of elemental magnesium a day or a placebo. At the end of only sixteen weeks, those who received the magnesium had improved metabolic control of diabetes (i.e., lower levels of hemoglobin A1c, an important marker for diabetes).

Energizer and Achy Muscle Reducer

Because magnesium is required in both the red blood cells and the muscles for energy production, low levels can easily sap your energy. If you've got any type of muscle aches or fatigue associated with conditions like tension headache, fibromyalgia, or chronic fatigue, consider the possibility that you're low in magnesium.

Magnesium is just all around great for cramps. Taking extra magnesium (and sometimes potassium) is one of the best ways I know of to ease leg cramps from exercise. It's also great for menstrual cramps, leg cramps from pregnancy, and virtually every other cramp you can think of. A great way to get its muscle-relaxing benefits is to take an Epsom salts bath. Not only will you absorb a ton of muscle-relaxing magnesium through your skin, you'll also lower your stress hormones. Try it!

Though oral magnesium supplements will help the huge majority of people, tough cases or people with specific health challenges may need magnesium intravenously. According to my friend Alan Gaby, M.D., an icon of integrative medicine, "approximately 50 percent of patients with chronic fatigue syndrome or fibromyalgia show considerable improvement after receiving several intravenous injections of a combination of magnesium, calcium, B vitamins, and vitamin C." In the same article, published in the *Townsend Newsletter for Doctors and Patients* in 2004, he goes on to mention a number of studies in which an average of 74 to 80 percent of patients improved with treatments such as this. He adds that in the majority of cases, "drug prescriptions for NSAIDS and muscle relaxants were virtually eliminated." (NSAIDs are over-the-counter nonsteroidal anti-inflammatory drugs like aspirin and ibuprofen.)

In addition to fibromyalgia, magnesium has been shown to affect kidney stones. In animal studies, you can induce kidney stones by reducing the amount of magnesium in the diet. Conversely, supplementing with magnesium—and ideally vitamin B6 at the same time—will prevent the recurrence of kidney stones. The citrate form of magnesium is best (see combo cure for kidney stones on page 154).

Bone Health

Ask the average American about bone health or the prevention of osteoporosis and the first thing that's likely to come up in the conversation is calcium. (Unfortunately, it's also the only thing that comes up, which makes me crazy—don't get me started.) This is more a triumph of marketing on the part of the dairy industry than anything else.

Don't get me wrong, calcium is very important, but it's fairly useless without a supporting cast of vitamins, minerals, and nutrients that help calcium be absorbed and utilized and stay where you want it to be (in the bones, not the arteries). This supporting cast is led by magnesium (and of course vitamin D). In animal studies, magnesium deficiency causes decreased bone strength and volume, poor bone development, and dysfunctions in bone formation and resorption (the process by which bone cells break down bone and release minerals like calcium into the blood).

Magnesium supplements are more important than calcium in reversing bone loss in postmenopausal women, one of the most vulnerable populations for osteoporosis, according to a May 1990 report in the *Journal of Reproductive Medicine*. The findings were so profound that the authors argued that the later development of osteoporosis may be due to a chronic magnesium deficiency. A second study done in 1998 suggested that magnesium consumed in levels higher than the recommended daily allowance is critical for preserving and slowing bone loss. And if you needed any further proof, the Framingham Heart Study found that men and women with the highest intakes of potassium and magnesium had the strongest bone density.

SAMe

DEPRESSION, ARTHRITIS, liver disease, and fibromyalgia. What could these four completely distinct conditions possibly have in common? Give up? All four can be treated with a wonderful compound called SAMe.

The Life Extension Foundation, an organization founded in 1980 that reports on the latest advances in life extension science, was first on the block to introduce a number of natural therapies to the public, including CoQ10 and melatonin. In 1997, the foundation announced that SAMe "promises to be the most potent, multipurpose, anti-aging, anti-disease therapy we have ever introduced." Powerful words.

Has the prediction held up?

In a word, yes. The Life Extension Foundation was on the money with this one. While I'm not a fan of hyperbole that sounds better suited to a late-night infomercial, this substance is pretty incredible.

SAMe: Your Energy "Spark Plug" to the Rescue

SAMe stands for the S-adenosylmethionine (you can see why it's easier to call it SAMe). And the secret to its effectiveness for so many disparate conditions is a process in the body called methylation.

Think back to your high school track meets and remember what it was like to watch a relay race. Remember how the stick was passed from runner to runner? Well, chains of molecules in your body perform that kind of activity every minute, and the "stick" they pass that keeps the chain running effectively is called a *methyl group* (a specific arrangement of hydrogen and carbon atoms). Think of the methyl group as a kind of spark plug that keeps the engines of the body firing cleanly and quickly. This constant transfer is called *methylation*. When methylation is compromised it's like having sticky, sludgy spark plugs. Everything slows down, energy is compromised, and things just don't work right.

Enter SAMe. SAMe is the ultimate "methyl donor." That means it literally donates a methyl group wherever it's needed, keeping the relay races running smoothly. It virtually passes a torch to whoever needs it so that the race never has to slow down or get derailed while someone goes looking for a torch.

A Natural Cure for Depression

Since the methylation process is so critical to a number of pathways in the body—including brain activity and joint activity—SAMe is able to act as a "natural cure" for a whole range of different problems that have, as a component, impaired methylation. Hence it's used as an antidepressant, a treatment for arthritis, and a tonic for a sick liver. The health of all those "systems" depends heavily on a well-oiled system of methylation.

SAMe is arguably the most effective "natural" antidepressant around. And one of the best things about it is that you'll know whether it's working within a week. (Actually this is true

WORTH KNOWING

SAMe should not be used for depression by people with bipolar disorders unless they're under medical supervision. It can make bipolar episodes worse.

SAMe is unstable at certain temperatures so needs to be kept dry. Some stable forms are now available, but just to be on the safe side, stick with the enteric-coated tablets available in a blister pack.

Take SAMe on an empty stomach, about an hour before a meal or two hours afterward. It's often possible to cut down the dosage once you start noticing a positive effect.

SAMe works best with adequate B vitamins, especially folate, B6, and B12, which also support the methylation process in the brain and elsewhere.

for the majority of people, but in some less common cases it may take up to five weeks to work, about the same as a pharmaceutical antidepressant in the SSRI class, which includes Prozac, Paxil, and Zoloft.)

A review of eleven research papers on SAMe, published in *Clinical Investigative Medicine* in June 2005, concluded that "there appears to be a role for SAMe in the treatment of major depression in adults." Note the qualifier "major." It's extremely hard to treat "major" depression, so the fact that the researchers were positive about SAMe says more than you might think on first glance. "Major depression" is one of three

Natural Prescription for SAMe

Doses and Precautions

SAMe has been used in doses ranging from 200–1,600 mg a day.

A common dose for depression is 800 mg a day, though people take up to 1,600 mg.

For liver problems, up to 1,600 mg a day.

For bone and joint health, the typical dose is between 200 and 1,200 mg a day.

SAMe is usually taken in divided doses. For example, 800 mg for depression would be divided into two 400 mg doses, one in the morning and the other at night.

Most commonly SAMe comes in 200 mg tablets in a blister pack.

It's frequently common to cut back the dosage after you feel the effect, but this is a personal decision. You can play with it.

There has never been a reported overdose, and there are no reported adverse interactions with other drugs, supplements, or foods. The *Physicians' Desk Reference* notes that there are no known contraindications, but warns—as I do—not to take SAMe if you're suffering from bipolar disorder (see page 309). Just to be safe, the same is probably true during pregnancy.

Do not discontinue conventional antidepressants and switch to SAMe without supervision. Most antidepressants should be discontinued gradually, and under the eye of a health-care provider.

categories of depression, but if you're reading this—and you're depressed—chances are you don't have "major" depression but instead have either "mild" or "moderate" depression, both of which respond even better to SAMe. About 70 percent of people with depression respond to SAMe, according to Richard Brown, M.D., author of *Stop Depression Now*.

Depression accompanies a lot of health conditions, and which comes first is a chicken-or-egg problem that no one has figured out. People with diabetes, fibromyalgia, Parkinson's disease, and other illnesses frequently suffer from depression, often at a higher rate than the general population. SAMe is a probably a valuable tool for treating depression in these folks, especially because there are no reported adverse interactions with SAMe and other drugs, dietary supplements, or foods.

In treating depression, SAMe works as well as certain standard antidepressants* and with fewer side effects. In a meta-analysis of twenty-eight studies done by the Agency for Healthcare Research and Quality, treatment with SAMe was associated with an improvement of about six points on the Hamilton Rating Scale for Depression after only three weeks, basically equal to treatment with conventional antidepressants and significantly better than treatment with a placebo. A paper in *Psychiatry Research* (1995) from researchers at the Depression Clinical and Research Program at Massachusetts General

---

*Standard antidepressants meaning the older tricyclic variety. Unfortunately, so far there are no head-to-head tests of SAMe and the newer antidepressants, like Prozac, Lexapro, etc.

Hospital concluded that "SAMe is a relatively safe and fast-acting antidepressant." A review of the evidence published in the *American Journal of Clinical Nutrition* in 2002 by two researchers affiliated with Harvard Medical School (Mischoulon and Fava) pointed out that SAMe may have a faster onset of action than conventional antidepressants and may even protect against the deleterious effects of Alzheimer's. This is good stuff.

The Best Liver Protection Around

SAMe is one of the most liver-friendly molecules on earth. The Life Extension Foundation calls it "serious medicine against liver disease," and I agree. The liver contains a high amount of SAMe, and one of the body's most important antioxidants—glutathione—is synthesized from it. Glutathione is absolutely central to keeping the liver healthy and helping it to do its many jobs, including detoxification. SAMe is seriously depleted in liver disease and has been shown in research to improve liver-function tests. And remember methylation (see page 309)? SAMe's outstanding properties as a methylating agent help keep liver membranes fluid. Anyone with liver disease or problems, such as hepatitis, should consider SAMe as an adjunct to treatment.

It's also been shown in research to significantly prevent or reverse the toxicity that can be induced in the laboratory by drugs, alcohol, or chemicals. And in one double-blind trial, people with cirrhosis of the liver due to alcoholism who took SAMe for two years had a 47 percent lower rate of death or need for liver transplantation,

compared with those who received a placebo. Great as the improvement was, it didn't quite achieve statistical significance, but the results were more impressive—and were statistically significant—in people with less severe cirrhosis.

Pain Relief from Arthritis

SAMe may be a great treatment for osteoarthritis. In one large randomized clinical trial, SAMe reduced the pain of osteoarthritis by 20 percent (about the same as nonsteroidal anti-inflammatories like ibuprofen, Advil, or Motrin, but with none of the side effects). There is reliable evidence going back to published studies in the late 1980s that SAMe possesses anti-inflammatory, pain-relieving, and tissue-healing properties that may help protect the health of joints. Several double-blind studies have shown that SAMe is useful for people with osteoarthritis because it can reduce pain, stiffness, and swelling better than placebos and equal to drugs such as ibuprofen and naproxen.

Although they're not frequently mentioned among the conditions SAMe can be used to help with, heart disease and stroke contain a potent risk factor that SAMe can reduce. That factor is homocysteine, a nasty and inflammatory metabolite that's produced as a by-product of methionine and that is ordinarily converted back to methionine. However, in many people, this process doesn't work too well, and they accumulate higher levels of this inflammatory metabolite than they should. High levels of homocysteine have been associated with a much greater risk for both heart disease and stroke in many different studies, including one in the prestigious *Journal of the American Medical Association* in 1992. High homocysteine levels are usually treated with extra B vitamins (folate, B6, and B12; see pages 35–41), but SAMe can help as well because it plays a critical role in helping to turn homocysteine back into the benign methionine so that large amounts don't build up in the system.

The Melatonin Matter

One important function of SAMe that's often overlooked is its connection to the synthesis of the important hormone melatonin. We think of melatonin as something you take for jet lag, but it's actually a powerful hormone that has multiple purposes in the body, one of which is to help regulate the sleep cycle. It may also have cancer-preventive properties. One interesting line of research has discovered that blind women almost never have breast cancer. It's believed that the connection is melatonin, which is only produced when it's dark (or at least when light does not get to the eyes, as should be the case when you sleep). Blind women evidentially have more of this hormone, hence the hypothesized connection. And SAMe is needed indirectly for the synthesis of melatonin.

Here's how it works. Serotonin is produced from tryptophan, both in the day and at night, in the gut and in the brain. At night, SAMe combines with two other compounds (hydroxyindole O-methyl transferase and N-acetylserotonin or NAS) to produce melatonin. Without enough SAMe around, melatonin production is compromised. In addition to whatever other benefits melatonin has (e.g., the possible anticancer activity), it definitely is needed for sound sleep, so if you don't have enough SAMe, your body's melatonin factory won't be working on all four cylinders and you'll be walking around bleary-eyed, wondering why you're irritated most of the time. Since disruption of sleep has a whole bunch of other nasty health consequences, this function of SAMe is an important but overlooked one.

Fibromyalgia in the Future?

There isn't a ton of evidence on SAMe and fibromyalgia, but there's enough to make it more than worth a try if you're suffering from this difficult disease, particularly since depression can so often accompany it. A couple of preliminary studies indicate it may be helpful, and my friend, naturopath Cathy Wong, N.D. (About.com's alternative medicine resident expert), puts it first on her list of supplements that may be useful for this condition. In one study, the number of tender points on the body decreased after using SAMe as did scores on two rating scales of depression.

Selenium

IF I WERE stuck on a desert island with only six supplements, I'd definitely want one of them to be selenium. This little trace mineral has more uses than you can shake a stick at. It's a powerful antioxidant, it's helpful for getting rid of toxic metals in the system, it's an antiviral agent, and it's shown the ability to protect against cancer. What's not to like?

I first started hearing about selenium's power at a Boulderfest conference on nutritional medicine, more than five or six years ago. As I recall, the great nutritionist and writer Robert Crayhon, M.S., C.N., mentioned that selenium status was a good predictor of how well a patient with AIDS would do; those with higher selenium intakes had better outcomes.

This was a textbook perfect example of something that has happened to those of us in nutritional medicine a thousand times—we hear about something, we know something works, and years later, the research catches up. Right before writing this section I went to the National Institute of Medicine's library, the main database for recognized, respected, peer-reviewed journal studies, and I typed in "Selenium and AIDS." The first entry, right off the bat, was from the January 2007 *Archives of Internal Medicine:* "Suppression of human immunodeficiency virus type 1 viral load with selenium supplementation." The researchers

concluded that "daily selenium supplementation can suppress the progression of HIV-1 viral burden and provide indirect improvement of CD4 count."

No one is saying selenium is a cure for AIDS, or cancer, or hepatitis C, or any of the other serious illnesses it seems to help protect against. But it's clear from the research that low levels of selenium depress both the immune system and antibody levels, making your body's defense system much less able to fight off challenges.

Sending your body out into the world with low levels of selenium is like sending an army to fight without proper armor (and, sad to say, we all know what happens when you do that). Selenium supplementation in humans has resulted in increased activity of natural killer cells—one of the most important weapons in your immune system's arsenal. For example, when it comes to the hepatitis C virus, Burt Berkson, M.D., Ph.D., calls selenium "a birth control pill for the virus."

A Weapon against Cancer

Low dietary intake of selenium is associated with increased incidence of several types of cancers, including lung, colorectal, skin, and prostate. Animal and human research shows that supplemental selenium can protect against certain cancers.

"Nearly 200 animal studies have been conducted to evaluate the effects of (supplemental) levels of selenium on experimental carcinogenesis. Of these, two-thirds have found that high levels of selenium reduced the development of tumors at least moderately and in most cases very significantly," writes P.D. Whanger, Ph.D., professor of agricultural chemistry at Oregon State University and an investigator at the Linus Pauling Institute.

Further, a study by Cornell University and the University of Arizona showed that men and women taking selenium supplements for ten years had 41 percent less total cancer than those taking a placebo. "Although more than a hundred of animal and dozens of epidemiological studies have linked high selenium status and cancer risk, this is the first double-blind, placebo-controlled cancer prevention study with humans that directly supports the thesis that a nutritional supplement of selenium, as a single agent, can reduce the risk of cancer," said Gerald F. Combs Jr., a nutritional biochemist and Cornell University professor of nutritional sciences.

Let me tell you about one other very interesting study on selenium and cancer before moving on to the many other things this miraculous supernutrient can do for you. In this study,

researchers wanted to see whether selenium supplementation had any affect on the incidence of skin cancer. Half the participants received one 200 mcg tablet of selenium a day, the other half got a placebo (an empty sugar pill). Turns out the selenium didn't have much of an effect on skin cancer.

But the story doesn't end there.

Midway through the study, the researchers noticed something else: The total cancer incidence in the selenium group was significantly

---

WORTH KNOWING

With selenium, more is not necessarily better. Though it's rare, there are reported cases of selenium toxicity. They involved nothing life-threatening: gastrointestinal upset, hair loss, white blotchy nails, and garlic breath. But why chance it? The Institute of Medicine set 400 mcg a day as a tolerable upper limit. The average stand-alone supplement is 200 mg, which is what usually produces great results in studies; you should be absolutely fine with that amount in a supplement.

One of my most trusted sources on vitamins and supplements, my dear friend Shari Lieberman, Ph.D., C.N.S., author of the definitive *Real Vitamin and Mineral Book,* told me: "Various studies have shown that long-term intakes of up to 500 to 750 mcg per day have produced no signs of toxicity in humans. Data extrapolated from animal studies suggests that toxicity does not occur in humans ingesting less than 1,000 to 2,000 mcg per day."

lower than the other group. There was a 37 percent reduction in total cancer incidence, a 63 percent decline in the incidence of prostate cancer, a 58 percent decrease in the incidence of colorectal cancer, and a 46 percent decline in the incidence of lung cancer. Oh yes, and a 50 percent decrease in total cancer mortality. (The authors speculate that the reason they didn't see results with skin cancer was because the nature of skin cancer is such that this study may have been too short to demonstrate a positive effect.)

An Antioxidant Superpower

Selenium is also one of the most powerful antioxidants on the planet. There's an inverse relationship between blood levels of selenium and the incidence of cardiovascular disease; selenium protects against oxidative damage to blood vessels—damage that probably plays a big role in the formation of dangerous plaque. Selenium is needed for regulating certain powerful enzymes in the body, the glutathione peroxidase enzymes, which figure prominently in various detoxification pathways. And selenium has anti-inflammatory properties as well. Supplemental selenium can help protect against Kashin-Beck disease, a form of arthritis that afflicts many people in China and other parts of Asia who live in selenium-deficient areas.

Then there are toxic metals like mercury. While this is yet to be "proven" conclusively, most nutritional experts I know believe that selenium is a powerful chelator, meaning it attaches to metals like mercury and helps to remove them from the body. Japanese researchers have found that adding selenium to the diets of birds gave them "complete protection" from large amounts of mercury. At a 2005 Washington conference sponsored by the governments of the United States, Norway, Canada, and Iceland, and assisted by the United Nations' food and agriculture organization, evidence was presented that showed that selenium helps neutralize the effects of mercury acquired from foods.

"This very important but little analyzed point helps us to understand how people from the Seychelles Islands can eat fish twelve times per week and show no toxic signs," said William E. M. Lands, a retired professor of biochemistry at the universities of Michigan and Illinois. No one is more concerned about mercury than me, and while I recommend you avoid it, it's nice to know that selenium can help mitigate at least some of the potential effects of this dangerous, neurotoxic metal.

I think taking a 200 mcg supplement of selenium every day is one of the most sensible things you can do. Many high-quality multiple supplements contain this much, or you can take it as a stand-alone pill. The very best food source is Brazil nuts, which are high in calories but a selenium bonanza. Canned clams, oysters, and tuna are also good sources, as are beef and lamb. Many areas of the world, including the United States, have soil that is selenium deficient, meaning you won't get much from the plants or grains that are grown there or the animals that eat them. Do yourself a favor and take a supplement, or eat at least one or two Brazil nuts every day.

Vitamin C

EVER WONDER why you have a sweet tooth? No, it's not just nature's way of playing a rather mean-spirited practical joke on you. There's an important functional reason for that sweet tooth. In fact, that sweet tooth probably kept your ancient prehistoric ancestors alive. Why? Because humans can't make vitamin C.

That's a weird feature we share with other higher primates (monkeys and apes), guinea pigs, the red-vented bulbul, and fruit-eating bats. Every other species in the world makes its own vitamin C. One theory is that since vitamin C is found in fruits and vegetables, and since fruits that are safe to eat are often sweet, nature in her wisdom gave us a sweet tooth so we would seek out the very foods without which we would die.

And make no mistake—without vitamin C we'd all be dead as doorknobs. Without vitamin C you can't form new collagen, the main protein in connective tissue. A deficiency of vitamin C results in a really nasty disease called *scurvy*.

The body breaks down cellular structures, flesh and bones decay, a baker's dozen of horrible symptoms manifest, and if scurvy is left untreated, you die a pretty horrible death. It was a particular problem for anyone separated from fruits and vegetables for long periods of time. Sailors who went on long voyages, for example, were at particular risk. In the 1400s and 1500s,

explorers like Magellan and Vasco da Gama would typically lose more than half their crew to the disease.

Then in 1747, James Lind, a ship's surgeon in the British Royal Navy, conducted a "cutting-edge" experiment that proved that lemon juice could prevent the disease. He published his findings in 1753. The legendary Captain Cook, who made three historic voyages between 1758 and his death in 1779, was credited with using cabbage and fruits to prevent anyone from dying of scurvy on his ships. Still, the British navy didn't make lemon or lime juice a standard requirement on ships until 1795. (This story is frequently used as an example of the "principle" that the establishment takes about fifty years to catch up with the cutting edge.)

From asthma to high blood pressure, from cancer to rheumatoid arthritis, vitamin C is one of those nutrients that is needed everywhere, and at any given time (and especially on a desert island). This powerhouse vitamin is required for at least 300 metabolic functions in the body. The body not only requires vitamin C, it demands it for proper functioning of virtually every organ system.

As mentioned, one of its primary functions is to produce collagen, which aids in wound healing, gum health, and the making of beautiful skin. But many studies prove that vitamin C benefits the body in numerous other ways, including protection from cancer, cardiovascular disease, and (maybe) the common cold. It also earns its place on the twenty-first-century desert island for its protection against environmental stressors like pesticides and toxins. And finally, its immune-enhancing properties make vitamin C one of the most useful nutrients for maintaining good health.

Vitamin C and the Immune System

Despite conventional wisdom to the contrary, quite a bit of controversy exists over whether vitamin C protects against colds. Numerous studies show that regular use of about 1,000 mg of vitamin C supplements can slightly reduce the symptoms of colds and shorten the length of the illness, albeit modestly.

Many studies have shown that taking vitamin C along with zinc will shorten the duration of respiratory tract infections like pneumonia. And a study of marathoners published in the *American Journal of Clinical Nutrition* showed that competitors taking 600 mg of vitamin C for twenty-one days prior to the race had significantly fewer cold symptoms within two weeks of completing it. Two other studies found that

Natural Prescription for Vitamin C

500–2,000 mg per day

A good starting point is 500 mg per day for good antioxidant protection. Plain old ascorbic acid is a sufficient, effective form. There is no need to buy an esterized form (e.g, Ester-C).

Bioflavonoids like quercetin and hesperidin also enhance vitamin C's effectiveness. Taking vitamin C with vitamin E and beta-carotene enhances its effects. Bioflavonoids like hesperidin and quercetin also enhance its absorption.

High doses of C can cause diarrhea, but that just means that you reduce your dose to 75 percent of the amount that gave you loose stools.

Tip: Stop smoking. It greatly depletes vitamin C stores.

Note: All dosages are daily dosages and in pill or capsule form unless otherwise noted.

vitamin C significantly reduced the number of colds experienced by people involved in rigorous exercise in very cold environments—for example, military men involved in training maneuvers in northern Canada during the winter and children attending skiing camp in the Swiss Alps.

That said, taking vitamin C at the onset of a cold, which is what a lot of people do, won't stop it. Personally, I say "Who cares?" The whole "controversy" over whether vitamin C can help with the common cold takes focus away from its far more important functions and uses.

Let's start with the immune system. Without vitamin C, your immune system is toast. When you've got an infection, your lymphocytes—white blood cells—kick in to defend the body. Lymphocytes use up a ton of vitamin C. So does a process known as phagocytosis, which is a mechanism used by the immune system to remove cell debris, bacteria, pathogens, and dead tissue cells. You need vitamin C for that "cleanup crew" to do its job properly. Vitamin C also increases *chemotaxis*, the rate at which white blood cells travel to the infection.

An Antioxidant for the Ages

Then there's vitamin C's powerful—and I mean *powerful*—activity as an antioxidant. If you're unfamiliar with what oxidative damage is, consider what happens when you leave a cut apple outside in the air—within half an hour it turns brown. That process is called *oxidation*. It's a kind of cellular aging, and it takes place inside your body all the time. While you're minding your own business, rogue oxygen molecules known as *free radicals* are attacking your cells and damaging your DNA at a frightening rate. The volume on that cellular assault is turned up even more when you're exposed to toxins, cigarette smoke, damaged fats from fried foods, car exhausts, overcooked barbecue, or any of the myriad sources of carcinogens that we come in contact with on a daily basis. All these exposures create free radical damage, also known as oxidative damage, which

is not only a big part of aging but also a component of absolutely every single degenerative disease you can think of (and many that you've never heard of).

An antioxidant acts like lemon juice on the apple slices—it protects against the damage of oxidation. Vitamin C is one of the most powerful antioxidants on the planet. To this extent it's a natural weapon against cellular damage from a host of enemies. It's also no accident that it's an important ingredient in so many high-end skin care products.

Vitamin C also boosts levels of a group of cells in the body that are programmed to target and kill tumors as well as protect against a variety of microbes that might be out to do you damage. These cells are called natural killer cells (NK cells), and they're one of the big guns of the immune system. In one study published in *Immunopharmacology and Immunotoxicology*, high doses of vitamin C enhanced natural killer cells by 78 percent. The authors also concluded that such levels of NK cells might help in the treatment of cancer.

Linus Pauling, Cancer, and Vitamin C

Speaking of cancer, let's talk for a minute about Linus Pauling.

Linus Pauling was the only person in history to win two unshared Nobel Prizes. In 1941 he was diagnosed with Bright's disease, a fatal kidney disease that experts believed was untreatable. Working with a doctor at Stanford University who used diet, vitamins, and minerals, Pauling was able to control his disease, and his interest and passion in vitamin therapy was born. (By the way, Pauling lived another fifty-three years, dying in 1994.) Pauling actually coined the phrase *orthomolecular medicine* referring to the practice of using substances—like nutrients—normally found in the body to prevent and treat disease.

Pauling was first introduced to the concept of high-dose vitamin C by a biochemist named Irwin Stone, and at Stone's suggestion, began taking several grams a day. Over the next three decades or so, he became an outspoken advocate for high-dose vitamin C, writing books like *Cancer and Vitamin C*, *Vitamin C and the Common Cold*, and the *New York Times* bestseller *How to Live Longer and Feel Better*, all of which sang the praises of vitamin C for just about everything. He eventually formed the Institute of Orthomolecular Medicine in 1973, which was soon renamed the Linus Pauling Institute and is now part of Oregon State University. The institute's major areas of research include heart disease, cancer, aging, and neurodegenerative diseases. Its basic premise is that "an optimum diet is the key to optimum health."

Pauling took a great deal of flack for his advocacy of high-dose vitamin C and was dismissed by much of the medical establishment as a nut job. But in 2005, researchers published a paper in the *Proceedings of the National Academy of Sciences* demonstrating that vitamin C killed cancer cells in test tubes.

Further, in the March 28, 2006, issue of the *Canadian Medical Association Journal*, researchers documented three cases of advanced cancers where patients had "unexpectedly long survival times after receiving high-dose vitamin C therapy." They concluded that "the role of intravenous vitamin C therapy in cancer treatment should be reassessed."

Another Vitamin C Backer

Pauling was not alone in supporting high-dose vitamin C therapy. One of the early advocates of this kind of treatment was a physician named Robert Cathcart. In 1981, Cathcart published a paper in the journal *Medical Hypotheses*, advocating the use of as much vitamin C as the patient could tolerate, "just short of the doses which produce diarrhea." He called this level "bowel tolerance."

"Bowel tolerance doses of ascorbic acid ameliorate the acute symptoms of many diseases," Cathcart wrote.

In several published papers, Cathcart argued that the amount of ascorbic acid a person can ingest orally without producing diarrhea was a good measure of how sick he or she was. His theory was that the amount of vitamin C needed to reach the level of bowel tolerance increases considerably the more toxic the illness.

"A person who can tolerate orally 10–15 grams of ascorbic acid within 24 hours when well might be able to tolerate 30–60 grams per 24 hours if he has a mild cold, 100 grams with a severe cold, 150 grams with influenza, and 200 grams per 24 hours with mononucleosis or viral pneumonia."

It should be pointed out that these are absolutely massive doses. But it should *also* be pointed out that holistic medical doctors practicing nutritional medicine and using vitamin drips intravenously think nothing of putting 10 to 20 g of vitamin C in a single intravenous drip, and 60 g is not unheard of, particularly when dealing with severe illness.

Cathcart has an interesting take on why some studies don't show great results with vitamin C supplements. He argues that "in all the studies yielding negative or equivocal results, inadequate doses were used. In some studies, doses barely bordering on adequate tease the investigator with statistically but not very impressive beneficial results."

The Vitamin C Foundation—a group of physicians and other health practitioners and advocates dedicated to promoting the therapeutic value of vitamin C—recommend that "every man, woman and child over the age of 3 consume at least 3 grams (3,000 mg) of vitamin C daily in order to enjoy optimum health." Hold on to your horses—it recommends even more during pregnancy (6,000 mg or 6 g) and "much, much more during periods of disease"— 20,000 mg and up.

Cardiovascular Health

Vitamin C also plays an important role in heart health. For one thing, it prevents oxidation (remember the apple) of LDL (the poorly named "bad" cholesterol). The thing about cholesterol is that it really isn't a problem until it gets oxidized (and then it's a *really* big problem). By helping to prevent this, vitamin C helps prevent problems that might be related to cholesterol. Vitamin C also strengthens collagen structures of the arteries.

And if that weren't enough, it can also benefit anyone with hypertension. Why? Because it helps lower levels of *thromboxane*, a major factor in blood clots. In one study, doses of 1 g of

WORTH KNOWING

As far as supplements go, plain old ascorbic acid is a sufficient, effective form. There is no need to buy an esterized form (e.g., Ester-C). Bioflavonoids like quercetin and hesperidin enhance vitamin C's effectiveness and increase its absorption. Taking vitamin C with vitamin E may enhance its effects in some cases. Very high doses of C can cause a little diarrhea, but that just means that you reduce your dose to 75 percent of the amount that gave you loose stools.

There was great anxiety recently in the United States over the well-publicized fact that most of the ascorbic acid in our supplements comes from China, and as of this writing, enormous concerns have been voiced over the safety of such imports. Fact is, most of the major manufacturers in the United States do their own testing for microbes, heavy metals, and toxins. If you buy any reliable brand from a well-known manufacturer, you should be fine. Any brand I list on my website, www.jonnybowden.com, is a brand almost exclusively sold through health practitioners, and virtually all of them are extremely thorough in their testing. Many even offer a certificate of analysis. You can trust them—I certainly do.

vitamin C per week showed a significant decrease in blood pressure for hypertensive patients. In another study, a vitamin C supplement of 3 g per day in divided doses was given to people who were stressed and anxious about speaking in public. Their blood pressure was significantly lower before, during, and after the presentations.

More evidence of vitamin C's "help for the heart" comes from the Framingham Nurses Study, which followed 85,000 women for more than sixteen years. In this study, a higher intake of vitamin C (in this case, more than 359 mg per day from dietary sources, or diet plus supplements) reduced the risk for cardiovascular disease by about 28 percent.

A pooled analysis of nine studies tracking 290,000 adults who were completely free of coronary heart disease at the beginning of the studies found that over the course of the next ten years, those who took more than 700 mg of supplemental vitamin C a day had a 25 percent reduction in risk for cardiovascular disease compared to those who took no vitamin C at all. In still another study, subjects taking the most vitamin C (in the highest quartile) had a stunning 80 percent lower risk of heart attack than those ranked in the lowest quartile for vitamin C intake. And a Finnish study examining the health of middle-aged men with no evidence of preexisting heart disease found that those who were deficient in vitamin C were 3.5 times more likely to suffer heart attack.

Not only does vitamin C decrease risk for heart attacks, it also seems to reduce damage following one. In a study called the *Myocardial Infarction and Vitamins Trial* (*MVIT*) researchers found that patients who suffered an acute heart attack and then supplemented with 1,200 mg of vitamin C (along with 600 mg of vitamin E) for one month had significantly lower rates of complications from the acute heart attack. Patients in the supplemented group also suffered fewer additional heart attacks, and few people in that group died compared to the other group.

The Three A's: Asthma, Arthritis, and Allergy

Because vitamin C is the major antioxidant in the lungs, it plays a critical role in protecting against oxidative damage. Low intakes of vitamin C from food or supplementation can lead to increased risks for asthma.

A 2005 study done by researchers from the Asthma and Allergy Research Institute in Australia found that the blood concentrations of vitamin C were markedly lower in patients with severe asthma compared to those who had mild asthma or were asthma-free. A review article in the *American Journal of Clinical Nutrition* concluded that "symptoms of ongoing asthma in adults appear to be increased by exposure to environmental oxidants and decreased vitamin C supplementation."

Asthmatics have a higher need for vitamin C than do members of the general population. One to two grams of vitamin C have been shown in studies to be the most helpful. This level is also helpful for those suffering from allergy or an excess production of histamine.

Because vitamin C has a variety of effects on histamine, it has also been shown to be beneficial in the management of allergic symptoms like rhinitis. And higher intakes (and blood levels) of vitamin C are related to decreased levels of histamine production.

There's some controversy when it comes to vitamin C and arthritis, but on closer examination the arguments against vitamin C supplementation appear to be bogus. No one contests the findings—published in the journal *Annals of Rheumatic Diseases*—that people who eat the least amounts of fruits and vegetables are twice as likely to develop inflammation in the joints, which is characteristic of rheumatoid arthritis. The researchers found that those who consumed the least amount of vitamin C in their diet had a whopping three times the risk of developing inflammatory arthritis than those who consumed the most. The controversy centers not on rheumatoid arthritis but on osteoarthritis, largely on the strength of one study with guinea pigs done at Duke University.

In this study, vitamin C supplements were given to forty-six guinea pigs (which, you may remember, are like us in that they're one of the few species that don't make their own vitamin C). The researchers found that a connection between high-dose vitamin C supplementation and the development of bony spurs in their knee joints. (The "high-dose" vitamin C given to the guinea pigs was the equivalent of about 1,500 to 2,500 mg in humans.) This led to much bad publicity about vitamin C and osteoarthritis.

But the issue is far from settled. An earlier study showed that the exact same amount of vitamin C *protected* guinea pigs against surgically induced osteoarthritis. (Remember that free radicals can and do damage collagen and connective tissue, and the antioxidant activity of vitamin C helps protect against this damage all the while helping collagen synthesis.) And a paper published in *Arthritis and Rheumatism* that looked at 640 human participants from the Framingham Osteoarthritis Cohort Study found a threefold reduction in the risk of osteoarthritis progression for those with higher intakes of vitamin C. This also translated into a reduced risk of cartilage loss. The researchers concluded that "high intake of antioxidant micronutrients, especially vitamin C, may reduce the risk of cartilage loss and disease progression in people with osteoarthritis."

The Ultimate Antiaging Vitamin?

Two major studies have associated vitamin C status with longevity. In a study of more than 19,000 adults, those with the lowest blood levels of vitamin C were twice as likely to die over the next four years as those with the highest levels of vitamin C in their blood. And a decade-long study from UCLA of more than 11,000 people showed that men who took 800 mg of vitamin C daily lived about six years longer than men who took only 60 mg of the vitamin. Just something to think about.

The National Health and Nutrition Examination Survey (NHANES) is an ongoing research project that looks at nutrition habits as they relate to health outcomes in a large population. An analysis of findings from the NHANES l looked at mortality from all causes and cross-referenced it with vitamin C intake. Researchers use a sophisticated predictive tool called the *standard mortality ratio*, which is the ratio of deaths observed in the study group compared to the number that would be expected in a similar, matched population. (For purposes of comparison, the similar population would have a standard mortality ratio of 1.00.) The NHANES l study found that among males with the highest vitamin C intake, mortality ratio was only .65 from all causes, only .78 from all cancers, and .58 from cardiovascular disease, a huge difference attributed to the vitamin C. Among females the reduction was slightly less dramatic but still significant.

Note also that vitamin C is an important part of the "antioxidant cocktail" shown in research to help prevent the deterioration of vision associated with macular degeneration (see page 169).

Vitamin C is found in virtually anything that grows. Berries, citrus fruits, kiwis, green vegetables—especially broccoli, cabbage, peppers, potatoes, and Brussels sprouts—all are loaded with the stuff. Fresh is best, as vitamin C content is reduced when vegetables are cut and left standing, sometimes in less than three hours. Frozen is right up there with fresh, but forget about canned fruits or vegetables (except maybe pumpkin). The top five foods containing vitamin C are acerola, red chile peppers, guavas, red bell peppers, and kale.

The bottom line: Vitamin C protects you. You'll definitely want it in your nutrient tool kit should you ever get stuck on a desert island—especially if you're not prone to eating a ton of fruits and vegetables.

GLOSSARY

ACE inhibitors—found in whey protein; reduce blood pressure and improve cardiovascular health

acemannen—starch or polysaccharide

acetylcholine—one of the major neuro-transmitters in the body, needed for memory and healthy brain function

acetylenics—component of celery that stops the growth of cancer cells

acidosis—depletion of the alkali reserve in the blood and tissues

acid rebound (or acid reflux)—a condition in which the stomach produces excess acid

adaptogen—any compound that has a normalizing influence on physiology, regardless of the direction of change caused by the stressor

adenosine triphosphate (ATP)—the body's energy molecule

alpha linolenic acid—omega-3 fatty acid that helps reduce inflammation

amino acids—molecules that link together to form proteins

angiotensin-converting enzyme (ACE) inhibitors—help reduce blood pressure by interfering with an enzyme that causes the constriction of muscles surrounding the arteries, thus raising blood pressure

anthocyanins—pigment molecules that make blueberries blue, red cabbage and cherries red; improve vision and brain function; guard against macular degeneration; help the body relieve inflammation

antioxidants—compounds in food that help fight the process of oxidation, or oxidative stress, a factor in virtually every degenerative disease

astaxanthin—antioxidant found in salmon

ataxia—shaky movements and unsteady gait

atherosclerosis—thickening of the arteries

benign prostatic hyperplasia (BPH)—annoying but essentially harmless condition characterized by frequent urination, especially in the middle of the night; hesitant, interrupted, or weak stream of urine; a pressing urgency to urinate; leaking; or dribbling

beta-carotene—carotenoid that converts in the body to vitamin A

betaine—metabolite that works synergistically with folate to reduce potentially toxic levels of homocysteine; also known as trimethylglycine (TMG); derived from sugar beets

beta-sitosterol—plant compound shown to significantly lower blood cholesterol as well as protect the prostate

bran—the main source of fiber in whole grains; can also contain nutrients

bromelain—proteolytic enzyme that breaks down amino acids; relives indigestion and is often extracted from pineapple

cardiac ischemia—a condition in which blood flow to the heart muscle is obstructed

carotenoid—antioxidant compound found in plants; associated with a wide range of health benefits

carpal tunnel syndrome—a painful disorder caused by compression of a nerve that passes between the bones and ligaments of the wrist

catechins—very powerful group of polyphenols; found in cranberry juice, green tea, and cinnamon

catecholamines—brain chemicals that improve mood and help fight depression

chalcone polymers—phytochemicals in cinnamon that increase glucose metabolism in the cells

chemotaxis—the rate at which white blood cells travel to the infection

cholecystokinin (CKK)—hormone in the gut that signals the brain when you've had enough to eat

choline—nutrient found in eggs, needed for healthy brain and liver function and fat breakdown; forms betaine in the body

chromium—trace mineral that helps insulin function

circulating immune complex—compounds responsibly for achy joints and general joint pain

citrate—compound that may help fight kidney stones

claudication—a painful cramping sensation in the muscles of the legs due to decreased oxygen supply

coenzyme Q10 (CoQ10)—ubiquinone found in most tissues in the body; essential for the manufacture of the body's energy molecule, ATP (adenosine triphosphate)

complement factor H (CFH) gene—strongly associated with macular degeneration

conjugated linoleic acid (CLA)—trans fat found naturally in grass-fed dairy and meat

cortisol—stress hormone that, in elevated levels, may ultimately age the brain by shrinking the hippocampus

COX-2 inhibitors—drugs that block pain and inflammation messages in the body

C-reactive protein—protein in the blood used as a measure of inflammation

curcumin—antioxidant and curcuminoid; has anti-inflammatory and antitumor effect; has positive effect on cholesterol

curcuminoids—family of compounds thought to be most responsible for turmeric's medicinal effects and bright yellow color

cyclooxygenase—a compound produced in the body in two or more forms, called COX-1 and COX-2

cynarin—active ingredient in artichokes that has demonstrated liver-protecting effects

cysteine—an amino acid needed to manufacture glutathione, arguably the most important antioxidant in the body

cytokines—inflammatory chemicals

dihydrotestosterone—testosterone metabolite partly responsible for hair loss and benign prostate hyperplasia

disaccharides—carbohydrate sugars

dopamine—"feel-good"neurotransmitter in the brain

D-ribose—molecule made in the body's cells and used for cellular function

eicosanoids—minihormones that control metabolic processes in the body; also called prostaglandins

ellagic acid—naturally occurring phenolic known to be both anticarcinogenic and antimutagenic; found in cherries and red raspberries; shown to inhibit tumor growth

Emotional Freedom Technique (EFT)—described by its founder, Gary Craig, as an emotional version of acupuncture, EFT is a technique that people use to liberate themselves from the energetic blocks caused by anger, grief, negative self-image, self-defeating beliefs, and even disease

endothelial dysfunction—dysfunction of the cells that line the inner surface of all blood vessels

epigallocatechin gallate (EGCG)—catechin believed to be responsible for the anticancer effects of green tea

escin—active ingredient in horse chestnut that helps strengthen vein valves, walls, and capillaries

essential fatty acids—"good fats" that must be obtained through diet; support many healthy body functions

estrogen dominance—condition associated with menopause in which both estrogen and progesterone decline, but progesterone declines more dramatically, throwing off the balance of the two hormones

fiber—indigestible component of food; associated with lower risks of heart disease, diabetes, obesity, and cancer

fibrin—sticky, weblike fibers that the body produces to form a structure that stops excess bleeding

fibrinogen—substance in the body that can cause blood clots and strokes

flavonoids—group of plant compounds with antioxidant, anticancer, and antiallergy properties; more than 4,000 have been identified

flavanols—flavonoids found in cocoa; prevent fatlike substances in the bloodstream from clogging the arteries and modulate nitric acid

folate—B vitamin that helps prevent neural tube defects and helps bring down homocysteine levels

free radicals—destructive molecules in the body; can damage cells and DNA

fructooligosaccharides—particularly healthy form of nondigestible carbohydrates that helps maintain healthy gut ecology

gamma-aminobutyric acid (GABA)—inhibitory neurotransmitter that also has significant calming effects in the brain

gamma-linolenic acid (GLA)—important "good" omega-6 found in hemp seed, primrose, and borage oils

gamma-tocopherol—component of vitamin E that neutralizes the perioxynitrite radical, which causes destruction to cellular endothelial membranes

glucose—plain blood sugar

glucose tolerance factor (GTF)—helps regulate blood sugar levels; found in brewer's yeast

glutathione—one of the body's premier antioxidants

glutathione peroxidase—enzyme critical in protecting against free-radical and oxidative damage associated with asthma; especially important in reducing the production of inflammatory compounds like leukotrines

glycemic index—measure of how much a given food (like fruit) raises blood sugar

glycemic load—measure of a food's effect on blood sugar that accounts for portion size

glycerophosphocholine (GPC)—phospholipid that has been extensively researched for its effect on mental performance, attention, concentration, and memory formation

glycogen—storage form of blood sugar

glyconutrients—active medicinal sugars

goiter—noncancerous enlargement of the thyroid gland due to iodine deficiency

gout—painful, largely inherited disorder in which the body can't properly metabolize uric acid; also known as metabolic arthritis

gut permeability—weakening of the lining in the gut that serves as a protective barrier for the bloodstream

helenalin—powerful anti-inflammatory agent contained in arnica

Helicobacter pylori (*H. pylori*)—common stomach bacterial infection that is a major cause of stomach ulcers

hesperidin—predominant flavonoid in oranges; strengthens capillaries and has anti-inflammatory, antiallergic, vasoprotective, and anticarcinogenic actions

hippocampus—area of the brain responsible for memory

homocysteine—amino acid, a natural product of metabolism, and an inflammatory biochemical that can increase risk of heart disease and stroke

hydrochloric acid (HCl)—activates enzymes in the stomach that allow protein breakdown

hydrolyzed whey protein—natural ACE inhibitor and a superb source of high-quality, absorbable protein

hydroxycitrate (hydroxycitric acid)—blocks a portion of an enzyme called citrate lyase, which helps turn sugars and starches into fat and may suppress the appetite

hydroxyl radicals—dangerous free radicals

hyperglycemia—high blood sugar

hypothyroidism—condition in which the thyroid gland fails to function adequately and which results in reduced levels of thyroid hormone in the body

immunoglobulin—protein fraction with important disease-fighting effects

inflammation—critical component of virtually all degenerative diseases

inositol—substance synthesized by the human body that is usually considered a member of the B vitamin family but is not technically a vitamin

insoluble fiber—indigestible part of foods that moves bulk through intestines

insulin—fat-storing hormone produced in the pancreas and released when blood sugar goes up

insulin resistance—associated with metabolic syndrome and type 2 diabetes

intrinsic factor—protein secreted in the stomach for vitamin B12 absorption

iodine—trace element required for production of thyroid hormones

isoflavones—phytochemicals in soy foods that may help ease menopause symptom

isomers—chemical compounds that have exactly the same number and type of atoms, but in different arrangements

L-arginine—amino acid shown to increase sperm production and motility and necessary for the creation of nitric oxide

lauric acid—fatty acid that is antiviral, antimicrobial, and important for immune function

lecithin—nutritional supplement that is 10 to 20 percent phosphatidylcholine

L-carnitine—a vitamin-like compound that escort fatty acids into the mitochondria of the cells where they can be "burned" for energy

L-glutamic acid—an excitatory neurotransmitter

L-glutamine—most abundant amino acid in the human body

linoleic acid—essential fatty acid with anticancer properties; also called omega-6 fatty acid

lutein—carotenoid that is a natural antioxidant and maintains eye and skin health

lysine—essential amino acid that works hand in hand with other essential amino acids to maintain growth, lean body mass, and the body's store of nitrogen, an essential part of all amino and nucleic acids

macula—central area of the retina that contain cone photoreceptors, which provide color sensitivity

manganese—trace mineral essential for growth, reproduction, wound healing, brain function, and metabolism of sugars, insulin, and cholesterol

magnesium—mineral that helps lower high blood pressure

malic acid—substance in vinegar important for fighting body toxins and inhibiting unfriendly bacteria

mast cells—storage sites for histamine

melatonin—powerful hormone that has multiple purposes in the body, one of which is to help regulate the sleep cycle; it may also have cancer-preventive properties

metabolic syndrome—a form of prediabetes that increases risk of heart disease

metabolite—by-product of the body's metabolic processes

methylation—chemical reaction in the central nervous system in which chains of molecules transfer methyl groups

methylhydroxychalcone polymer—active ingredient in cinnamon; seems to mimic insulin function, increasing glucose uptake by cells and signaling certain kinds of cells to turn glucose into glycogen

monounsaturated fats—fats central to the Mediterranean diet, associated with lower rates of heart disease; found in nuts and olive oil; also called omega-9s

myelin sheath—insulation that surrounds nerves

N-acetyl-cysteine (NAC)—antioxidant that can protect the liver; derivative of the amino acid L-cysteine that is a precursor to the formation of the powerful antioxidant glutathione

nattokinase—fibrinolytic enzyme that can help reduce and prevent clots; found in natto

natural killer cells—cells in the body that are programmed to target and kill tumors as well as protect against a variety of microbes

neurotransmitter—chemical produced in the brain that transmits information

neutrophils—most abundant kind of white blood cell in the body and an important part of the immune system

NF-kappa B—protein that controls the expression of genes that produce an inflammatory response

nitric oxide—compound in the body that helps relax constricted blood vessels and ease blood flow; synthesized from arginine

oleic acid—omega-9 fat that is found in high amounts in olive oil and macadamia nut oil and many nuts; increases the incorporation of omega-3 fatty acids into the cell membrane

oleuropein—active ingredient in olive leaf extract

omega-3 fats—ALA (alpha-linolenic acid), found in flaxseed; DHA (docosahexaenoic acid) and EPA (eicosapentaenoic acid), found in fish like wild salmon; keep cell membranes fluid

orthomolecular medicine—term used by Linus Pauling to refer to the practice of using substances normally found in the body to prevent and treat disease

osteocalcin—compound that anchors calcium molecules inside the bone; activated by vitamin K

osteoarthritis—chronic condition in which cartilage in the joints wears thin

osteocalcin—protein that helps get calcium into the bones where it's needed

oxalate—substance that inhibits calcium absorption

oxidative stress—the damage done to cells by free radicals of oxygen molecules

oxidization—damage with free radicals that leads to cellular aging

oxymel—combination of apple cider vinegar and honey widely used to dissolve painful calcium deposits in the body

papain—one of a class of enzymes called proteolytic enzymes that help to break down or digest protein; extracted from papaya and used in digestive enzyme supplements as well as in enzyme supplements used for pain

pectin—type of fiber that helps relieve constipation, reduce cholesterol, and regulate blood sugar; found in apples and quince

peelu—natural twig fortified with minerals that help clean the teeth and other inhibitors that prevent gums from bleeding

pepsin—major protein-digesting enzyme in the stomach

perillyl alcohol—compound that may inhibit tumor growth; found in cherries

phagocytosis—mechanism used by the immune system to remove cell debris, bacteria, pathogens, and dead tissue cells

phenolic acids—block the action of compounds in the body known to encourage the growth of cancerous tumors

phenolic compounds—natural antioxidants that help neutralize harmful free radicals in the body that are thought to be linked to most chronic diseases including cancer, heart disease, and diabetes; most belong to the flavonoid group

phenylalanine—amino acid that is a primary building block for pain control

phenylbutazone—anti-inflammatory medicine with effects similar to curcumin

phosphatidylcholine—active ingredient in the popular supplement lecithin. In animal research, it protects against cirrhosis and fibrosis and is essential for normal liver function.

phosphatidylserine—phospholipid and naturally occurring nutrient that's found in the cell membranes but most concentrated in the brain

phthalides—group of phytochemicals that relax muscle tissue in artery walls and lower stress hormones

phytates—substances that block the absorption of minerals

phytic acid—phytochemical that decreases the absorption of chromium (and other minerals)

phytoestrogens—weak estrogenic compounds from plants

phytonutrients—nutrients from plants

pineal gland—a gland in the brain that helps regulate circadian rhythm and produces melatonin

plasmin—enzyme in the body that dissolves and breaks down fibrin

p-methoxybenzyl isothiocyanate—chemical in maca root reputed to have aphrodisiac and cancer-preventive qualities

polyphenols—powerful antioxidants, many of which have anticancer activity. There are more than 4,000 of these compounds, and they fall into many classes and subclasses including flavonoids, anthocyanins, and isoflavones. Polyphenols, like other antioxidants, help protect cells from the normal, but damaging, physiological process known as oxidative stress

polysaccharide—long string of glucose molecules

polyunsaturated fats—large class of fatty acids with many members, including both the omega-6s and the omega 3s; found in vegetable oils, nuts, and fish

proanthocyanidins—plant compounds helpful in preventing degenerative disease; powerful antioxidants that are several times more potent than vitamins C and E. They help protect against the effects of internal and environmental stresses (cigarette smoking, pollution)

probiotics—good bacteria in the gut; found in yogurt

prostaglandins—known to encourage the growth of cancerous tumors

proteolytic enzymes—animal-derived enzymes that break down proteins

punicalagins—most abundant tannins in pomegranates; believed to be one of the major reasons why pomegranate juice packs such a powerful antioxidant wallop

pyridoxal-5-phosphate—active form of vitamin B6

quercetin—flavonoid that is a natural anti-inflammatory

resveratrol—compound found in grapes and blueberries, associated with antiaging effects

rhizome—part of turmeric that is actually used

rutin—flavonoid that helps protect blood vessels

saponin—phytochemical in beans that inhibits the reproduction of cancer cells and slows the growth of tumors

selenium—cancer-fighting trace mineral and antioxidant

serotonin—neurotransmitter for relaxation

silicon—important nutrient for bone health

silymarin—active ingredient in milk thistle

soluble fiber—breaks down as it passes through the digestive tract, forming a gel that traps some substances related to high cholesterol; also helps control blood sugar by delaying the emptying of the stomach and retarding the entry of sugar into the bloodstream

sterols—fats that serve as the basic molecule for important hormones like the sex hormones

subluxation—degenerative condition in which one or more of the spinal vertebrae are out of place

substance P—chemical that transmits pain messages to the brain

superoxide dismutase (SOD)—important antioxidant enzyme found in cereal grasses

systemic enzymes—break down a number of biochemicals that are intimately involved in pain and inflammation

tannins—bitter-tasting plant compounds found in tea, wine, and certain fruits, notably pomegranate

tartaric acid—found in vinegar, important in fighting body toxins and inhibiting unfriendly bacteria

taurine—amino acid and natural diuretic

theanine—substance in green tea that induces the release of a brain neurotransmitter called GABA, which tends to calm down the brain; also triggers the release of dopamine in the brain, one of the main brain chemicals associated with well-being

theobromine—compound that occurs naturally in many plants such as cocoa, tea, and coffee plants and is known for relaxing the lower esophageal sphincter

thrombosis—formation of a clot (or thrombus) inside a blood vessel that winds up obstructing the flow of blood

thromboxane—major factor in blood clots

thyroid—small, butterfly-shaped gland that wraps around the windpipe

tocopherols—beneficial plant compounds found in olives; part of the vitamin E family

triglycerides—main form of fat found in the body and are nearly always measured on a standard blood test

triterpenoids—active ingredient in Reishi mushrooms

trivalent chromium—chromium found in foods and supplements

tryptophan—raw material from which the body makes the neurotransmitter serotonin

turmeric—anti-inflammatory spice

tyramines—chemicals derived from the amino acid tyrosine; cam be a huge trigger for migraines

tyrosine—amino acid found in oysters that the brain converts to dopamine

zeaxanthin—carotenoid related to lutein; important to eye health

RECOMMENDED READING AND RESOURCES

VITAMINS, MINERALS, AND SUPPLEMENTS

Most of the products and supplements mentioned can be purchased through links on my website, www.jonnybowden.com, by clicking on "shopping." These are the brands and products I most recommend and that I use myself. Everything mentioned in this book is available there.

Alternately, you can go to the website of Designs for Health at www.designsforhealth.com or call 800.847.8302 to order their products, or to Emerson Ecologics at www.emersonecologics.com or 800.654.4432, which carries a full line of products from all of the companies I recommend. Both of these companies deal only with health-care providers, so the first time you order, they will ask you for a referring doctor or nutritionist. You are welcome to give my name, which will allow you to set up an account.

BOOKS

General Health

The following books are terrific additions to the general library of anyone concerned about health and wellness.

Eat, Drink, and Be Healthy: The Harvard Medical School Guide to Healthy Eating by Walter Willett, M.D., and P. J. Skerrett.
Willett, one of the most respected nutritional researchers in the world, explains why the U.S. Department of Agriculture's guidelines for eating are not only wrong but dangerous.

Ending the Food Fight: Guide Your Child to a Healthy Weight in a Fast Food/Fake Food World by David Ludwig and Suzanne Rostler.
An absolute must-have book on how to guide your child to a healthy weight in a fast food/fake food world, by the director of the Optimal Weight for Life Program at Children's Hospital in Boston.

The 150 Healthiest Foods on Earth: The Surprising, Unbiased Truth about What You Should Eat and Why by Jonny Bowden, Ph.D., C.N.S.
Everything you need to know about the best foods in the world for health and longevity and weight control, plus some good "myth-busting" essays.

The Real Vitamin and Mineral Book: The Definitive Guide to Designing Your Personal Supplement Program by Shari Lieberman, Ph.D., C.N.S., and Nancy Pauling Bruning, M.P.H.
A terrific reference book on vitamins and minerals.

You: An Owner's Manual: An Insider's Guide to the Body that Will Make You Healthier and Younger by Mehmet Oz, M.D., and Michael F. Roizen, M.D.
An all-around great book for the general public. Anything that has Mehmet Oz's name on it is worth reading.

Natural Medicine, Optimal Wellness: The Patient's Guide to Health and Healing by Jonathan Wright, M.D., and Alan Gaby, M.D.
This is a great reference book by two of the iconic figures in complementary medicine. Folksy, engaging success stories from Wright's practice complemented by scientific analysis by Gaby. Great for everyone's library.

Healing from the Heart: A Leading Heart Surgeon Combines Eastern and Western Traditions to Create the Medicine of the Future by Mehmet Oz, M.D., and Dean Ornish, M.D.

Staying Healthy with Nutrition: The Complete Guide to Diet and Nutritional Medicine by Elson Haas, M.D.
One of the foundations of a good library on nutritional medicine.

The Extraordinary Healing Power of Ordinary Things: Fourteen Natural Steps to Health and Happiness by Larry Dossey, M.D.
A terrific book by one of the great pioneers of mind-body medicine.

Train Your Mind, Change Your Brain by Sharon Begley.
My friend Sharon Begley, one of the best science writers in America, has written a superb guide to what's possible in the human brain.

Food, Health, and Medicine

For anyone interesting in digging deeper into the forces that shape how we look at medicine, food, and health in this country, here are some books that may forever change the way you see natural medicine, health advice, the U.S. Food and Drug Administration, drug safety, and the business of drug (and food) marketing. Read them in the spirit of "information is power." Warning: Don't even dabble in these excellent books unless you're willing to have some cherished myths and beliefs about health and medicine challenged.

The Republican War on Science by Chris Mooney.
Though this book focuses on the recent administration, don't let the title fool you. You'll find meticulously documented examples of how "independent" research can be molded to fit a political agenda, regardless of what that agenda happens to be.

The Hundred-Year Lie: How Food and Medicine Are Destroying Your Health by Randall Fitzgerald.
This book is well documented and well researched. Be prepared to be scared, and with good reason.

Overdosed America: The Broken Promise of American Medicine by John Abramson, M.D.
My friend, Harvard professor of medicine John Abramson—hardly a wild-eyed radical—has written an amazingly well-researched, readable book that should be read by everyone.

The Truth About the Drug Companies: How They Deceive Us and What To Do About It by Marcia Angell, M.D.
Written by someone who ought to know—the former editor-in-chief of the prestigious *New England Journal of Medicine* and a senior lecturer in the department of social medicine at Harvard Medical School. 'Nuf said.

Inside the FDA: The Business and Politics Behind the Drugs We Take and the Food We Eat by Fran Hawthorne.
A terrific and well-researched book that also happens to be a page-turner!

Generation Rx: How Prescription Drugs Are Altering American Lives, Minds and Bodies by Greg Critser.
Michael Pollan—one of my favorite authors—says "What *Fast Food Nation* did for the way Americans eat, *Generation Rx* does for the way we medicate ourselves." Right on.

Food Politics: How the Food Industry Influences Nutrition and Health by Marion Nestle, Ph.D.
I don't agree with Nestle about everything, but she sure got it right in this terrific book. Dense, but important.

RESOURCES FOR SPECIFIC CONDITIONS

Acne

Books

The Dietary Cure for Acne by Loren Cordain, Ph.D.
This book, by the respected researcher Loren Cordain, is the original "Paleo Diet" for acne on which I based my work in this book. It's backed by solid research and is a great nuts-and-bolts approach, complete with an actual diet plan. Highly recommended. Available only as a download at www.dietaryacne.com.

Healing Adult Acne: Your Guide to Clear Skin and Self-Confidence by Richard Fried, M.D., Ph.D. Fried is both a dermatologist and a psychiatrist whose unique approach addresses both the physical and emotional components of acne.

Skin Deep: A Mind/Body Program for Healthy Skin by Ted Grossbart, Ph.D., and Carl Sherman. A Harvard psychologist's unique approach to treating acne by addressing the emotional connection.

Asthma and Allergies

Books
Reversing Asthma: Breathe Easier with This Revolutionary New Program by Richard N. Firshein, D.O.

Asthma Survival: The Holistic Medical Treatment Program for Asthma by Robert S. Ivker, D.O.

Sinus Survival: The Holistic Medical Treatment Program for Allergies, Colds and Sinusitis by Robert S. Ivker, D.O.

Asthma Free in 21 Days by Kathryn Shafer, Ph.D.

Clinics
The Palm Beach Holistic Center for Natural and Integrative Medicine
Jupiter, Florida
561.799.6789
This is where you'll find Kathryn Shafer, who is the founder of *image therapy* for asthma, discussed in the book. If you want to try image therapy with the originator of the technique, this is the place to go.

Online Resources
The Buteyko Breathing Method
The Buteyko method is a highly regarded, drug-free approach to the management of asthma and other breathing-related health problems. If you want to find out more about it, a good place to start is at www.buteyko.com.

ADD and ADHD
Healing ADD: The Breakthrough Program That Allows You to See and Heal the Six Types of ADD by Daniel Amen, M.D. Groundbreaking book by the great psychiatrist that will change forever how you conceptualize, and deal with, attention deficit disorder.

Alcoholism and Addiction

Clinics
The Health Recovery Center
Minneapolis, Minnesota
800.554.9155 and 612.827.7800
www.healthrecovery.com
Founded in 1980 by Joan Mathews-Larson, Ph.D., the Health Recovery Center in Minneapolis is a program for recovery that uncovers and treats the true physical underpinnings that drive addictions.

Tai Sophia Institute
Laurel, Maryland
800.735.2968
The Tai Sophia Institute is an accredited and highly respected graduate school for acupuncture and other healing arts located between Baltimore and Washington. It has been innovative in the use of acupuncture as an adjunct to addiction treatment programs, having created the Penn North Neighborhood Center as a community-based wellness center for those "seeking to recover their lives by understanding their relationships with substances." The Penn North center provides ongoing access to the wellness program, including a six-month outpatient substance abuse program and is well worth checking out.

Recovery Systems
Mill Valley, California
415.383.3611
Recovery Systems is the excellent, twelve-week outpatient clinic program designed by Julia Ross, M.A., author of *The Mood Cure* and *The Diet Cure*. It's a nutritionally based program for a variety of issues, but particularly for mood disorders, addictions (alcohol, substance abuse addictions, and sugar addiction) and depression.

Alzheimer's Disease

The Alzheimer's Research and Prevention Foundation
Tucson, Arizona
520.749.8374
www.alzheimersprevention.org
A charitable organization that advocates a complete prevention program for memory loss and Alzheimer's, mixing complementary and conventional medical modalities.

Brain Health
Books

Making a Good Brain Great: The Amen Clinic Program for Achieving and Sustaining Optimal Mental Performance by Daniel Amen, M.D.
Daniel Amen is one of the leaders in the field of brain imaging, brain nutrition, and brain performance. This is his holistic program for keeping the brain sharp for the rest of your days on the planet.

Change Your Brain, Change Your Life: Conquering Anxiety, Depression, Obsessiveness, Anger, and Impulsiveness by Daniel Amen, M.D.
More wisdom from the master.

The Brain Trust Program: A Scientifically Based Three-Part Plan to Improve Memory, Elevate Mood, Enhance Attention, Alleviate Migraine and Menopausal Symptoms, and Boost Mental Energy by Larry McCleary, M.D.
A neurosurgeon shares his wisdom on the care, feeding, and preservation of the most important organ in the body.

BrainRecovery.com: Powerful Therapy for Challenging Brain Disorders by David Perlmutter, M.D.

The Better Brain Book: The Best Tools for Improving Memory and Sharpness and Preventing Aging of the Brain by David Perlmutter, M.D., and Carol Colman.
Perlmutter, a superb nutritionist and a board-certified neurologist, is one of the sharpest minds around and always worth reading when it comes to natural treatments for brain disorders.

Brain Longevity: The Breakthrough Medical Program That Improves your Mind and Memory by Dharma Singh Khalsa, M.D.
Khalsa, president of the Alzheimer's Prevention Foundation, was the first physician in the world to formulate a holistic medicine program for the prevention and treatment of Alzheimer's disease and memory loss. Brain Longevity has been translated into more than twelve languages.

Clinics

The Amen Clinics
4019 Westerly Place, Suite 100
Newport Beach, CA 92660
949.266.3700
(other locations around the country)
www.brainplace.com
The Amen Clinics are dedicated to optimizing brain health and using the latest medical advances in the treatment of psychiatric diseases.

Cancer
Books

Natural Strategies for Cancer Patients by Russell Blaylock, M.D.
Blaylock is a neurosurgeon, professor of medicine, and an outstanding nutritionist. This book is well researched and very thorough. Covers foods, supplements, and much more.

Beating Cancer with Nutrition by Patrick Quillin, Ph.D., R.D., C.N.S., and Noreen Quillin.
This is a classic by a Ph.D. nutritionist who specializes in nutritional protocols for cancer.

Clinics

Cancer Treatment Centers of America
800.615.3055
www.cancercenter.com
Personally, I would never decide on a treatment plan for cancer without consulting with the Cancer Treatment

Centers of America. It is unique in that it offers a complete integration of treatment modalities under one roof—from surgery, radiation, and chemotherapy to naturopathy, mind-body medicine, and nutrition. It has some of the best practitioners I have ever met, including one of my most respected resources, Tim Birdsall, N.D., a naturopathic oncologist. It has hospitals in Philadelphia; Tulsa, Oklahoma; Zion, Illinois; and Seattle, and its staff is friendly, supportive, and welcoming.

Online Resources

The Moss Reports

www.ralphmoss.com

If you or someone you love has a diagnosis of cancer and you're overwhelmed with the options and opinions at a time when you're most vulnerable, Ralph Moss can be your secret weapon. Ralph Moss, Ph.D., is a recognized expert on treatment options, including (and especially) alternative treatments, and a tireless investigator about who's doing what, what works, and what doesn't. His "Moss Reports" are expensive, but worth it. Complete, unbiased, well-researched specific reports on any cancer you can think of, how it's treated, where it's treated, and the pros, the cons, the successes, the options, and the alternatives. Don't make a move without at least checking out what Ross has to say. Also check out his many books on amazon.com.

Chronic Fatigue Syndrome

See *Fibromyalgia*.

Depression And Mood

Books

Depression-Free Naturally: 7 Weeks to Eliminating Anxiety, Despair, Fatigue, and Anger from Your Life by Joan Mathews-Larson, Ph.D.

Mathews-Larson has a long history of successfully treating addiction with a multifaceted, nutritionally based program, and she takes a similar approach to depression in this book.

The Mood Cure by Julia Ross, M.A.

One of the best nutritional programs for mood disorders.

See also *Alcoholism and Addiction*.

Digestion and Gastrointestinal Health

See *Gastrointestinal Issues*.

Emotional Freedom Techniques (EFT)

Online Resources

www.emofree.com

Emofree.com is the website of EFT's founder, Gary Craig. You can find out all about EFT as well as order instructional DVDs from this website.

www.mercola.com

Joseph Mercola's site is another valuable resource for a baker's dozen of subjects having to do with complementary healing, nutrition, and health. His endorsement of EFT was one of the things that brought EFT to national attention. His website offers some excellent information on EFT, as well as a free guide to how to perform it on yourself.

Eye Movement Desensitization and Reprocessing (EMDR)

Books

EMDR: The Breakthrough Therapy for Overcoming Anxiety, Stress, and Trauma by Francine Shapiro, Ph.D., and Margot Silk Forrest.

Shapiro is the originator of this innovative therapy. If you want the story straight from the horse's mouth, this is it.

Transforming Trauma: EMDR: The Revolutionary New Therapy for Freeing the Mind, Clearing the Body, and Opening the Heart by Laurel Parnell.

An excellent introduction for the general public.

Online Resources

www.emdr.com
The best place to find out about EMDR is to go to the home base website for the EMDR institute, where you'll find an excellent explanation, the story of how it was created, FAQs, information about training, and a ton of research.

www.emdrhap.org
EMDR also has a wonderful nonprofit organization (EMDR Humanitarian Assistance Program) that could well be described as a mental health equivalent of Doctors Without Borders. It's a global network of clinicians who travel anywhere there is a need to stop suffering and prevent the aftereffects of trauma and violence.

Fibromyalgia and Chronic Fatigue Syndrome

Books

From Fatigued to Fantastic!: A Clinically Proven Program to Regain Vibrant Health and Overrcome Chronic Fatigue and Fibromyalgia, revised third edition by Jacob Teitelbaum, M.D.

Pain Free 1-2-3 by Jacob Teitelbaum, M.D.

The above two—especially the first one—are Teitelbaum's classic books on the subject of treating fibromyalgia and chronic fatigue syndrome in an integrative, holistic way.

Clinics

Jacob Teitelbaum, M.D.
Teitelbaum is the go-to guy for fibromyalgia and chronic fatigue syndrome (FMS/CFS). He's an M.D. who himself came down with FMS/CFS in medical school and is the leading expert on integrative protocols for fibromyalgia. He's the author of a groundbreaking study showing that FMS/CFS patients can have an average 91 percent improvement rate with an integrated treatment protocol.

Although he no longer treats patients as a physician, he now does life and wellness consulting in Kona, Hawaii, where he helps people from all around the world get a life they love! His website has a program that will analyze your symptoms and lab test results to tailor a treatment protocol to your case. You'll receive a free e-mail newsletter, too. All of the information you need to get well now is at www.Vitality101.com.

To find a medical expert to treat your CFS or fibromyalgia, go to:

Fibromyalgia and Fatigue Centers, Inc.
866-443-4276
www.fibroandfatigue.com
These clinics are located throughout the United States.

Online Resources

www.Vitality101.com
The above website has Teitelbaum's entire protocol, a free e-mail newsletter to keep you up to date, and all the resources you need to get well. Simply follow the four-step program on his home page. The research studies (also on his site) show that you will have a greater than 90 percent chance of getting your life back! The site also has a Q&A section.

www.co-cure.org/drt.htm
The above website is a good introduction to some of Teitelbaum's writings on CFS and FMS.

Gastrointestinal Issues

Books

Guess What Came to Dinner?: Parasites and Your Health by Ann Louise Gittleman, Ph.D.
An excellent book on an often overlooked topic of importance.

The Gluten Connection: How Gluten Sensitivity May Be Sabotaging Your Health and What You Can Do To Take Control Now by Shari Lieberman, Ph.D., C.N.S.
This is an important book that details the connection between gluten sensitivity—often overlooked and undiagnosed—and a host of symptoms and conditions.

Online Resources

www.irritable-bowel-syndrome.ws
www.helpforibs.com
Two wonderful self-help websites for those with irritable bowel syndrome (IBS).

www.ibstales.com
This personal site, lovingly maintained by a British woman named "Sophie" is a great resource for information, shared experiences, and support.

www.healthy.net/scr/Recipes.asp?RCId=17
Some amazing recipes for inflammatory bowel disease (IBD) can be found at this site.

www.ibsaudioprogram100.com
The hypnosis audio program mentioned in the text, developed by clinical hypnotherapist Michael Mahoney specifically for IBS sufferers, is available at this site.

Hypertension and Heart Disease
Books
What Your Doctor May Not Tell You about Hypertension by Mark Houston, M.D., with Barry Fox, Ph.D., and Nadine Taylor, M.S., R.D.
The best go-to sourcebook for a holistic and nutritional approach to hypertension.

Reverse Heart Disease Now by Stephen Sinatra, M.D.

The Sinatra Solution: Metabolic Cardiology by Stephen Sinatra, M.D.
Read these two books or at least give them to your doctor!

Clinics
Hypertension Institute of Nashville
Nashville, Tennessee
615.297.2700
info@hypertensioninstitute.com
This is my most recommended resource for anything to do with hypertension.

Meditation and Stress Reduction
www.drdharma.com
I'm a big fan of the meditation CDs put out by my friend Dharma Singh Khalsa, M.D., a brain specialist and the author of *Meditation as Medicine*. You can find his CDs, including "Wake up to Wellness," at this site.

See also *Relaxation Response*.

Menopausal Issues and Hormones
Books
The Wisdom of Menopause: Creating Physical and Emotional Health and Healing During the Change by Christiane Northrup, M.D.

Women's Bodies, Women's Wisdom: Creating Physical and Emotional Health and Healing by Christiane Northrup, M.D.
Absolutely anything by Northrup is worth reading—twice—but the first one listed above is a classic.

The Hormone Solution: Naturally Alleviate Symptoms of Hormone Imbalance from Adolescence through Menopause by Erika Schwartz, M.D.

The 30-Day Natural Hormone Plan: Look and Feel Young Again—Without Synthetic HRT by Erika Schwartz, M.D.
Schwartz is a really smart endocrinologist and one of my favorite hormone specialists on the East Coast. This is her program.

Get Off the Menopause Roller Coaster: Natural Solutions by Shari Lieberman, Ph.D.
Out of print, but if you can find it, grab it!

Before the Change: Taking Charge of Your Perimenopause by Ann Louise Gittleman, Ph.D.
Wonderful advice on diet and lifestyle for the pre-menopausal woman by the First Lady of Nutrition!

Pregnancy and Postpartum
Books
Natural Guide to Pregnancy and Post-Partum Health by Dean Raffelock, D.C., C.C.N., and Robert Roundtree, M.D.
This is the book I give everyone in my life who is either pregnant, thinking about becoming pregnant, or has just had a baby. It's that important.

Reflexology
Online Resources
www.americanacademyofreflexology.com
For anyone interested in reflexology, there is no better resource than Bill Floco, one of the top practitioners in the country, and a gentle and healing man who likes nothing better than to share his knowledge. You can find him—and a ton of information about reflexology—at The American Academy of Reflexology.

The Relaxation Response and Mind-Body Medicine
www.mbmi.org
The author of *The Relaxation Response* and arguably the dean of mind-body physicians in America is Herbert Benson, M.D., an associate professor of medicine at Harvard Medical School. He cofounded the institute that bears his name, The Benson-Henry Institute for Mind-Body Medicine, which is a part of Massachusetts General Hospital. For more information about their programs, including a mind-body cancer program and a mind-over-menopause program, go to the site above.

See also *Meditation and Stress Reduction.*

Sugar Addiction
Radiant Recovery
www.radiantrecovery.com
Radiant Recovery is an online community developed by addiction specialist Kathleen DesMaisons, Ph.D.

See also *Alcoholism.*

Weight Loss and Diet
Books
Living the Low Carb Life: Choosing the Diet That's Right for You from Atkins to Zone by Jonny Bowden, Ph.D., C.N.S.
A guidebook to the theory and practice of low carb—what works and what doesn't.

Sugar Shock by Connie Bennett and Stephen Sinatra, M.D.
A wonderful book about breaking the sugar habit. Well-researched information about what sugar does to your body, your health, and your life.

The Inside Out Diet by Cathy Wong, N.D., C.N.S.
A thoughtful and smart book that takes a holistic approach to weight loss and health by about.com's alternative medicine expert.

The Fat Resistance Diet by Leo Galland, M.D.
A unique approach to weight loss, and an original contribution by one of the great icons of integrative medicine.

Ultrametabolism by Mark Hyman, M.D.
Terrific, useful information on metabolism, sugar, diet, hormones, weight control, and stress.

Dare To Lose by Shari Lieberman, Ph.D., C.N.S.
My friend Dr. Shari lays it all out for you in this women-centric and excellent, down-to-earth book on weight loss.

FINDING A DOCTOR OR HEALTH PRACTITIONER

I'm often asked about finding a doctor or a medical facility where they "speak" nutrition and integrative medicine. This is an incomplete list, and I apologize for the many great docs and health practitioners I've left out. But here are some of the ones you can absolutely rely on. If none of these excellent practitioners are near you, I recommend going to the Institute of Functional Medicine website (www.functionalmedicine.org) and clicking on "find a practitioner."

Jonathan Wright, M.D.
Tahoma Clinic
801 S.W. 16th Street, Suite 121
Renton, WA 98057
425.264.0059

David Leonardi, M.D.
Leonardi Executive Health Center
8400 E. Prentice Avenue, Suite 700
Greenwood Village, CO 80111
303.462.5344
www.go2lehi.com

Julian Whitaker, M.D.
Whitaker Wellness Institute
4321 Birch Street
Newport Beach, CA 92660
800.488.1500

Leo Galland, M.D.
Foundation for Integrated Medicine
156 Fifth Avenue
New York, NY 10021
212-989-6733

Woodson Merrell, M.D. and staff
The Continuum Center for Health and Healing
Beth Israel Medical Center
245 5th Avenue, 2nd floor
New York, NY 10016

Mehmet Oz, M.D.
Director, Integrative Medicine Program
Columbia University Medical Center
Milstein Hospital Building, 7-435
177 Fort Washington Avenue
New York, NY 10032
212.342.0002

Joseph Brasco, M.D.
(nutrition and gastrointestinal disease)
Center for Colon and Digestive Disease, P.C.
19 Longwood Drive
Huntsville, AL 35801
256.533.6488

Elson Haas, M.D.
Preventive Medical Center of Marin
25 Mitchell Blvd., Suite 8
San Rafael, CA 95903
415.472.2343
www.elsonhaas.com/medcenter.html

Hyla Cass, M.D.
(psychiatry)
Pacific Palisades, CA 90272
310.459.9866
Call or write for appointment
Hyla@drcass.com
www.drcass.com

Mark Hyman, M.D.
The UltraWellness Center
45 Walker Street
Lenox, MA 01240
413.637.9991

Decker Weiss, N.M.D., F.A.S.A.
(integrative cardiology)
9755 North 90th Street, Suite A210
Scottsdale, AZ 85258
480.767.7119

Bijan Pourat, M.D.
(cardiology and anti-aging medicine)
125 North Robertson
Beverly Hills, CA 90211
310.289.3679

Andrew L. Rubman, N.D.
Southbury Clinic for Traditional Medicines
900 Main Street South
Southbury, CT 06488
203.262.6755
www.naturopath.org

Sonja Peterson, N.M.D.
16601 N. 90th Street
Scottsdale, AZ 85260
480.502.5398

Prudence Hall, M.D.
Howard Leibowitz, M.D.
The Hall Center for Rejuvenation and Vitality
1148 4th Street
Santa Monica, CA 90403
310.458.7979
info@thehallcenter.com

John Hernandez, M.D.
Medical Director
Center for Health and Integrative Medicine
2235 Thousand Oaks Drive, Suite 102A and B
San Antonio, TX
210.495.3055

Joseph Mercola, D.O.
Optimal Wellness Center
1443 W. Schaumburg, Suite 250
Schaumburg, IL 60194
847.985.1777

Al Sears, M.D.
Center for Health and Wellness
12794 Forest Hill Blvd., Suite 16
Wellington, FL 33414
866.792.1035 (toll-free)

Andrew Larson, M.D.
(surgery)
142 JFK Drive
Atlantis, FL 33462
561.439.1500

Allen E Sosin, M.D.
Institute for Progressive Medicine
4 Hughes, Suite 175
Irvine, CA 92618
www.iprogressivemed.com

Richard Firshein, D.O.
Firshein Center for Comprehensive Medicine
1226 Park Avenue
New York, NY 10128
212.860.0282

Erika Schwartz, M.D., P.C.
10 West 74th Street
New York, NY 10023
212.873.3420
866.373.7452
office@drerika.com

ACKNOWLEDGMENTS

Writing a book like this requires many things, but chief among them is an amazing Rolodex (okay, make that a Palm Pilot). I've got one of the best. Even though I don't always make use of every name that's in it for every book I write, the fact that these folks are there and available to me, and that I know they will—and have, and do—give generously of their time and their information, makes it much easier to proceed with a project like this. So for all of those who contributed your time and energy so willingly and graciously, I thank you enormously.

Stephen Sinatra, M.D., read and critiqued the "Awesome Foursome" chapter on heart disease. Mark Houston, M.D., M.S., gave me his always invaluable input on the hypertension section. Acupuncturist Cindy Lawrence, LAc, was essential for the section on acupuncture and fertility, ditto Matthew Mannino, D.O., for the section on chiropractic and back pain. Kathryn Shafer, Ph.D., helped enormously with the section on image therapy for asthma, as did Bill Flocco with the section on PMS and reflexology, and Harry Preuss, M.D. with the section on weight loss supplements. Bert Berkson, M.D., Ph.D., gave generously of his time and was essential to the section on hepatitis C. Joe Brasco, M.D. ("GI Joe") was as always a rich source of information on everything to do with gastrointestinal illness. Robbie Dunton, M.D., was kind enough to proofread the EMDR chapter, and Joan Mathews-Larson, Ph.D. could not have been more gracious in offering her input for the section on addiction. Others who contributed their time, valuable info, and input include Daniel Amen, M.D., Hyla Cass, M.D., Shari Lieberman, Ph.D., Parris Kidd, Ph.D., Andrew Rubman, N.D., Robert Portman, Ph.D., and Al Sears, M.D.

And for all my "rolodex regulars" who I didn't call on this time, I still appreciate you for being there in case I needed you: Jacob Teitelbaum, M.D., Timothy Birdsall, N.D., David Ludwig, M.D., Ph.D., Evelyn Tribole, M.S., R.D., Regina Wilshire, N.D., David Leonardi, M.D., C. Leigh Broadhurst, Ph.D., Dharma Singh Khalsa, M.D., Jeffrey Bland, Ph.D., Alan Gaby, M.D., Elson Haas, M.D., Ann Louise Gittleman, Ph.D., Barry Sears, Ph.D., Fred Pescatore, M.D., Colette Heimowitz, M.S., Oz Garcia, John Abramson, M.D., Robert Crayhon, M.S., Sonja Petterson, N.D., Charles Poliquin, Richard Firshein, D.O., J. J. Virgin, Ph.D., Linda Lizotte, R.D., David Brady, N.D., Esther Blum, R.D., Liz Neporent, M.S., C.S.C.S., Michael Eades, M.D., Mary Dan Eades, M.D., Cathy Wong, N.D., Karl Knopf, Ph.D., Kilmer McCully, M.D., Ron Rosdale, M.D., Robert Roundtree, M.D., Walter Willett, M.D., Ph.D., Mehmet Oz, M.D., and Christiane Northrup, M.D.

And don't think you'll get away without a call next time.

I'd also like to thank and acknowledge the most comprehensive and thorough database on natural medicine in the world, The Natural Standard, whose staff generously allowed me access to their subscription-only website, www.naturalstandard.com. Their assistance was invaluable and was greatly appreciated, and I recommend them highly. And each year, Tod Cooperman, M.D., is kind enough to give me free access to www.consumerlab.com, for which I am grateful as well.

But wait, there's more!

I've said it before and I'll say it again—I have the best literary agent in the world. Coleen O'Shea nurtures, protects, fertilizes, and germinates ideas and projects and then goes out and makes them happen. And takes my calls at all hours of the night. She's an endless source of support. I'm lucky to have her.

My editor, Cara Connors, did the best thing in the world an editor can do for a writer: She "got" me. And she edited in the smartest way possible for an editor who has to deal with a writer (like me) who doesn't like being edited—selectively and judiciously and intelligently, making every change count and winning my respect and admiration in the process. Great job.

My publishers, Will Kiester and Ken Fund, who believe in the Jonny Bowden brand, and the amazing editors, designers, and copyeditors at Fair Winds Press—especially John Gettings, Tiffany Hill, and Dutton and Sherman Design, and Megan Cooney who make each of my books look so gorgeous I almost can't believe it.

My Web designer, Christopher Loch, who designed my website, made it beautiful, and best of all, has made it possible for me not to ever have to learn anything about html. You can contact him at www.whatismysecret.com, but don't even think about trying to steal him away from me.

The many teachers who continue to inspire me on a daily basis—Jack Canfield, Mark Victor Hanson, Les Brown, Armand Moran, and especially to my good friends, Alex Mandossian and T. Harv Eker.

To Werner Erhard, who started me on a path that changed my life and continues to influence me—almost forty years later—to this day. Wherever you are, I love you.

My editors at my "day jobs" who keep me up to my neck in interesting and challenging projects when I'm not writing books—especially Nicole Wise and Sarah Hiner at Boardroom, Colette Heimowitz at Atkins Nutritionals, Kalia Donner at Remedy, Lyle Hurd at Total Health, Adam Campbell and Jeff O'Connell at Men's Health, and Tanya Mancini and the gang at America Online. All the folks at Greenstone media—especially Heather Cohen—deserve a special smile. Mo Gaffney, Shana Wride, and Sally Jesse Raphael always make my radio appearances a pleasure.

My publicists, Mary Aarons at Fair Winds Press, and Melissa McNeese and Leslie McClure, for doing such a great job of getting me out there.

Hollywood stars have their stylists, their hair people, and their makeup artists to make them look as good as they do when they walk down the red carpet. I, on the other hand, have "The Sues."

Suzanne Copp and Susan Mudd are two of the smartest and most dedicated nutritionists I know, and I could not have written this book—at least and have it finished in less than a decade—without their tireless support.

Suzanne Copp, M.S., is a clinical nutritionist who has maintained a private practice in Connecticut that focuses on health conditions such as weight loss, women's issues, hypoglycemia, diabetes, gastrointestinal ailments, and eating disorders. A former adjunct professor in the nutrition department at the prestigious University of Bridgeport, she now works as a consultant for Crayhon Research focusing on writing and editorial projects.

Susan Mudd, M.S., C.N.S., is a clinical nutritionist practicing in Gaithersburg, Maryland. She maintains a busy client practice, is a sought-after speaker and consultant and writes a monthly column called "Edible Insights." She is also a licensed provider of "Shapedown," a program focused on child and adolescent obesity counseling.

I am eternally grateful for their enormous contributions to this project.

My writing style would not be what it is without the input of an eclectic group of writers, some of whom have delighted me since I was old enough to read (Harold Pinter, Tennessee Williams) others of whom I discovered later but whose work has shaped mine as surely as if I had sat at their feet in an imaginary classroom. One in particular stands out in this eclectic group, and his name is William Goldman. I would not be the writer I am today if William Goldman hadn't enriched my life with his every written word. He's simply not capable of writing anything bad. Thanks are also due to the late Ed McBain (Evan Hunter). And to the best science writer in America, Robert Sapolsky, whose writing serves as a model for anyone wanting to educate and entertain at the same time. There is no one alive who does it better.

My love and gratitude goes out to my family—Jeffrey Bowden, Nancy Fiedler, Pace Bowden, and Cadence Bowden for, well, being my family. Which can't always be easy, hard as that is to believe. And as always, to the people and animals I love who make my life wonderful: Susan Wood and Christopher Duncan, my partner-in-crime Jackie (Sky London) Balough, my brother Peter Breger, my sisters Randy Graff and Lauree Dash, Kimberly Wright the Sushi Goddess, my lifelong friend Jeanette Lee Bessinger, Scott Ellis, Ron Ellison, Dr. Richard Lewis, Gina Lombardi and Kevin Sizemore, Anita Waxman, Diane Lederman, Oz Garcia (when I can find him), Billy Stritch, Liz Neporent, Zack Kleinmann, Marlon Reveche, Oliver Becaud, Jennifer Schneider, and Leslie.

And to Howard, Robin, Gary, Fred, and Artie for continuing to make me smile every single morning since 1995.

And to Woodstock and Emily the Second for whom I am grateful on a daily basis.

And of course, to Anja, my muse, the love of my life … in all ways and for always.

ABOUT THE AUTHOR

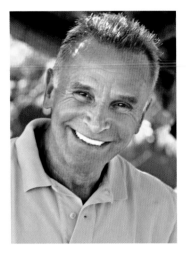

Jonny Bowden, Ph.D., C.N.S., a board-certified nutrition specialist with a master's degree in psychology, is a nationally known expert on weight loss, nutrition, and health. A motivational speaker and former personal trainer with six national certifications, he was the acclaimed "Weight Loss Coach" on iVillage for twelve years, and is now a contributing health writer for America Online.

His book, *Living the Low-Carb Life: Choosing the Diet that's Right for You from Atkins to Zone*, has more than 100,000 copies in print. His most recent book, *The 150 Healthiest Foods on Earth: The Surprising Truth About What to Eat*, has been endorsed by a virtual who's who in the world of integrative medicine and nutrition, including Christiane Northrup, M.D., Mehmet Oz, M.D., Barry Sears, Ph.D. (who calls him "one of the best"), and Ann Louise Gittleman, Ph.D., (who calls him "the personal health coach I would want in my corner no matter what").

He has been featured in *The New York Times*, *The New York Post*, *Chicago Sun Times*, *Chicago Tribune*, *Time Magazine*, *GQ*, *Muscle and Fitness*, *Cosmopolitan*, *Oxygen*, *Seventeen*, MSNBC Online, MSN Online, *Self*, *Fitness*, *Oxygen*, *Family Circle*, *Marie Claire*, *Allure*, *Men's Health*, *Ladies Home Journal*, *Prevention*, *Personal Trainer Magazine*, *Woman's World*, *Weight Watchers*, *In Style*, and *Shape*, and has appeared on Fox News, CNN, MSNBC, ABC, NBC, and CBS as an expert on nutrition, weight loss and fitness.

He lives in Los Angeles with his beloved life companion, Anja Christy, and as many dogs as possible.

His DVD "The Truth About Weight Loss," as well as his popular motivational CDs, and many of the supplements recommended in this volume can be found at www.jonnybowden.com.

INDEX

apples, 102, 103
arginine. *See* L-arginine
Aricept, 248
Armour thyroid, 59
arnica, 227–229
arthritis, refer to page 357
Arthritis Foundation, 100
artichokes, 149
ascorbic acid, 319, 320. *See also* vitamin C
ashwagandha, 67
Asian ginseng (Panax ginseng), 237.
   See also ginseng
aspartame, 99–100, 158
astaxanthin, 61–62
asthma, refer to page 357
athletes, 143, 227
Atkins diet, 181
Atkins, Robert, 49
ATP. *See* adenosyntriphosophate (ATP)
ATTICA studies, 302
Ausubel, Kenny, 17
autism, refer to page 357
Aviram, Michael, 207
azelaic acid, 204, 257, 259

B

B vitamins. *See also specific B vitamins*;
   vitamin B complex
   for brain health, 116
   doses of, 35
   folic acid and, 126, 128
   S-adenosyl-methionine (SAMe)
      and, 309
back pain, refer to page 357
bad breath, refer to page 357
Baird, Douglas, 93
Bartter, Fred, 147
Baylock, Russell, 111
BDNF. *See* brain-derived neu-
   rotrophic factor (BDNF)
Beltsville Human Nutrition
   Research Center, 193–194
Benadryl, 166
benign prostatic hyperplasia, refer to
   page 357
Benson, Herbert, 291, 293
Benson-Henry Institute for Mind
   Body Medicine, 293
bentonite clay, 182

benzoyl peroxide, 259
Berkson, Burt, 146–148, 313
Berkson, D. Lindsey, 130
berries, 114, 117, 188, 196, 245, 246,
   323. *See also specific berries*
beta-amyloid, 248
beta-carotene, 38, 170, 317
betaine-HCl, 140
beta-sitosterol, 258, 261
bifidus, 107, 179, 180–181. *See also*
   probiotics
Big Pharma. *See* pharmaceutical
   industry
bilobalides, 236
biochemical individuality, 49
biofeedback, 201
bioflavonoids, 166–167, 168, 245,
   317, 320
   for asthma, 102–103
   in ginkgo, 236
   for herpes simplex virus, 52
   in horny goat weed, 241
   quercetin, 101–106
   for varicose veins, 245, 246
biotin, 47, 193, 200, 202
Birch, Patricia, 33–34
bitters. *See* digestive enzymes
black cohosh, 131, 132
black currant seed oil, 124
Bland, Jeffrey, 133
Blask, David, 64
bloat, refer to page 357
blueberries, 114, 117
Blumenthal, Mark, 236
borage oil, 124
boric acid, 180, 182
boric acid douches, 180
Bortz, Walter, 28–29
boswellia, 67, 100, 216
Bragg, Patricia, 298
brain health, 117
   acetylcholine and, 112
   alpha lipoic acid for, 114, 115
   antioxidants and, 114, 115
   B vitamins for, 114, 116
   berries and, 114, 117
   Combo Cure for, 109–119
   CoQ10 for, 114
   dementia, 109
   diet and, 114, 117, 118
   eggs and, 118
   exercise for, 114, 118–119

fish and, 114, 118
fish oil for, 117, 300–301
folic acid for, 116–117
free radicals and, 115
glycerophosphocholine (GPC) for,
   113–115
homocysteine and, 116
huperzine A for, 114
inflammation, 117
inflammation and, 117
iodine and, 59–61
L-carnitine for, 111–112, 114, 115
liver and, 118
magnesium for, 114
mild cognitive impairment (MCI),
   110
mitochondrial dysfunction,
   111–112
multivitamins for, 114
myelin sheath and, 116
neurons, 110, 117
neurotransmitters and, 112
niacin and, 118
nutrition and, 111
omega-3 fatty acids for, 114, 117
phosphatidylserine (PS) for,
   112–113, 114
polyphenols and, 117
spinach and, 114, 117
stress and, 119
vegetables and, 114
vinpocentine for, 114, 116
vitamin B12 for, 116, 116–117
vitamin B6 for, 36, 116–117
vitamin C for, 114
brain imaging, 292
brain-derived neurotrophic factor
   (BDNF), 282–283
Brasco, Joseph, 9, 218, 231
Bratman, Steven, 113, 235, 237, 254
Bray, George, 105
Brazil nuts, 315
bread, zinc in, 83
breastfeeding, ginseng and, 240
Brekhman, Israel, 238
Broadhurst, C. Leigh, 193
Brody, Jane, 13
bromelain, 75, 98, 99, 102, 105, 140,
   167
Brooks, David, 110
Brown, Richard P., 250, 310
burns, refer to page 357

Bush, George W., 110
Buteyko therapy, 104
butterbur, 158

C

caffeine, 15, 135, 139, 155, 156, 158, 164, 165, 231, 233
calcium, 79, 152, 154, 155, 298
  food sources of, 164
  in green leafy vegetables, 164
  for high blood pressure, 153
  hydrochloric acid (HCI) and, 138
  for irritable bowel syndrome (IBS), 233, 234
  kidney stones, 155–156
  for pain, 74
  for PMS (premenstrual syndrome), 163–164
  in sardines, 164
  in seeds, 164
  taurine and, 41
cancer, refer to page 357
candied citrus peels, 168
caprylic acid, 180, 181–182
carbaryl, 20
carbohydrates, 14, 71, 107, 151. *See also specific carbohydrates*
  asthma and, 104
Candida-albicans, 181
  disaccharides, 217
  eczema and, 122
  food allergies and, 168
  irritable bowel syndrome (IBS) and, 231
  magnesium and, 306
  migraines, 160
  yeast infections, 181
  zinc in, 83
cardiovascular health. *See also* cardio-vascular health
  black cohash for, 132
  L-arginine and, 41
  magnesium for, 306
  omega-3 fatty acids for, 299
  stress and, 304–305
  taurine for, 41
  vitamin C for, 320–321
carnitine. *See* L-carnitine
carnosine, 84–87
carotenoids, 38, 170, 317
cartilage, 96, 97–98, 99

Cass, Hyla, 94
catechins, 196
catecholamine metabolism, 44
catecholamines, 304
Cathcart, Robert, 149, 319–320
CCK. *See* cholecystokinin (CCK)
CDC (Centers for Disease Control and Prevention), 43, 56
Celebrex, 97
celecoxib. *See* Celebrex
celery, 27, 152, 153, 186
Centers for Disease Control and Prevention. *See* CDC (Centers for Disease Control and Prevention)cetyl myristolate (CMO), 98, 100
chamomile, 122, 166
chasteberry, 164. *See also* vitex
chemotherapy, melatonin and, 64–65
Cheraskin, Emanuel, 93
cherries, 187–188
chi, 266
Chicago Health and Aging Project, 111
chicken pox, 51
chicken soup, 189–191
Chinese club moss plant. *See* huperzine A
Chinese medicine, 8, 133, 186, 241, 245, 247, 266
chiropractic, 27, 269–272
chlorophyll, 107
cholecystokinin (CCK), 87–89
choline, 150
chondrocytes, 97
chondroitin, 74, 97–98
Chopra, Deepak, 272
ChromeMate, 47, 175
chromium, 47
  for alcoholism, 95
ChromeMate, 47
  for diabetes, 46–48
  for high blood sugar, 193
  insulin and, 177
  for polycystic ovary syndrome (PCOS), 200, 202
  for weight loss, 48, 175, 177–178
chronic conditions, 18
chymotrypsin, 75
CIC. *See* circulating immune complexes (CICs)
cinnamon, 47, 194

circadian rhythms, 64
circulating immune complexes (CICs), 75
circulation, 236, 243, 245
Citrin K, 175
CLA. *See* conjugated linoleic acid (CLA)
clams, 38, 61, 315
Clearogen, 204, 256, 257, 258–259
Clorets, 107
CMO. *See* cetyl myristoleate (CMO)
coconut oil, 147, 181, 218
coenzyme Q10. *See* CoQ10
coffee, 139, 164, 165. *See also* caffeine
cognitive function, ginkgo for, 235
colds, refer to page 357
collagen, 316, 317
colloidal oatmeal bath, 122
coloring agents, eczema and, 122
Colpo, Anthony, 70
combo cures, 10, 27, 91–183
combo douches, 182
combo herbs, 158
Combs, Gerald F., 314
complement H factor (CFH) gene, 169
computational units, 118
concentration, rhodiola for, 250–252
conjugated linoleic acid (CLA), 174–176
connective tissue, 96
Continuing Survey of Food Intakes by Individuals (1994-96 CSFII), 126
conventional medicine. *See also* Western medicine
Copp, Suzanne, 35, 55, 67, 83, 84, 123, 182, 297
copper, 94, 259, 298
CoQ10
  for aging complications, 38
  for brain health, 114
  for energy, 144
  for heart disease, 141–143, 144
  for high blood pressure, 151, 152, 153
  L-carnitine and, 144
  for migraines, 158, 160–161
  for varicose veins, 245
Cordain, Loren, 204–205
coriander, 108
cortisol, 68, 291–292

COX inhibitors, 97, 187–188
Craig, Gary, 273
cranberry juice, 195–198
cravings, refer to page 357
Crayhon, Robert, 23, 24, 301, 313
C-reactive protein, 220, 302
cumin, 108
curcuminoids, 147, 220. *See also* turmeric
cyclic mastalgia, 61
cynarin, 149
cysteine. *See* L-cysteine
cytokines, 76, 103

D

dairy products. *See also specific dairy products*
    acne and, 257
    allergies to, 168
    asthma and, 104
    eczema and, 122, 123
    heartburn, 139
    high blood pressure and, 152
    inflammatory bowel disease (IBD) and, 218
    iodine in, 60
    irritable bowel syndrome (IBS) and, 231–232, 233
    lysine in, 52
    zinc in, 83
dandelion root, 149
dandelion tea, 146
DASH (Dietary Approaches to Stop high blood pressure) diet, 150–153
deglycyrrhizinated licorice (DGL) powder, 85, 135
delta-6-desaturase, 123–124
dementia, refer to page 357
depression, refer to page 357
desert island cures, 27, 295–323
Designs for Health, 39
detoxification, 34, 147, 297, 315
DHA. *See* docosahexaenoic acid (DHA)
DHT. *See* dihydrotestosterone (DHT)
diabetes, refer to page 357
Diao Yuan Kuang, 241
Diehl, Harry W., 100
digestion, apple cider vinegar for, 297

digestive enzymes, 74, 85, 106–108, 135, 140, 216. *See also specific enzymes*
dihydrotestosterone (DHT), 257–258, 260, 262
DIM (diindolylmethane), 131
disaccharides, 217
diuretics, glucosamine and, 99
DLPA, 99
DL-phenylalamine, 98, 99
docosahexaenoic acid (DHA), 117, 300, 301. *See also* omega-3 fatty acids
dong quai, 131, 133
dopamiine, 44
douches, 182
D-ribose, 141, 142–143, 144
drugs. *See* pharmaceutical medicines
dual attention stimulus, 276
Duggan, Robert, 94
Duke University, 322
Dulloo, Abdul, 177
Durlach, Jean, 305

E

Eaton, Boyd, 306
echinacea, 81
eczema, refer to page 357
EFT (Emotional Freedom Technique), 272–274
EGCG. *See* green tea extract (EGCG)
eggs, 38, 118, 122
eicosapentaenoic acid (EPA), 300, 301. *See also* omega-3 fatty acids
Eli Lilly, 12
elimination diet, 104, 121–123, 168, 233
ellagic acid, 188
EMDR (eye movement desensitization and reprocessing) technique, 15, 274–277
EMDR Humanitarian Assistance Program (HAP), 276
Emotional Freedom Technique. *See* EFT (Emotional Freedom Technique)
emotional relief, 272–274
EMS (eosinophilia myalgia syndrome), 43–44
endocrine system, 252

endothelial dysfunction, 153, 282
energy, 144, 238–240, 267, 268, 306–309
enteric-coated peppermint oil, 230–234
enzymes, 47, 74–76, 77, 85, 107, 123–124, 134–141, 216, 315. *See also specific enzymes*
epigallocatechin gallate (EGCG), 176–177. *See also* green tea extract (EGCG)
epimedium sagittatum. See horny goat weed
Epsom salts baths, 304, 307
erythromycin ointment, 259
escin, 245
essential fatty acids, 11, 299–302. *See also* fish oil; omega-3 fatty acids; omega-6 fatty acids; omega-9 fatty acids
    for acne, 204, 257
    for Alzheimer's disease, 248
    for autism, 34
    for blood clots, 77
    for cardiovascular disease, 77
    for cholesterol, high, 71
    for cognitive decline, 248
    for dementia, 248
    for HDL cholesterol, low, 71
    for hot flashes, 131
    for inflammatory bowel disease (IBD), 216
    for menopause symptoms, 131
    for stroke prevention, 77
    for triglycerides, high, 71
estrogen, 129, 130
ethyl larueate, 258
European Congress of Allergology and Clinical Immunology, 213
evening primrose oil, 122–124
    for eczema, 122, 123
    gamma-linolenic acid (GLA) in, 124, 163
    for hot flashes, 131
    for menopause symptoms, 131
    for PMS (premenstrual syndrome), 27, 163, 164
excitotoxins, 158
exercise, 27, 280–283
    aerobic exercise, 280–281
    for arthritis, 98, 100, 280
    for brain health, 114, 118–119,

247, 280, 282–283
brain-derived neurotrophic factor
(BDNF), 282
for cardiovascular health, 280, 281
for cholesterol, high, 71
for depression, 44, 280
for diabetes, 47, 280
erectile disfunction and, 282
fartlek training, 284
for high blood pressure, 151, 152
for high triglycerides, 71
for hot flashes, 131
IGF-1 and, 282
interval training for fat loss,
284–288
for low HDL cholesterol, 71
for menopause symptoms, 131
for migraines, 160
for osteoporosis, 280
PACE (Progressively Accelerating
Cardiopulmonary Exertion),
288–289
pregnancy and, 282
sex and, 282
for varicose veins, 245
water aerobics, 98, 100
for weight loss, 175
weight training, 281–282
eye movement desensitization and
reprocessing technique. *See*
EMDR (eye movement desensitization and reprocessing) technique
eyebright, 166, 167

F

fartlek training, 284
fat loss, interval training for,
284–288
fats, 104, 151, 152. *See also* essential
fatty acids
fatty acids. *See* essential fatty acids
FDA. *See* U.S. Food and Drug
Admininstration
fennel *seed*s, 108
fenugreek, 202
fermented food, 159, 218
fermented soy, 131, 133–134
feverfew, 158
fiber, 152, 155, 233, 246
for diabetes, 47
for hot flashes, 131

for irritable bowel syndrome
(IBS), 234
for menopause symptoms, 131
for varicose veins, 245, 246
for weight loss, 175, 178
fibrin, 77
fish, 61
for acne, 257
for arthritis, 61, 100
for brain health, 114, 118
eczema, 122
high blood pressure, 152
for high cholesterol, 71
inflammatory bowel disease (IBD),
218
iodine in, 61
niacin in, 71
vitamin B6 in, 38
fish oil, 299–302. *See also* omega-3
fatty acids
for acne, 257
for anger, 301
anti-inflammatory properties of,
301–302
for arthritis, 100
for attention deficit disorder
(ADD), 301
for brain health, 117, 300–301
for cardiovascular disease, 143,
300
for cholesterol, 71
for depression, 301
for high blood pressure, 300
insulin and, 302
for stroke prevention, 300
flavonoids. *See* bioflavonoids
flax, 131
Flocco, Bill, 288–290
flour, 71, 104
fluoxetine, 254
fluvoxamine, 44–45
folacin. *See* folic acid
folate. *See* folic acid
folic acid
for aging complications, 38
Alzheimer's disease, 116
B vitamins and, 126, 128
for brain health, 116–117
in citrus fruits, 128
deficiency in, 126
dosages of, 127
folic acid deficiency, 126

food sources of, 128
for hearing loss, 125–129
hydrochloric acid (HCl) and, 138
neural tube defects, 125
pregnancy, 125
sperm counts and, 82
vitamin B12 and, 37, 126, 127,
128
vitamin B6 and, 126, 128
food cures, 8, 27, 186–221
food diaries, 233
food elimination trials, 68
food pyramid, 14
FOS. *See* fructoogliosaccharides
(FOS)
Fosamax, 23
Foster, Harold, 305
Framingham Heart Study, 308
Framingham Nurses Study, 320
free radicals, 115, 128–129, 318
Freud, Sigmund, 17
Fried, Richard, 203, 258–259
fructoogliosaccharides (FOS), 107
fructose, 225
fruits, 151–152, 153, 181, 188, 196,
257, 323. *See also specific fruits*
Fulton, James, 203, 226
functional medicine, 18

G

GABA (gamma aminobutyric acid),
32
Gaby, Alan, 104, 156–157, 218, 232,
259, 262, 307
galactose, 225
Galland, Leo, 141
gamma aminobutyric acid. *See*
GABA (gamma aminobutyric acid)
gamma-linolenic acid (GLA),
123–124, 163
for acne, 204, 257
for alcoholism, 95
anti-inflammatory properties of,
163
eczema, 123–124
in evening primrose oil, 163
for hot flashes, 131
for menopause symptoms, 131
for pain, 74
PMS (premenstrual syndrome),
163

infections, refer to page 358

infertility, refer to page 358

inflammation, refer to page 358

inflammatory bowel syndrome, refer to page 358

Ingram, Cass, 182

inositol, 44, 56–58, 72

insomnia, 25, 64, 65

Institute of Medicine, 48, 54

insulin, 46–47

    acne, 205

    acne and, 205

    apple cider vinegar and, 298

    chromium and, 177

    fish oil and, 302

    high blood sugar and, 192

    omega-3 fatty acids and, 302

    polycystic ovary syndrome (PCOS) and, 198, 199, 200–201

integrative medicine, 14, 18

International Council for the Control of Iodine Deficiency Disorders, 60

International Foundation for Functional Gastrointestinal Disorders, 231

interval training, 284–288

intervertebral foramin (IBF), 270

intrinsic factor, 37

iodine, 58–61

iodized salt, 58, 60

Iowa Women's Study, 306

irritable bowel syndrome, refer to page 358

isoflavones, 133–134

isomers, 175

Ivker, Robert, 206

J

Jackson, Carole, 278

Jacques, Jacqueline, 68

James, William, 28–29

jet lag, refer to page 358

Joseph, James, 117

junk food, 15

K

Kashin-Beck disease, 315

kefir (fermented milk), 181

kelp, 60

Kennedy, John F., 37

keratin, 203–204, 256, 257

Kevala Center for Holistic Health, 263

Khadavi, Alex, 258

Khalsa, Dharma Singh, 292

Kidd, Parris, 111, 113, 114, 115

kidney stones, refer to page 358

Kilham, Chris, 241, 243

Kramer, Arthur, 118, 283

krill oil, 15, 61–63, 164

Kriya Kirtan, 292

Kroon, Mark, 73–74

kundalini yoga, 292

L

Lactobacillus acidophilus, 179, 180–181

Lactobacillus rhamnosus GG, 124

Lamm, Steven, 40

Lands, William E.M., 315

L-arginine, 41, 52–53, 152, 208, 242, 243

lauric acid, 147, 218

Lawrence, Cindy, 267

L-carnitine, 38, 71, 111–112, 114, 115, 141, 142, 143, 144, 152, 175, 236

L-cysteine, 40, 148, 154, 171

leaky gut, 86, 137

LEAP (Lifestyle, Eating, and Performance) test, 123

Lee, Sophie, 234

lemon balm, 52

lemon juice, 154

LES. *See* lower esophageal sphincter (LES)

leukotrines, 103

Lexapro, 42, 43

L-glutamine, 49–50, 85, 94, 95, 216, 233

licorice root gel, 52

Lieberman, Allan D., 212

Lieberman, Shari, 72, 132, 173, 177, 314

Life Extension Foundation, 308, 311

Lind, James, 316

Linde, Klaus, 254

Linus Pauling Institute, 319

Lipitor, 23, 71

lipoic acid, 38

lithotripsy, 155

Little, Tanya, 88–89

liver, 38, 118

liver disease, refer to page 358

liver health

    acetaminophen (Tylenol) and, 147

    alcohol and, 147

    alpha lipoic acid for, 145–150

    choline for, 150

    coconut oil for, 147

    dandelion root for, 149

    dandelion tea for, 146

    detoxification and, 147

    diet and, 147, 149

    milk thistle for, 145–150

    N-acetyl-cysteine for, 145–150

    oleuropein for, 146

    olive leaf extract for, 146, 149

    phosphatidylcholine for, 146, 149–150

    Reishi mushrooms for, 149

    S-adenosyl-methionine (SAMe) for, 149, 308, 309, 311

    selenium for, 145–150

    shiitake mushrooms for, 149

    turmeric for, 147, 219, 220–221

    vegetable juices for, 147–148

    vitamin C for, 149

    vitamin E for, 149

    wheatgrass juice for, 147

    whey protein powder for, 146, 148

Lizotte, Linda, 35

lobster, 61

Lombard, Jay, 112–113

Lonsbury-Martin, Brenda, 128

low-carbohydrate diet, 14

    for acne, 205–206

    for cholesterol, high, 71

    for diabetes, 47

    for HDL cholesterol, low, 71

    for high blood sugar, 193

    for high triglycerides, 71

    for polycystic ovary syndrome (PCOS), 198–202

    for weight loss, 175

lower esophageal sphincter (LES), 137–139

L-theanine, 32–33

L-tryptophan, 35, 43–44, 64, 159, 163, 312

Ludwig, David, 178

lutein, 170, 196

Lutein Antioxidant Supplementation Trial (LAST), 170

Luvox, 58
lymphocytes. *See* white blood cells
Lynch, Darren M., 196
Lyon Diet Heart Study, 28, 70
lysine, 51–53

M

Maalox, 85, 134
maca, 241–243
macadamia nut oil, 71
macaenes, 242
macamides, 242
macular degeneration, refer to page
    358
magnaflorine, 241
magnesium, 144, 152, 154, 155,
    303–308
    for allergies, 105
    in apple cider vinegar, 298
    for asthma, 105, 106
    for autism, 34
    for bone health, 307–308
    for brain health, 114
    carbohydrates and, 306
    for cardiovascular disease, 77, 305
    for cardiovascular health, 77, 141,
        143, 144, 303, 304, 305, 306
    for cramps, 307
    deficiency in, 303, 307
    for diabetes, 47, 303, 306
    dosages of, 305
    for energy, 306–307
    Epsom salts baths, 304, 307
    for fibromyalgia, 307
    food sources of, 304
    forms of, 305
    for high blood pressure, 153, 303,
        305
    for high blood sugar, 193, 303,
        306
    for immune system, 304
    for irritable bowel syndrome
        (IBS), 233
    for kidney stones, 10, 156–157,
        197, 307
    for low HDL cholesterol, 305
    for menstrual cramps, 307
    for migraines, 158, 161
    for muscle pain and inflammation,
        306–307
    for osteoporosis, 307–308

for pain, 74
for PMS (premenstrual syn-
    drome), 10, 27, 162–163, 164,
    303, 307
potassium and, 305
for sleep, 303
sodium and, 305
stress, 304–305
stress and, 304–305
for stroke prevention, 77
taurine and, 40
vitamin B6 and, 307
water and, 305
Mahady, Gail, 132
Maharishi Mahesh Yogi, 292
Mahoney, Michael, 233–234
Malabar tamarind, 172–173
Mannino, Matthew, 270–271
mannose, 225
mast cells, 103, 166
Mathews-Larson, Joan, 49, 92–95
Mayer, Jean, 13
McCleary, Larry, 109
McDaniel, H.R., 225
McDougall, John, 203, 206
McNaughton, Carly, 215
meat, 71, 152, 218, 257
media, testing and the, 21–22
medical specialization, 16
medicines. *See* pharmaceutical
    medicines; specific medicines
meditation, 201, 292. *See also* yoga
Mediterranean diet, 28
melatonin, 44, 57
    for alcoholism, 95
    as "antiaging" supplement, 65–66
    breast cancer and, 63–65
    chemotherapy and, 64–65
    depression and, 65
    driving and, 65
    drug interactions and, 65
    for headaches, 65
    for jet lag, 27, 63–66
    for migraines, 65
    for PMS (premenstrual
        syndrome), 164
    radiation therapy and, 64–65
    S-adenosyl-methionine (SAMe)
        and, 312
    for sleep disorders, 64, 65
Melissa officinalis, 52
Melzer, Jörg, 228

memory, 37
    ginkgo for, 235–237
    glycerophosphocholine (GPC) for,
        236
    huperzine A for, 236
    L-carnitine for, 236
    phosphatidylserine (PS) for, 236
    rhodiola for, 250–252
    vinpocentine for, 236
    vitamin B12 for, 37, 38–39
men, 82
    vitamin D and, 54–55
    zinc for, 82
Mercola, Joe, 193, 272, 273
mercury, 69, 315
meridians, 266
Metagenics, 84
Metagenics Ultra-Clear, 147
metformin (Glucophage), 201–202
methionine, 40
methyl group, 309
methyl sulfonylmethane. *See* MSM
    (methyl sulfonylmethane)
methylation, 38, 309
methylhydroxychalcone polymer
    (MHCP), 193
Meyerowitz, Steve, 226
migraine, refer to page 358
milk. *See* dairy products
milk thistle, 145–150
Miller, Donald, 60–61
mind-body feedback loop, 18–21
minerals, 8, 26. *See also* specific
    minerals
    for alcoholism, 92–93, 95
    in apple cider vinegar, 298
    for immune support, 81
    research on, 11
Minnesota Model, 92
mint, 108
misalignment, 270–271
Mischoulon, David, 254
miso, 133
mitochondrial dysfunction, 111–112
moldy foods, 180
mollusks, 38
Money, Nisha, 292
MSM (methyl sulfonylmethane),
    67–69, 98, 99
Mudd, Susan, 41, 84, 122, 123, 182
multivitamins. *See also* specific
    vitamins

for blood clots, 77
for brain health, 114
for cardiovascular disease, 77
for heart disease, 143
for high blood pressure, 152
for immune support, 81
for macular degeneration, 170,
171
for stroke prevention, 77
for vision, 170, 171
Murray, Michael, 102, 197, 218, 257
muscle pain, refer to page 358
myelin sheath, 37, 116
Mylanta, 85, 134

N

NAC. *See also* N-acetyl-cysteine
N-acetyl-cysteine, 126, 128,
145–150
N-acetylgalactosamine, 225
N-acetylneuraminic acid, 225
Napoli, Claudio, 209
nasal decongestants, 166
National Academy of Sciences, 161
National Eye Institute, 169–170
National Health and Nutrition
Examination Survey (NHANES),
126, 322–323
National Health and Nutrition
Survey, 195–196
National Institute of Mental Health,
253
National Institute on Aging (NIA),
247National Institutes of Health
(NIH), 255, 304
natto, 77–79
nattokinase. *See* natto
Natural Health Encyclopedia, 113
natural medicine, 8, 14–18. *See also*
nutritional medicine
definition of, 24–26
guiding principles of, 18–29
risks of, 10
Natural Medicines Comprehensive
Database, 41
Natural Standard, The, 240
natural treatments, 27, 265–293
neominophagen, 149
Neptune Krill Oil, 62, 63, 164. *See
also* krill oil
Neptune Technologies and

Bioresources, 63
nervous system function, 39, 236
Neto, Catherine, 197
neural tube defects, folic acid and,
125
neurons, 110, 117
neuropathy, 39
neurotransmitters, 42–43, 112, 247,
248, 249
neutrophils, 190
New York Heart Association, 41
Newbold, H.L., 36–37
Nexium, 134
NF-kappa B, 103, 220, 228
niacin, 70–73, 118
niacinamide, 72
nicotinamide, 72
nicotinic acid, 72
Nieman, David, 103
nitric oxide, 103, 208
NK cells, 318
nonsteroidal anti-inflammatory
drugs (NSAIDS). *See* NSAIDS
(nonsteroidal anti-inflammatory
drugs)
noradrenaline, 176–177
norepinephrine, 44
Northrup, Christiane, 132
NSAIDS (nonsteroidal anti-inflammatory drugs), 76, 86, 97, 155
Nurses' Health Study, 28, 156, 306
nutritional medicine, 8, 13, 18–29,
111. *See also* natural medicine
nuts, 71, 83, 122, 152, 155, 180, 181,
257
NWFP Agricultural University,
193–194

O

oil of oregano, 107, 108, 180,
182–183
oils, 151, 152
oleuropein, 146
olive leaf extract, 146, 149
olive oil, 71, 152
omega-3 fatty acids, 10, 299–302. *See
also* essential fatty acids; fish oil
for acne, 258–259
for arthritis, 98
for brain health, 114, 117, 248
for cardiovascular health, 77, 299

cell membranes and, 77, 302
for cognitive decline, 248
C-reactive protein and, 302
for dementia, 248
for depression, 44
for diabetes, 47, 193
for eczema, 123–124
for high blood pressure, 152, 153
for high cholesterol, 71
for high triglycerides, 71, 300
insulin and, 302
in krill oil, 62, 164
for low HDL cholesterol, 71
for macular degeneration, 170,
170–171
for pain, 74
phosphatidylserine (PS) and, 113
for PMS (premenstrual syndrome), 164
for stroke prevention, 77
for vision, 170–171
omega-6 fatty acids, 299. *See also*
essential fatty acids
for acne, 258–259
for blood clots, 77
for cardiovascular disease, 77
for eczema, 122
gamma-linolenic acid (GLA),
123–124
for stroke prevention, 77
omega-9 fatty acids, 71, 299. *See also*
essential fatty acids
onions, 139
oral tetracycline, 259
Oregon State University, 319
organic foods, 104
Ornish, Dean, 208, 209
orthomolecular medicine, 26, 319
osteocalcin, 79
osteoporosis, refer to page 358
oxalates, 155, 197
oxidation, 318, 320
oxidative stress, 105
oxymel, 297
oysters, 38, 61, 83, 315

P

PACE (Progressively Accelerating
Cardiopulmonary Exertion),
288–289
Pacific Health, 88

DISEASE/AILMENT/CONDITION INDEX

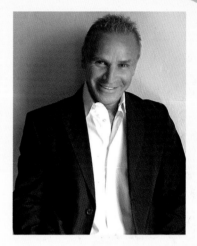